# TRAINING
## Scientific Basis and Application

"LIVING MODERN FITNESS"
*From* "TRIANGLE FITNESS"
*By*
Arthur H. Steinhaus

We take coffee to wake up,
  Pep pills to stay awake and
    Barbiturates to fall asleep.
With vitamins we increase our appetites,
  With special tablets we shut them off and
    Slenderella must make up the difference.
With uplifts and girdles we keep shape up front
  With arch supports we hold up our feet.
We steer with power, shift gears with buttons,
  And tune TV by remote control and an EZ chair.
For pleasure we smoke something up front of a filter
  That protects us from the irritation that's up front.
We drown our worries in alcohol,
  Reduce our tensions with tranquilizers,
    And deaden our pains with aspirin by the bottle.
For tired blood its Geritol, for nagging back aches
  Doane's Pills.
And we don't even have the guts to move our bowels
  Without Serutan.
And for quality we move up to Schlitz.

         ✿    ✿    ✿

It is said that Europe is more fit than America
  And India more spiritual than the USA.
There is little virtue in FITNESS with POVERTY
  In spirituality without temptation of diversion.
America must learn the habits of FITNESS IN PLENTY
  OF STRENGTH—with automobiles
    Of spiritual discipline with TV to distract and
      Ease to deter.
For it is easier for a camel to enter through the eye of a
  Needle than for a Nation of affluence to enter the
    Kingdom of Fitness—Physical, Mental, and Spiritual.

# TRAINING
## Scientific Basis and Application

A Symposium Conducted by the
Canadian Association of Sports Sciences
at the
Pavilion de L'Education Physique et des Sports
Laval University, Quebec City
Province of Quebec, Canada

*Compiled and Edited by*

ALBERT W. TAYLOR, Ph.D.

*Surgical-Medical-Research Institute and
Faculty of Physical Education
University of Alberta
Edmonton, Canada*

*With a Foreword by*

Maxwell L. Howell, Ed.D., Ph.D.

*Chairman
Department of Physical Education
University of Alberta
Edmonton, Canada*

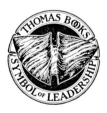

CHARLES C THOMAS • PUBLISHER
*Springfield • Illinois • U.S.A.*

*Published and Distributed Throughout the World by*
CHARLES C THOMAS • PUBLISHER
Bannerstone House
301–327 East Lawrence Avenue, Springfield, Illinois, U.S.A.
Natchez Plantation House
735 North Atlantic Boulevard, Fort Lauderdale, Florida, U.S.A.

© *1972, by* CHARLES C THOMAS • PUBLISHER
ISBN 0–398–02428–6
Library of Congress Catalog Card Number: 70–172467

*With THOMAS BOOKS careful attention is given to all details of
manufacturing and design. It is the Publisher's desire to present books
that are satisfactory as to their physical qualities and artistic possibilities
and appropriate for their particular use. THOMAS BOOKS will be true
to those laws of quality that assure a good name and good will.*

*Printed in the United States of America*

*BB-14*

# Contributors

**J.G. Albinson, Ph.D.:** *School of Physical Education, Queens University, Kingston, Canada.*

**R.D. Bell, Ph.D.:** *School of Physical Education, University of Saskatchewan, Saskatoon, Canada.*

**M. Booth, M.Sc.:** *Department of Physical Education, University of Alberta, Edmonton, Canada.*

**C. Bouchard, M.Sc.:** *Departement D'Education Physique, Université Laval, Quebec, Canada.*

**R. Carrier, M.D., D.Sc.:** *Hopital Saint-Francois-d'Assise, Quebec, Canada.*

**B.J. Cratty, Ed.D.:** *Department of Physical Education, University of California at Los Angeles, Los Angeles, U.S.A.*

**G.R. Cumming, M.D.:** *The Children's Hospital of Winnipeg, and Department of Medicine, University of Manitoba, Winnipeg, Canada.*

**D.A. Cunningham, Ph.D.:** *Department of Physical Education and Department of Physiology, University of Western Ontario, London, Ontario.*

**J. Damoiseau, Ph.D.:** *Institut Superieur d'Education Physique, Universite de Liege, Belgium.*

**S. Dulac, M.Sc.:** *Laboratoire D'Endocrinologie, Departement De Physiologie, Faculte De Medecine, Université Laval, Quebec, Canada.*

**D.H. Elliott, Ph.D.:** *Department of Physical Education, Dalousie University, Halifax, Canada.*

**R.B. Eynon, M.Sc.:** *Department of Physical Education, University of Western Ontario, London, Canada.*

**J. Falize, Ph.D.:** *Institut Superieur d'Education Physique, Universite de Liege, Belgium.*

**R.J. Ferguson, Ph.D.:** *Departement De Cardiologie Et Ecole D'Education Physique, Université De Montreal, Montreal, Canada.*

**P. Gauthier, M.Sc.:** *Ecole D'Education Physique, Université De Montreal, Montreal, Canada.*

**J.A. Gibbins, M.Sc.:** *Department of Physical Education, University of Western Ontario, London, Canada.*

**N. Gledhill, M.Sc.:** *Department of Physical Education, York University, Toronto, Canada.*

**C.F. Grindstaff, Ph.D.:** *Department of Sociology, University of Western Ontario, London, Canada.*

**R.T. Hermiston, Ph.D.:** *Faculty of Physical Education, University of Windsor, Windsor, Canada.*

**P. Houssière, Ph.D.:** *Institut Superieur d'Education Physique, Universite de Liege, Belgium.*

**M.E. Houston, Ph.D.:** *Department of Kinesiology, University of Waterloo, Waterloo, Canada.*

**J.E. Howell, M.Sc.:** *Department of Physical Education, Dalhousie University, Halifax, Canada.*

**M.L. Howell, Ph.D., Ed.D.:** *Chairman, Department of Physical Education, University of Alberta, Edmonton, Canada.*

**G. Hunnebelle, Ph.D.:** *Institut Superieur d'Education Physique, Universite de Liege, Belgium.*

**M. Jetté, Ph.D.:** *Department of Kinanthropology, University of Ottawa, Ottawa, Canada.*

**P. King, Ph.D.:** *Department of Kinesiology, University of Waterloo, Waterloo, Canada.*

**D.M. Landers, Ph.D.:** *Department of Physical Education, State University of New York, Brockport, U.S.A.*

**F. Landry, Ph.D.:** *Departement D'Education Physique, Université Laval, Quebec, Canada.*

**L. Leger, M.Sc.:** *Ecole D'Education Physique, Université De Montreal, Montreal, Canada.*

**J.P. Maréchal, M.Sc.:** *Institut Superieur d'Education Physique, Universite de Liege, Belgium.*

**D. Massicotte, M.Sc.:** *School of Physical Education, University of Ottawa, Ottawa, Canada.*

**S. Mendryk, Ph.D.:** *Department of Physical Education, University of Alberta, Edmonton, Canada.*

**K. McBean (Hopkins), M.Sc.:** *Department of Physical Education, University of Alberta, Edmonton, Canada.*

**T.D. McIntyre, Ph.D.:** *Department of Men's Physical Education, State University of New York, Brockport, New York, U.S.A.*

**M. Nadeau, M.Sc.:** *Ecole D'Education Physique, Université De Montreal, Montreal, Canada.*

**M.E. O'Brien, M.Sc.:** *Faculty of Physical Education, University of Windsor, Windsor, Canada.*

**R. Potvin, M.D.:** *Hopital Saint-Francois-d'Assise, Quebec, Canada.*

**R.L. Rasmussen, M.Sc.:** *School of Physical Education, St. Francis Xavier University, Antigonish, Canada.*

**J.B. Redford, M.D.:** *School of Rehabilitation Medicine, University of Alberta, Edmonton, Canada.*

**D.C. Reid, M.C.S.P., Dip. T.P.:** *School of Rehabilitation Medicine, University of Alberta, Edmonton, Canada.*

**H. Reindell, M.D.:** *Department of Cardiology, University of Freiburg, Freiburg, in Breisgau, West Germany.*

**H. Roskamm, M.D.:** *Department of Cardiology, University of Freiburg, Freiburg in Breisgau, West Germany.*

**B. Roy, Ph.D.:** *Departement D'Education Physique, Université Laval, Quebec, Canada.*

**D. B. Shaw, M.D., Ph.D.:** *St. Joseph's Hospital, London, Canada.*

**R.J. Shephard, M.D., Ph.D.:** *Department of Environmental Health, School of Hygiene, University of Toronto, Toronto, Canada.*

**R. Simmons, M.Sc.:** *Department of Environmental Health, School of Hygiene, University of Toronto, Toronto, Canada.*

**K.H. Sidney, M.Sc.:** *School of Physical Education and Department of Physiology, University of Western Ontario, London, Canada.*

**G. Smith, M.A.:** *Department of Physical Education, University of Western Ontario, London, Canada.*

**A.W. Taylor, Ph.D.:** *Surgical-Medical-Research-Institute and Faculty of Physical Education, University of Alberta, Edmonton, Canada.*

**J. Thoden, Ph.D.:** *Department of Kinanthropology, University of Ottawa, Ottawa, Canada.*

**G.B. Thompson, M.Sc.:** *Bio-Engineering Institute and Department of Physical Education, University of New Brunswick, Fredricton, Canada.*

**G. Tomlinson, Ph.D.:** *Department of Chemistry, University of Waterloo, Waterloo, Canada.*

**R. Vanroux, M.D.:** *Charleroi, Belgium.*

**E.W. Vaz, Ph.D.:** *Department of Sociology, University of Waterloo, Waterloo, Canada.*

**R.R. Wallingford, Ed.D.:** *Physical Education Division, Laurentian University, Sudbury, Canada.*

Dedicated to

CASS/ACSS

An association grouping professional persons from various disciplines interested in the scientific aspects of sports, training, and physical activity.

BOARD OF DIRECTORS OF CASS/ACSS 1970–71

| | | | |
|---|---|---|---|
| President | Roy S. Shephard | M.D., Ph.D. | Toronto |
| Past President | Max Avren | M.D. | Winnipeg |
| President Elect | F. Landry | Ph.D. | Quebec City |
| Secretary | D. Clement | M.D. | Vancouver |
| Treasurer | C. Bouchard | M.Sc. | Quebec City |
| Membership and Credentials | P. Godbout | M.Sc. | Quebec City |
| Programme | T. Fried | M.D. | Downsview |
| Publications | A.W. Taylor | Ph.D. | Edmonton |
| Research | R.J. Ferguson | Ph.D. | Montreal |
| Nominating | R. Osborne | M.A. | Vancouver |
| Medical Aspects of Sports | G. Cumming | M.D. | Winnipeg |
| Public Relations | G. Kenyon | Ph.D. | Waterloo |
| Director | M.L. Howell | Ed.D., Ph.D. | Edmonton |
| Director | S. Landa | M.D. | Saskatoon |

# Foreword

It is indeed a very great honor to be asked to open the Symposium on "Training—Scientific Basis and Application."

May I be permitted, however, to make a few remarks of a broad nature, because of the importance of the occasion, and perhaps because these occasions occur for me so rarely.

The first comment is obvious—to congratulate the organizers on the excellence of their program and preparation for what is, after all, only the fourth annual meeting of the C.A.S.S. Close to forty papers will be presented, and one must be impressed with the range of studies being delivered—a most encouraging sign. We are witnessing C.A.S.S. coming of age. We see papers on physiology of exercise, such as Dr. Taylor's and Dr. Cumming's; we see the papers by Smith and Grindstaff on "Race and sport in Canada" and by Vaz on "The culture of young hockey players" and we enter the realm of sociology of sport; we see the papers by Albinson on "The relationship of need achievement and test anxiety to performance of physical tasks" and McIntyre on "A field experimental study of attitude change in four biracial small sport groups" and the psychology of sport is envisaged; the paper by Elliot, Howell and Whitehead, "Causes and consequences of differential leisure participation among females in Halifax, Nova Scotia" is in the area of recreation research; papers by such as Reid, Redford and King on the "Rate of absorption of experimental hematomas: Influence of ultrasound and high frequency radio waves" can be considered as embracing the field of sportsmedicine; papers such as that by De Lisle, *et al.* are in the field of work capacity; papers such as Hermiston's and Wallingford's are in the area of measurement; papers by Thompson and Roy are in the area of biomechanics and kinesiology, and, of course, all the papers to come are in the area of training, its scientific basis and application.

May I also be permitted to reflect a little. This begins my seventeenth year in Canada, and the changes have been remarkable in the scientific area in our field in that time. No casual relationship is, however, inferred. The Research Committee of C.A.H.P.E.R., at the McMaster Biennial Convention some twelve years ago, had its formative meetings, and research papers were given for the first time. When I think of the quality of the papers, my own included, I can see how far we have come. The papers were products of the limited knowledge of the time, by dedicated workers with a belief in examining the scientific aspects of the total field, and must be appreciated in their historical perspective. Most of us thought variance was something to do with a woman's menstrual cycle, and that covariation smacked of homosexuality. There were no research laboratories in physical education—the sum total of equipment at my own institution was a beautiful C.H. Stoelting grip dynamometer purchased for $120. Now our laboratories have become more sophisticated, our methods more scientific—our young people are better trained than we were. Many of our peers seventeen years ago could not keep the pace of the scientific explosion and many of us had to learn "on the run." Ah, the good old days, when a "t" ratio was the sum total of man's knowledge, and you could impress the locals with a $120 dynamometer!

Then the need for a link with medicine, in particular, became more apparent as mutual interests were revealed. C.A.H.P.E.R. and the C.M.A. formed a joint committee, and meetings began. I can always remember going to the first one in Toronto. There were no travel funds then, and so I caught a train to and from Toronto, with lots of sandwiches and a little liquid refreshment in the briefcase. Ah, the good old days! And this body, the C.M.A.-C.A.H.P.E.R. Committee led to the formation of the Canadian Association of Sports Sciences, and the variety and number of papers attests to the successful merging of the various scientific fields.

The impetus in the field was assisted by Bill C-131, particularly with the availability of research grants and financial assistance for so many of our bright, young people to go on to ad-

vanced degrees. The success of this program is best illustrated
by the appearance of so many new faces at these meetings, and
though research grants have in the main temporarily been
stopped, it is anticipated that, in the near future, such policies
will be reviewed. And it is hoped there will be renewed funding.
This part of the Symposium, with the emphasis on training and
practical research, attests to the need to continue such aid. Not
all the research is "pure," whatever that really means. Much of
it in our field has immediate or near-immediate applicability,
and as this is a reminiscence, may I offer a word or two of
advice to those presenting papers for the first or second time.
Your paper will, doubtless, not shake the foundations of science,
and must often be viewed as a learning experience. Your work
is best a fragment of a total problem, and must be recognized
as but a fragment. As I view such contributions over the large
haul, they too often, as one writer said, are but bricks thrown
randomly in a brickyard. Your challenge, essentially, is to place
those bricks in a more ordered manner, reducing the chaos in
the brickyard—indeed, the aim should be to build houses, perhaps castles in the brickyard.

There is a delusion, among the young, that the statistical hypothesis is the ultimate, the end point. I would suggest that in
the main it is fragmentary, incomplete, a random brick. The
fragmentary studies need to be directed to larger and more encompassing hypotheses, but may take a lifetime to affirm or
reject. The aim of success is to develop laws. Hypotheses of
greater scope will assist us in moving towards such laws. We
have neglected, I feel, the literary hypothesis in our scramble
to produce papers for symposia such as this. It is interesting to
me to hear hypotheses in so many papers at this convention. We
see them in sociology and psychology, we hear of models as well,
but in physiology, particularly, they are too often neglected.
Too often we are faced solely with a conclusion such as that
seventh grade girls, following six weeks of training with six
isometric contractions of six seconds duration, improved their
flexor strength at the .01 level of confidence. Our perspectives
should be broader, our aims higher, and we should direct our
attentions to major hypotheses. If not, the studies will be viewed

as darts going on a dart board, some falling, and all arriving at different places on the board. And then the darts are taken off the board, and the game starts again.

What are some hypotheses that may bind our studies together? Let us try a few:

1. Fitness tends to be specific.
2. A general fitness results from habitual repetition of vigorous activity.
3. Fitness is transitory.
4. Fitness may be improved by many different methods.

Many others can be suggested and it would be interesting to brainstorm the hypotheses that are apparent in our fields.

As such hypotheses are affirmed or rejected, they may become laws, and in this manner knowledge in our field can continually advance. Without such attempts to draw knowledge together, to generalize, without concerted efforts by teams of investigators to examine a particular problem, our field will never achieve a high measure of scientific acceptance. The formulation of generalizations that explain phenomena is one of the aims of science.

Hypotheses, theories and laws are generalizations of increasing generality. Since the generalization that offers the most comprehensive explanation is of the greatest value, a law is of greater importance than a theory or hypothesis.

We owe it to the progressive scientific development of our field to consider this question, to contemplate the interrelationship of studies, their repetition, the similarities that have appeared. We need to see beyond the study.

For science aims at the progressive unification of the generalizations. The ultimate goal of science is to seek laws of the higher generality—laws of the utmost comprehensiveness.

Our challenge, as we sit listening to these papers, is to think beyond the particular to more encompassing generalities. Our challenge, as we direct our reseach, is to increasing generality. Our challenge is to suggest hypotheses for training, theories and perhaps ultimately laws. This is our challenge, and we should not be lost in the maze of 1 and 5 percent levels of confidence, in statistical jargon, in the "ready mix" study. The bricks are important, but let us aim to build houses and castles. Then we can justly chaim to be a science—A Sports Science.

It is a great honor to declare the Symposium on Training—Scientific Basis and Application open.

MAXWELL L. HOWELL

# Preface

This book compilates the papers presented at the fourth annual meeting of the Canadian Association of Sports Sciences held at Laval University in Quebec City, October 28–31, 1970, under the theme "Training—Scientific Basis and Application." The Association was established in July, 1967, after many years of earnest endeavor by the Joint Committee composed of representatives of "The Canadian Medical Association" and of the "Canadian Association for Health, Physical Education and Recreation." The major objectives of CASS/ACSS are the following:

1. To promote and advance medical and other scientific studies dealing with the effects of sports and physical activity on the health of human beings at various stages of life.
2. To cooperate with other organizations, physicians, physical educators, physiologists and scientists concerned with the various aspects of human fitness.
3. To encourage the collection and circulation of information and literature related to fitness and physical activity.

At this meeting the papers of Vanroux, Massicotte, Roy, Hunnebelle, Damoiseau, Dulac and Carrier were presented in French. The authors are gratefully acknowledged for permitting their papers to be translated into English for this publication. A great deal of thanks must go to the organizing committee—Michele Fleury, Claude Bouchard, Paul Godbout and Fern Landry for translation and assistance with the editing of these papers.

A.W. Taylor

# Contents

|  | Page |
|---|---|
| *Contributors* .......................................... | v |
| *Foreword* ........................................... | xi |
| *Preface* ........................................... | xvii |

## A.  PHYSIOLOGICAL–CLINICAL ASPECTS

*Chapter*

*1.* THE HEART AND CIRCULATION OF THE SUPERIOR ATHLETE— *H. Roskamm and H. Reindell* ........................ 5

*2.* EPIDIDYMAL FAT PAD REGENERATION AND FREE FATTY ACID MOBILIZATION WITH EXERCISE AND TRAINING—*Albert W. Taylor, Marilyn Booth and Katherine McBean* ........... 21

*3.* THE FREQUENCY AND POSSIBLE SIGNIFICANCE OF ISCHEMIC S-T CHANGES IN THE EXERCISE ELECTROCARDIOGRAM—*G.R. Cumming* .......................................... 39

*4.* METABOLIC ACIDOSIS DURING MUSCULAR EXERCISE, ITS REPERCUSSIONS ON VENTILATION—*R. Vanroux* .................. 60

*5.* THE EFFECTS OF THREE TYPES OF WARM-UP ON THE TOTAL OXYGEN COST OF A SHORT TREADMILL RUN—*R.T. Hermiston and M.E. O'Brien* ....,............................. 70

*6.* APPLICATION OF A PRACTICAL TEST TO PREDICT THE MAXIMAL OXYGEN INTAKE OF HIGH SCHOOL BOYS—*Denis Massicotte* .. 76

*7.* MAXIMAL CARDIAC OUTPUT BY "$CO_2$ REBREATHING"—*R.J. Ferguson, L. Léger, M. Nadeau and P. Gauthier* ......... 87

*8.* THE INTENSITY OF TRAINING—*Norman Gledhill and Robert B. Eynon* ............................................. 97

*9.* LABORATORY MEASUREMENTS APPLIED TO THE DEVELOPMENT AND MODIFICATION OF TRAINING PROGRAMS—*James S. Thoden and Maurice Jetté* ................................... 103

*Chapter*                                                                    *Page*

10. A Profile of the Canadian National Cross-Country Ski
    Team—*Maurice Jetté and James S. Thoden* .............. 115

11. Exercise and the Myocardial Fiber Capillary Ratio—
    *R.D. Bell and R.L. Rasmussen* ......................... 123

12. The Influence of Training Upon the Distribution of
    Cardiac Output—*R. Simmons and Roy J. Shephard* ....... 131

13. The Effect of Swimming Training on Selected Aspects
    of the Pulmonary Function of Young Girls—A Pre-
    liminary Report—*J.A. Gibbins, D.A. Cunningham, D.B.
    Shaw and R.B. Eynon* .................................. 139

14. The Effect of Frequency of Exercise Upon Physical
    Work Performance and Selected Variables Representa-
    tive of Cardiorespiratory Fitness—*K.H. Sidney, R.B.
    Eynon, and D.A. Cunningham* .......................... 144

15. Characterization of Physiological Modifications Occur-
    ring During Interval Training—*Jacques Damoiseau, Gi-
    nette Hunnebelle and Paul Houssiere* .................. 149

16. The Urinary Elimination of Vanilmandelic Acid Before
    and After a Standard Exercise in Trained and Untrained
    Men—*Serge Dulac* .................................... 166

17. Effect of an Anabolic Steroid at the Molecular Level
    *M.E. Houston and G.T. Tomlinson* ..................... 175

18. Comparisons Between Athletes, Normal and Eskimo Sub-
    jects from the Point of View of Selected Biochemical
    Parameters—*Robert Carrier, Fernand Landry, Robert Potvin
    and Claude Bouchard* ................................. 180

### B.  PSYCHO–SOCIOLOGICAL ASPECTS

19. Psychology of the Superior Athlete—*Bryant J. Cratty* ... 189

20. Race and Sport in Canada—*Garry Smith and Carl F. Grind-
    staff* ............................................... 197

21. The Relationship of Need Achievement and Test Anxiety
    to Performance of Physical Tasks—*J.G. Albinson* ...... 207

*Chapter* *Page*

22. CAUSES AND CONSEQUENCES OF DIFFERENTIAL LEISURE PARTICIPATION AMONG FEMALES IN HALIFAX, NOVA SCOTIA—*David H. Elliott, and Janet E. Howell* .................. 213

23. THE CULTURE OF YOUNG HOCKEY PLAYERS: SOME INITIAL OBSERVATIONS—*Edmund W. Vaz* ...................... 222

24. THE EFFECTS OF ORDINAL POSITION AND SIBLING'S SEX ON MALES' SPORT PARTICIPATION—*Daniel M. Landers* ......... 235

25. A FIELD EXPERIMENTAL STUDY OF ATTITUDE CHANGE IN FOUR BIRACIAL SMALL SPORT GROUPS—*Thomas D. McIntyre* ..... 242

APPENDIX A ........................................ 261

## C. SPORTS MEDICINE AND KINESIOLOGY

26. THE INFLUENCE OF ULTRASOUND AND HIGH FREQUENCY RADIO WAVES ON THE RATE OF REABSORPTION OF EXPERIMENTAL HEMATOMAS—*David C. Reid, John B. Redford and Peter King* ............................................... 267

27. AN ELECTROMYOGRAPHIC TECHNIQUE FOR COMPARING THE RELATIVE INVOLVEMENT OF SKELETAL MUSCLES DURING EXERCISE—*G.B. Thompson* ............................... 282

28. KINEMATICS OF THE STANDING LONG JUMP IN SEVEN, TEN, THIRTEEN AND SIXTEEN-YEAR-OLD BOYS—*Benoit Roy* ........ 290

29. RELATIONSHIPS BETWEEN AMPLITUDE OF HIP MOVEMENTS AND JUMPING PERFORMANCES—*Ginette Hunnebelle, Jean Paul Maréchal and Julien Falize* .......................... 305

30. THE EFFECTS OF ISOMETRIC, ISOTONIC, AND SPEED CONDITIONING PROGRAMS ON SPEED OF MOVEMENT, REACTION TIME, AND STRENGTH OF COLLEGE MEN—*Stephen Mendryk* ........... 320

## D. STATISTICS AND COMPUTERIZATION

31. STATISTICAL ANALYSES OF HOCKEY—*R.T. Hermiston* ....... 333

32. APPLICATION OF A COMPUTER RETRIEVAL SYSTEM FOR EXERCISE PHYSIOLOGY—*R.R. Wallingford* .......................... 338

33. CLOSING REMARKS—*Claude Bouchard* ................... 349

*Index* ................................................ 355

# TRAINING

## Scientific Basis and Application

# A. PHYSIOLOGICAL—CLINICAL ASPECTS

# Chapter 1

# The Heart and Circulation
# of the Superior Athlete

H. Roskamm
H. Reindell

G eneral circulatory adjustment to exercise in well-trained subjects may be evaluated (a) from comparative studies between athletes and untrained persons and (b) from follow-up studies during a training period of formerly untrained persons. A point of criticism against the first approach is the fact that different results in athletes may not only be affected by training but may also be a matter of primary selection.

## Heart Volume

In comparison with untrained normal persons of the same age, well-trained weight lifters and gymnasts showed no increase of heart volume. Only athletes in endurance competitions, such as bicyclists, showed significantly increased heart volumes (Fig. 1–1).

Not only all parts of the heart, but also the pulmonary veins are enlarged. This can be demonstrated by tomographic studies, that is, x-ray exposures focused at different depths in the chest.

## Maximum Oxygen Uptake

Well-trained athletes have an elevated maximum oxygen uptake; the highest values reported are 6.17 l/min or 85l ml/min/kg.[19] Sportsmen in endurance competitions such as bicycling or cross-country skiing have the highest increases compared with untrained persons. Sportsmen with the most pro-

5

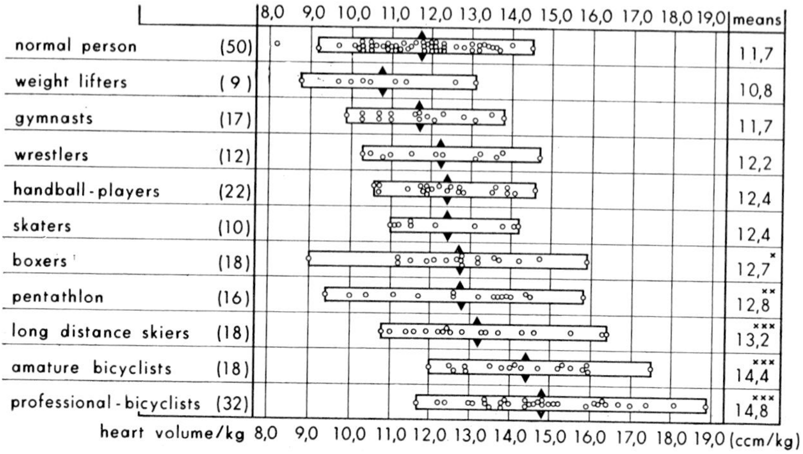

Figure 1–1. Heart volume per kg/body weight in untrained persons and members of different national teams in West Germany.

nounced increases of heart volume have the highest values of maximum oxygen uptake, as shown by Israel[9] in 471 well-trained athletes of Eastern Germany. 

## Heart Rate at Submaximal Exercise

Athletes have lower heart rates than untrained persons during standardized submaximal exercise. The lowest individual heart rate values in different watts steady state exercise were found in bicyclists (Fig. 1–2).

## Maximum Heart Rates

Maximum heart rate during exercise decreases with increasing heart volume, as shown by Israel[9] in 471 well-trained athletes of Eastern Germany.

## Heart Volume, Maximum Oxygen Uptake and Maximum Heart Rate in Follow-up Studies

Six healthy men aged twenty-two to thirty-five years were trained daily except Sundays by a stepwise increased bicycle

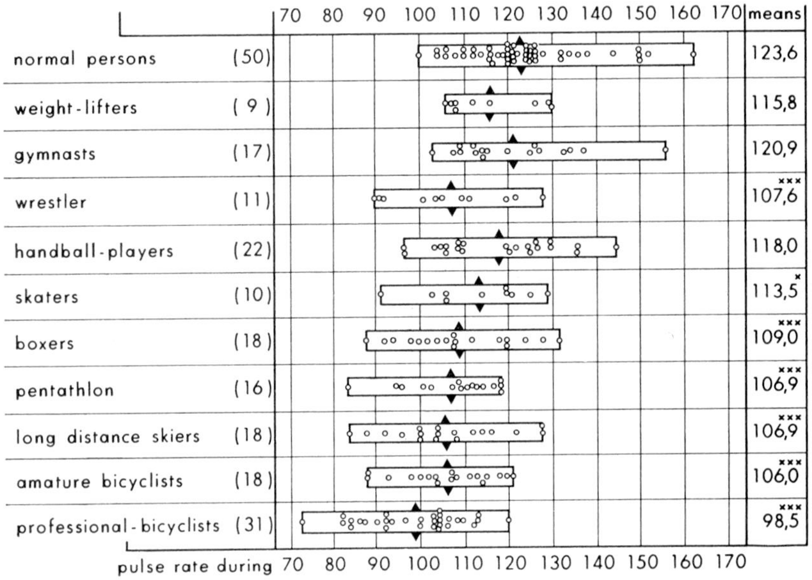

| | | means |
|---|---|---|
| 70 80 90 100 110 120 130 140 150 160 170 | | |
| normal persons | (50) | 123,6 |
| weight-lifters | (9) | 115,8 |
| gymnasts | (17) | 120,9 |
| wrestler | (11) | 107,6 ××× |
| handball-players | (22) | 118,0 |
| skaters | (10) | 113,5 × |
| boxers | (18) | 109,0 |
| pentathlon | (16) | 106,9 ××× |
| long distance skiers | (18) | 106,9 ××× |
| amature bicyclists | (18) | 106,0 ××× |
| professional-bicyclists | (31) | 98,5 ××× |

pulse rate during 70 80 90 100 110 120 130 140 150 160 170

Figure 1–2. Heart rate during 100 watts steady state bicycle-ergometer exercise in lying position in untrained persons and members of different national teams in West Germany.

ergometer exercise. This training was also used to measure maximum oxygen uptake. $Vo_2$ max. increased significantly from 3034 to 3486 $cm^3$ on the average that is 18.8% ($p < 0.01$). The increase is linear during four weeks. Heart volume did not change. In the same study we found a significant linear decrease of maximum heart rate from 192 to 186 ($p < 0.01$). In another study sixteen students were trained daily on bicycle-ergometers for one hour for half a year. The heart rate during the one hour training period was on the average 155, in the process of training increasing work loads were necessary to raise the heart rate to the demanded value. After two months of training the increase of $Vo_2$ max. became less steep (Fig. 1–3). After 4½ months the maximum of the half a year period was reached, the increase was 22 percent of the pretraining value. This program will be continued for a further 2½ years. Probably a much more pronounced increase in intensity and duration of training is necessary to reach further improvement. Maximum heart rate was reduced from 194 to 188 on the average ($p < 0.01$). In

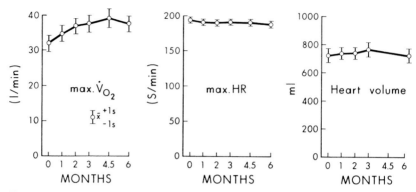

Figure 1–3. Maximum oxygen uptake, maximum heart rate and heart volume during a six-month period of heavy physical training in sixteen men aged eighteen to twenty-four years (mean values and standard deviation).

spite of the marked increase in $V_{O_2}$ max., there was no increase of heart volume after six months of training.

A surprising result could be found: the 4½ months value was significantly increased compared with the pretraining value, but the six months value was significantly reduced again.

## Cardiac Output, Stroke Volume and Arteriovenous Oxygen Difference (avD)

According to results of Bevegard and co-workers,[4] the increase of cardiac output with increasing oxygen uptake follows about the same relationship as in untrained persons, both in lying and in sitting position. A slightly hyperkinetic circulation was found. That means that the avD were slightly reduced at different levels of oxygen uptake, the maximum avD was enlarged compared with untrained persons. On transition from rest to exercise the stroke volume increased, similar to untrained persons, 9 percent in the supine and 48 percent in the sitting position, but starting, of course, from a higher level. The higher oxygen transport capacity in the athletes can be explained predominantly by a larger stroke volume. The avD during maximum exercise is only slightly higher, the maximum heart rate is a little reduced.

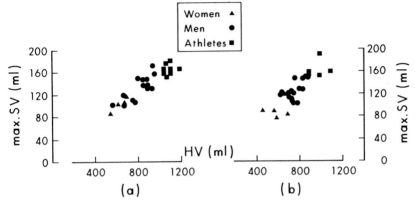

Figure 1–4. The relationships between maximum stroke volume and heart volume in untrained women and men and in athletes. The left panel shows results from Bevegard *et al.*, and Holmgren *et al.*, the right panel from Reindell *et al.*

A good correlation between maximum stroke volume and heart volume could be found by many authors[2,4,11] (Fig. 1–4).

In contrast to the comparative studies in athletes, follow-up studies after weeks or months of training in formerly untrained persons could demonstrate an enlarged avD at different levels of oxygen uptake.[1] During maximum exercise only an increase in avD or both increases in maximum stroke volume and maximum avD could be found.

In our own three years study, which runs now for six months, the first systematical reinvestigation of cardiac output will be performed after one year of training. Samples taken offhand showed both possibilities, increases in maximum stroke volume and in maximum avD, without any increase of heart volume.

## Pressures in the Systemic and Pulmonary Circulation

In relation to work load or oxygen uptake there is no significant difference of pressures in the systemic and pulmonary circulation compared with untrained persons.

In relation to heart rate systolic pressures are elevated as a consequence of the larger stroke volumes.[4] The increase of pulmonary wedge pressure during exercise was found to be more pronounced, possibly caused by a reduced compliance of the hypertrophied athlete's heart.

In untrained persons, there is no increase of pulmonary wedge pressure during exercise. In summary, the capacity of the oxygen transport system may be increased through several factors (including the results from following and comparative studies):

1. Increase of avD at rest, during submaximum and maximum exercise.
2. Increase of ejection fraction (SV/EDV) at rest, and especially during exercise. This can be derived from significant increases of stroke volumes and constant total heart volumes.
3. Further increase of stroke volume by increase of the heart volume.

The lower the pretraining values, the more pronounced are the training effects. Factors 1 and 2 are functional factors which take place after short and not extremely severe training periods. These factors are temporary in the training process. They vanish partly after long periods of severe training, especially when an anatomical factor, the increase of heart volume, comes into play. The enlarged hearts of athletes may be predominantly developed by early training, particularly in the growth years. This may be derived from the results of a three years longitudinal study from Cermak.[5] After one year of training for swimming there was a marked increase in heart volume/kg body weight.

That would imply that mechanisms of increasing oxygen transport capacity by training are age dependent.[7,12,13,14]

## Heart Weight

In individual cases, even in the age between twenty and thirty years, marked increases of heart volume can be seen in a relatively short time after severe physical training. It is possible that hearts which have been large at one time will increase more rapidly.

It was once believed that the oxygen supply to the hypertrophied heart of the athlete would become more and more critical. Linzbach[10] demonstrated that 500 g is a critical weight of a heart with normal coronary arteries. That is, hearts which weighed more than 500 g showed morphological signs of coronary insufficiency. The heart weights of forty athletes who died by accidents during their active career were classified by Reindell *et al.*[11]

It could be seen that only in three cases the heart weights were more than 500 g. In two of these three cases, however, epicardial fat and intraepicardial vessels were also weighed. That means that the heart weight of athletes usually is not more than 500 g. Moreover, hypoxia tolerance of athletes was found to be the same as in untrained hearts.[11]

Figure 1–5 is a schematic representation of the relationships between heart weight, enddiastolic and endsystolic volumes in a normal heart, a pressure overloaded heart, an athlete's heart and a volume overloaded heart. The heart of the athlete adapts the same as a volume overloaded heart, so long as there is no structural damage, for example in a case with aortic regurgitation.

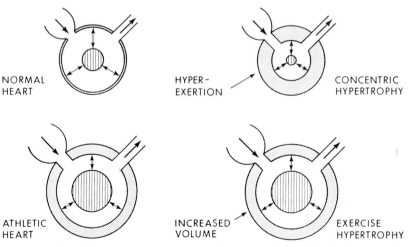

Figure 1–5. Schematic representation of ventricular wall thickness, end-diastolic and end-systolic volumes in a normal heart, a pressure overloaded heart, an athlete's heart and a volume overloaded heart.

## Mechanical Activity of the Heart

Sympathetic stimulation during exercise is about the same as in an untrained heart. In untrained persons—the investigations in athletes are not yet completed—maximum dp/dt measured with a catheter tip manometer Stratham $SF_1$ increased about three times during exercise with 150 watts (Fig. 1–6). This sympathetic stimulation may not be so important as believed up to now. After $\beta$—receptor—blocking with propranalol, maximum dp/dt/p, as contractility indices, increased only little; there remained only a frequency related increase. But

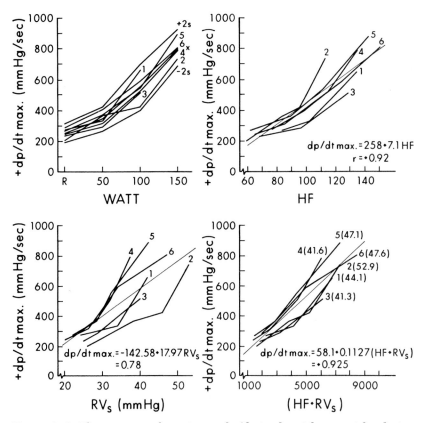

Figure 1–6. The increase of maximum dp/dt in the right ventricle, during stepwise increased exercise in six untrained normal persons. The relationships to the work intensity in watts, the heart rate (HF), the systolic pressure in the right ventricle ($RV_s$) and HF × $RV_s$ are demonstrated.

in spite of eliminating sympathetic stimulation during exercise $VO_2$ maximum decreased only about 10 percent.

Cardiac output during 200 Watts exercise decreases as a consequence of reducing maximum heart rate. Maximum stroke volume remains the same. The most important fact is the elevation of diastolic pressure in the pulmonary artery, which corresponds with the mean pressure in the left atrium (Fig. 1–7).

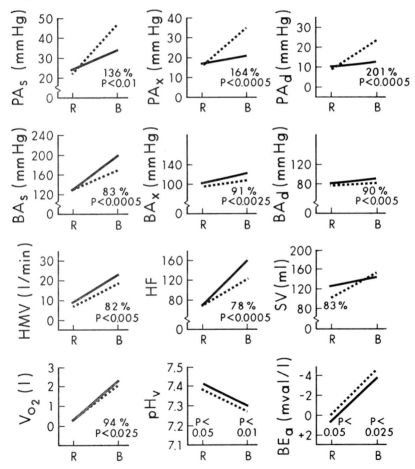

Figure 1–7. Pressures in the pulmonary artery ($PA_s$, $PA_x$, $PA_d$), pressures in the brachial artery ($BA_s$, $BA_x$, $BA_d$), cardiac output (HMV/1/min), heart rate (HF), stroke volume (SV), oxygen uptake ($VO_2$, 1/min), pH of mixed venous blood ($pH_v$) and base excess (BE, mval/1) at rest (R) and during six minutes of 200 watts exercise (B) before (uninterrupted line) and after 60 mg Propranolol in six untrained normal persons.

But this is not incipient heart failure, it only means switching from predominantly sympathetic activation to the mere operation of Starling mechanism.

## Electrical Activity of the Heart

In about 9 percent of athletes, electrocardiographic signs of increased vagotonia are found, as prolongation of PQ-interval or even Wenckebach phenomenon.

The amplitudes of the R waves in $V_4$, $V_5$ and $V_6$ are larger in athletes than in untrained persons; this is a sign of left ventricular hypertrophy.[11]

A relationship between heart volume and the frequency of incomplete right bundle branch block in athletes could be found.[13] 40 percent of the athletes with a heart volume between 1200 and 1300 ccm have this ECG pattern.

In another study we reinvestigated former athletes, who up to ten years ago had had an incomplete right bundle branch block.[14] At the present time half of them no longer show this ECG pattern. The others show an incomplete right bundle branch block.

In cardiology, an incomplete right bundle branch block is usually associated with a pressure or volume overloaded right ventricle.

Therefore, we thought that perhaps people with an incomplete right bundle branch block would show increased pressures in the pulmonary artery at rest and/or during exercise.

In six subjects with an incomplete right bundle branch block we measured pressures in the pulmonary artery and cardiac output at rest and during exercise. A normal increase in pulmonary artery pressures was found with increasing exercise as shown in Figure 1–8. The pulmonary vascular resistance decreased with increasing exercise in a normal way.

## Effects of Altitude

To complete the discussion of the circulatory system of the athletes we would like to add some results about the perform-

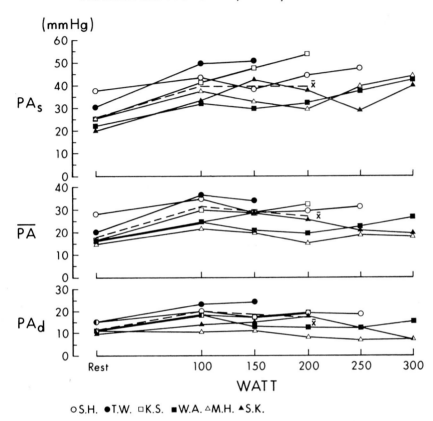

Figure 1–8. Pressures in the pulmonary artery ($PA_s$, $\overline{PA}$, $PA_d$) at rest and during stepwise increased bicycle ergometer exercise in lying position in six men with an uncomplete right bundle branch block.

ance at altitude, which we did together with the president of this session, Dr. Landry, during his stay in Germany.

With increasing altitude there is a decrease of $Vo_2$ max. At an altitude of 2250 m, that is the altitude of Mexico City, there is an decrease of $Vo_2$ max. of about 10 percent. In spite of a significant increase in hemoglobin, there is only a little change in $Vo_2$ max, during a prolonged stay at altitude (Fig. 1–9). This is also true at higher altitudes, as shown by many authors (summary of references in Roskamm *et al.*, 1968[16]).

In another study, the author has investigated whether a rigorously standardized exercise program, performed daily at

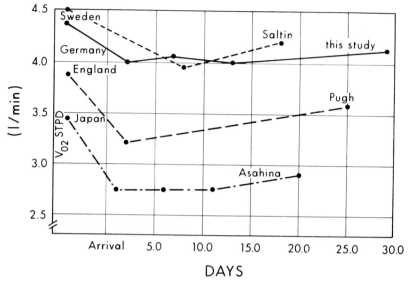

Figure 1–9. Maximum oxygen uptake of four national teams at sea-level (Sweden, Germany, England, Japan) and during an up to four weeks stay in Mexico City (mean values).

barometric pressures of 580 and 500 mm Hg (simulated altitudes of 2,500 and 3,450 m, respectively), was able to trigger the process of acclimatization, and if such a training program performed at two different altitudes could produce significantly different training effects than if it was done at sea level.

In conclusion we found greater increases of the posttraining mean values for maximum oxygen uptakes in the two altitude trained groups than in the sea-level trained one.[15,16,17]

It has been suggested that there may be a risk in exercising at altitude for example from pulmonary hypertension or pulmonary edema, which is associated with pulmonary hypertension.

In order to study these problems we exposed normal persons to different levels of hypoxia.[17] The decrease of oxygen saturation was found to be the same as in high altitude residents as reported by Hultgren *et al.*[8] But the increase of mean pulmonary artery pressure was found to be less (Fig. 1–10).

During exercise with 50 watts the increase of mean pulmonary

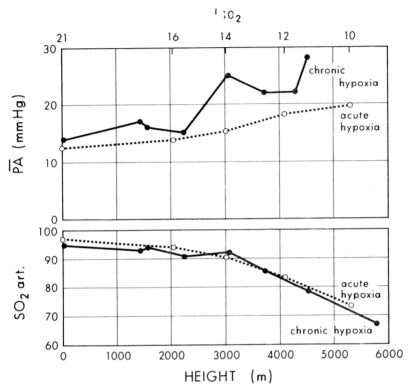

Figure 1–10. Mean pressure in the pulmonary artery ($\overline{\text{PA}}$ mm Hg) and arterial oxygen saturation (SO₂ art.) in high altitude residents (Hultgren *et al.*) and during acute exposure to hypoxia in ten sea-level residents (mean values).

artery pressure is the same as at rest (Fig. 1–11). The absolute values are higher because of a higher cardiac output. However with maximum exercise there is no increase of mean pulmonary artery pressure with increasing hypoxia, that means that the pulmonary vasoconstriction caused by hypoxia is eliminated by heavy physical exercise. This is in contrast with the behavior of altitude residents as reported by Banchero and coworkers.[3] Figure 1–12 shows the increase of mean pulmonary artery pressure in relationship to the decrease of arterial oxygen saturation. With increasing acidosis the increase in mean arterial pulmonary pressure is steeper, as shown by many authors. It can

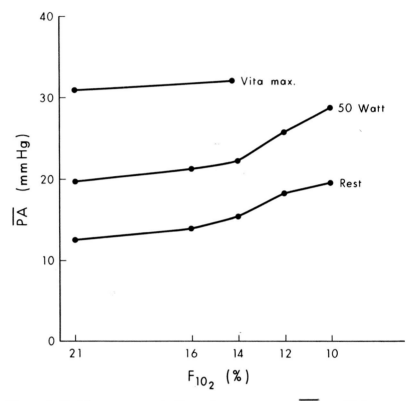

Figure 1–11. Mean pressure in the pulmonary artery ($\overline{\text{PA}}$ mm Hg) at rest, during 50 watt and during maximum exercise (mean values of ten sea-level residents at rest, six during 50 watt exercise and six during maximum exercise), steady state exercise in 21, 16, 14 (13, 8), 12 and 10% $O_2$ in $N_2$.

be seen, however, that acidosis induced by heavy physical exercise has no potentiating effects on the pulmonary vasoconstriction caused by hypoxia.

## Conclusion

In conclusion the athlete's heart reacts at rest and during exercise under normoxic and hypoxic conditions in quite the same way as an untrained heart; its increased oxygen transport capacity is mainly caused by its larger stroke volume which is enabled by the enlarged heart volume.

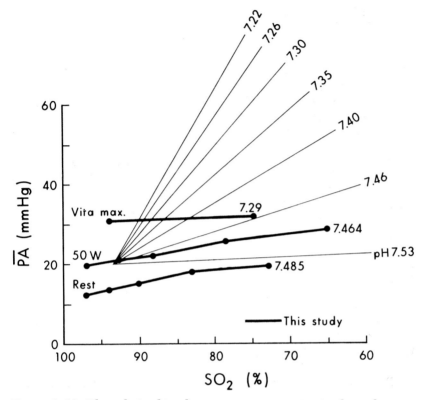

Figure 1–12. The relationships between mean pressure in the pulmonary artery ($\overline{PA}$ mm Hg) and arterial oxygen saturation [$SO_2$ (%)]. The lower the pH, the more pronounced is the increase of $\overline{PA}$. (According to results of Enson *et al.*, *J Clin Invest*, 43, 1146 (1964).

Our results (see Fig. 1–11) and the corresponding pH values are added.

It is understandable that I could not discuss all aspects of the circulation of the superior athletes, for example the peripheral circulation and changes at the cellular level which have and will be stressed by other speakers.

## References

1. Andrew, G.M., Guzman, C., and Bechlake, M.R.: *J. Appl. Physiol.* *16:* 603–608, 1966.

2. Astrand, P.O., Cuddy, T.E., Saltin, B., and Stenberg, J.: *J Appl. Physiol.* 2: 268–274, 1964.
3. Banchero, N., Sime, F., Penalozo, D., Cruz, J., Gamboa, R. and Marticorena, E.: *Circulation* 33: 249–262, 1966.
4. Bevegard, S., Holmgren, A., and Jonsson, B.: *Acta Physiol Scand.* 57: 26–50, 1963.
5. Cermak, J.: *XVIIIth World Congress of Sports Medicine.* (OXFORD : 6–11 September 1970).
6. Ekblom, B., Astrand, P.O., Saltin, B., Stenberg, I., and Wallström, B.: *J. Appl. Physiol.* 24: 518–528, 1968.
7. Hartley, L.H., Grimby, G., Kilbom, A., Nilsson, N.J., Astrand, I., Bjure, J., Ekblom, B., and Saltin, B.: *Scand. J. Clin. Lab. Invest.* 4: 335–344, 1969.
8. Hultgren, H.N., Miller, H., and Kelly, J.: *J. Appl. Physiol.* 20: 233–238, 1965.
9. Israel, S.: *Sport, Herzgrösse und Herz-Kreislauf-Dynamik.* Johann Ambrosius Barth Verlag, Leipzig, 1968.
10. Linzbach, A.J.: *Virch. Arch.* 314: 534, 1947.
11. Reindell, H., Klepzig, H., Steim, H., Musshoff, K., Roskamm, H., and Schildge, E.: *Herz, Kreislauf und Sport.* Johann Ambrosius Barth Verlag, München, 1960.
12. Roskamm, H., Brandts, N., and Reindell, H.: *Cardiologia* (Basel) 58: 441–460, 1966.
13. Roskamm, H., Weidenbach, J., Reindell, H.: *Sportarzt und Sportmedizin,* 6: 251–260, 1966.
14. Roskamm, H., Weidenbach, J., and Reindell, H.: *Zschr. f. Kreislaufforschg.,* 55: 783–794, 1966.
15. Roskamm, H., Landry, F., Samek, L., Schlager, M., Weidemann, H., Reindell, H.: *J. of Appl. Physiol.* 27: 840–847, 1969.
16. Roskamm, H., Samek, L., Weidemann, H., and Reindell, H.: *Leistung und Höhe.* Knoll, AG, Ludwigschafen, 1968.
17. Roskamm, H., Petersen, J., Weidemann, H., Blümchen, G., Landry, F., and Reindell, H.: *Zschr. Kreislaufforsch,* (im Druck) 1970.
18. Rowell, L. B.: Factors affecting the prediction of maximal oxygen uptake from measurements made during submaximal work with observations related to factors, which may limit maximal oxygen uptake. Minneapolis: Thesis, 1962.
19. Saltin, B., and Astrand, P.O.: *J. Appl. Physiol.* 3: 353–358, 1967.

*Chapter 2*

# Epididymal Fat Pad Regeneration and Free Fatty Acid Mobilization with Exercise and Training

ALBERT W. TAYLOR
MARILYN BOOTH
KATHERINE McBEAN

## Abstract

This study was undertaken to investigate the effects of exercise and training upon the regeneration of epididymal fat tissue and the possible effects upon free fatty acid (FFA) mobilization. The investigation was divided into three experiments in which animals had either the epididymal fat pads bilaterally lipidectomized or the right epididymal fat pad unilaterally lipidectomized for the measurement of FFA mobilization and *in vitro* release of FFA from adipose tissue in intact and regenerating lipid tissue. The third aspect of the experiment measured the DNA content per gram of fresh adipose tissue in regenerating and intact fat pads. Epididymal fat pads were found to regenerate as measured by total pad weight and as indicated by total DNA content. The regenerating fat pads were unable to mobilize FFA or release FFA *in vitro* after exercise to fatigue, whereas the mobilization and release of FFA from the fat pads of nonlipidectomized fatigued animals increased as expected. The total DNA content of the regenerating fatty tissue decreased for twelve to twenty-four weeks after lipidectomy and at twenty-eight to thirty weeks of age the DNA content of all fat tissue approached that of control animals.

*Note:* This study was supported by University of Alberta grants GR 55–32185 and GR 32322 and The Department of National Health and Welfare Grant DNHW 55–04021.

A.W. Taylor is the recipient of a research associateship from the Department of National Health and Welfare, Ottawa, Canada.

We gratefully acknowledge the technical assistance of Miss Diane Tougas, Miss Deloras Franz and Miss Nancy Smith.

21

Much uncertainty exists about the growth and regeneration of adipose tissue. During the period 1903–1912 numerous investigators denied the ability of the fat cell to regenerate. More recently Cameron and Seneviratne[8] have demonstrated that a local stimulus after partial resection does not stimulate compensatory hypertrophy in the fat organ but that new fat cells are produced through differentation of precursors in close association with an expanding vascular framework. Hausberger[26] on the other hand noted that for lipid transplants random development of new adipose tissue played a definite role during excessive fat storage which was primarily dependent upon the amount of immature adipose tissue transplanted. The size of the adipose depot is dependent upon the number and size of the constituent cells but little is known about the factors that determine total adipose cell number or size in the immature or adult rat fat pad, although each cell, regardless of size, converts glucose at comparable rates.[37] Hirsch and Han[31] most recently have indicated that with age, adipose tissue progressively loses the ability to grow by hyperplasia of the adipocytes. That adipose tissue is not continuously capable of regeneration was also noted by Goss.[25]

Until recently, white fat tissue has been regarded as a storage organ for fatty acids synthesized in the liver.[30] It is becoming more evident that the fat cells actively participate in fat metabolism.[27] Experiments with dogs,[33,34] horses,[10] rats[20,22] and man[3,4,5,9,11,12,13,18,19,28,29] have demonstrated that fat in the form of free fatty acids serves as a major source of energy for muscular contraction. It has been estimated that fat oxidation may contribute approximately 90 percent of endurance exercise metabolism.[9,29,34] Fat used during exercise is supplied to the muscles by adipose tissue via the blood and not from lipid stores of the muscle.[42] Since the rate of oxidation of fat is closely related to the plasma FFA level[4] a rise in FFA must take place during exercise if use of fat is to increase. Such an increase in the mobilization of fat during exercise has been shown to occur.[4] However, the mechanism by which the mobilization of lipid is controlled during exercise is obscure.[22,53]

Most of the knowledge concerning adipose tissue metabolism

is derived from studies on the epididymal fat pad of the rat.[39,57,58] In general, the metabolism of the tissue at this site is similar to that in other depots such as the mesenteric, inguinal, perirenal, and subcutaneous areas.[52] Lipid deposition is a result of two processes: incorporation of preformed lipid from the circulation and "de novo" synthesis of lipid from carbohydrate directly in the adipose cell itself.[52] The present investigation was divided into three separate studies and was undertaken to determine what effect the removal of one or both of the epididymal fat pads had on the regeneration of the tissue and in initiating FFA mobilization during exercise and training.

## Methods and Materials

### Bilateral Epididymal Lipidectomy

All animals were housed in individual $7 \times 10 \times 7$ inch self-cleaning cages in an air-conditioned room maintained at 24.5°C. The animals were fed a complete, synthetic diet for rats as described by Allison *et al.*[1] This diet was prepared as previously related by Gollnick and Taylor.[23] Each animal received daily food and water *ad libitum.* All animals in the study were 180–200 grams and six to eight weeks of age at the initiation of each experiment.

One hundred and four male Wistar rats were allocated into a control group of thirty-two animals and an exercise group of seventy-two respectively. The exercised rats were trained to run on a motor-driven treadmill (Collins Company) and after four weeks were capable of running continuously for one hour at 1 mph. Prior to the exercise regimen, bilateral lipidectomy of the epididymal fat pads was performed upon one half of the controls and one quarter of the exercise group. When the exercised group attained the required training speed and duration, the fat pads were removed from a second set of eighteen rats. The other half of the exercised animals were either sham operated upon or trained to run with no surgical operation being performed upon them. One quarter of each group was sacrificed at four week intervals with one-half of each exercise group being run to exhaustion immediately prior to death. All remaining animals were killed at rest.

The rats were sacrificed under light ether anesthesia. Eight to 10 ml of blood were withdrawn from the bifurcation of the abdominal aorta into heparinized syringes and the epididymal fat pads were quickly removed and weighed on a Roller-Smith torsion balance. Plasma and adipose tissue FFA levels were estimated as well as the *in vitro* release of FFA by adipose tissue.[16,50] Nile Blue A was used as the titration indicator in place of Thymol Blue as it gave a more reproducible end-point.

## Unilateral Epididymal Lipidectomy

Thirty-five Wistar rats were divided into an exercise group of eighteen and a control group of seventeen animals. Nine animals of the exercise group had the left epididymal fat pad removed prior to training. Six animals had the fat pad removed upon attaining the required training regimen and a further three (FRLLT) animals had unilateral lipidectomy performed upon them after four weeks of training. One-third of each exercise group was exercised to fatigue prior to sacrifice. Unilateral lipidectomy was performed upon control animals numbering eight (FRIC), six (FRLC) and three (FRLLC) at similar times.

## DNA Content of Epididymal Fat Pads

One hundred and sixty male Wistar rats 180–200 grams were divided into three groups of which sixty-eight were bilaterally lipidectomized, sixty were unilaterally lipidectomized (left pad) and thirty-two served as controls. Fifty-two of the bilaterally and forty-eight of the unilaterally lipidectomized animals were trained to run as described in Study I. DNA content of regenerating and intact fat pads was measured by a modification of the method of Wannemacher *et al.*,[55] Robinson[47] and Robinson and Bradford[48] at four week intervals after lipidectomy.

Fat samples were homogenized at medium speed on a Virtis homogenizer for five minutes in 0.14M KCl (5% homogenate W/V). Two ml of cold (4° C) 1.2N PCA and 5 ml of the ethanol/ether/acetate solution were added to 4 ml of the tissue homogenate, mixed well, and centrifuged. The supernatant was removed by section and discarded. The precipitate was then washed twice with 5 ml of the ethanol/ether/acetate solution and twice with 5 ml of 0.2N PCA (4° C). Each time the supernatant was removed and discarded after centrifugation. Four ml of 0.3N KOH was added to the precipitate, mixed, and incubated at 37° C for one hour. Two ml of cold (4° C) 0.2N PCA was then added to the test tube, centrifuged and the supernatant discarded. The precipitate was washed twice with 0.2N PCA (4° C) and the supernatant discarded. Exactly 5 ml 0.2N PCA was added to the precipitate mixed, and incubated in 70° C waterbath for one hour. Tubes were cooled and centrifuged at 3000 rpm for ten minutes. Contents were transferred to another tube and respun if necessary to obtain a clear supernatant. The test solution was then read at 265 mu and 290 mu. A 0.2N PCA blank was used.

A standard curve was obtained by dissolving 10 mg DNA (corrected for moisture) in 10 ml 0.3N KOH and incubated at 37° C for one hour. DNA was precipitated with cold (4°C) 1.2N PCA and centrifuged. Five ml 0.2N PCA was added to the precipitate and incubated at 70° C for one hour. Tubes were read at 265 mu and 290 mu when cool. A standard curve was made plotting ($OD_{265}$–$OD_{290}$) versus DNA concentration.

## Results

### Bilateral Epididymal Lipidectomy

Plasma FFA levels were elevated in all groups of animals exercised to fatigue (Fig. 2–1). Adipose tissue FFA values were elevated in only the control trained groups which were run to fatigue (Fig. 2–2). A similar finding was evident for the release of FFA by the adipose tissue *in vitro* (Fig. 2–3). The unexpected findings that regenerating fat pads do not mobilize FFA nor release FFA from adipose tissue *in vitro* is made evident in Table 2-I.

Table 2-II contains the data representative of body weights for the eight groups. All animals were of the same relative

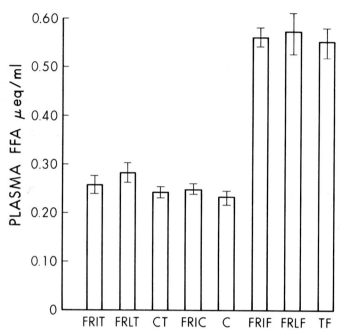

Figure 2–1. Effects of exercise on plasma FFA in epididymal bilaterally lipidectomized and control rats.

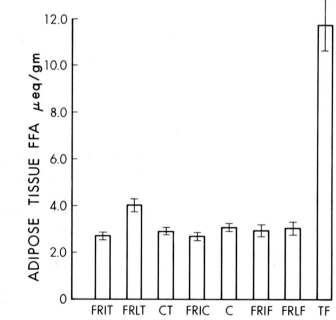

Figure 2–2. Effects of exercise on adipose tissue FFA in epididymal bilaterally lipidectomized and control rats.

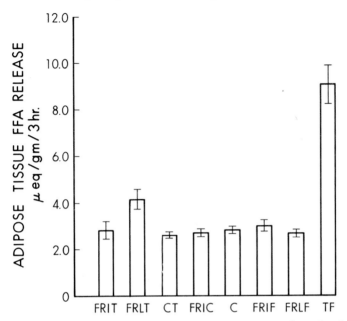

Figure 2–3. Effects of exercise on *in vitro* release of FFA from lipid tissue in bilaterally lipidectomized and control rats.

TABLE 2-I

EFFECTS OF EXERCISE ON PLASMA AND ADIPOSE TISSUE FFA AND
*IN VITRO* RELEASE OF LIPID TISSUE FFA IN EPIDIDYMAL
BILATERALLY LIPIDECTOMIZED AND CONTROL RATS

| Group[a] | Plasma FFA ueq/ml | Adipose Tissue FFA ueq/gm | Adipose Tissue FFA Release ueq/gm/3 hr |
|---|---|---|---|
| Fat Removed Initially Trained— Rest (10)[b] | .257 ± .014 | 2.71 ± .156 | 2.84 ± .374 |
| Fat Removed Late—Trained— Rest (10) | .283 ± .018 | 4.02 ± .285 | 4.16 ± .447 |
| Control—Trained—Rest (18) | .247 ± .011 | 2.93 ± .119 | 2.63 ± .120 |
| Fat Removed Initially— Fatigue (8) | .563 ± .019[c] | 2.98 ± .228 | 3.02 ± .216 |
| Fat Removed Late— Fatigue (8) | .571 ± .043[c] | 3.05 ± .230 | 2.69 ± .171 |
| Trained—Fatigue (18) | .554 ± .030[c] | 11.77 ± 1.12[d] | 9.99 ± .841[d] |
| Fat Removed Initially— Control—Rest (16) | .246 ± .011 | 2.71 ± .138 | 2.72 ± .159 |
| Control—Rest (16) | .238 ± .010 | 3.08 ± .151 | 2.86 ± .118 |

[a] Values are means ± S.E.M.
[b] Numbers in parentheses are animals per group
[c] Exercised to fatigue vs. rested or control animals $P < 0.01$ or less
[d] Trained intact exercised to fatigue vs. lipidectomized animals $P < 0.01$ or less

TABLE 2-II
ANIMAL (WEEKLY) MEAN BODY WEIGHTS
AFTER BILATERAL LIPIDECTOMY

| Group[a] | 0[b] | 4 | 8 | 12 | 16 |
|---|---|---|---|---|---|
| FRIT (10)[c] | 225.4 | 302 | 331 | 377 | 419 |
| FRLT (10) | 224.2 | 275 | 326 | 392 | 412 |
| TC | 224.6 | 355 | 360 | 426 | 436 |
| FRIF (8) | 225.3 | 270 | 298 | 391 | 456 |
| FRLF (8) | 224.7 | 301 | 425 | 428 | 431 |
| TF (18) | 225.0 | 327 | 361 | 445 | 464 |
| FRIC (16) | 225.8 | 365 | 404 | 463 | 534*[d] |
| C (16) | 225.0 | 408 | 401 | 501 | 513*[d] |

[a] Values are group means in grams
[b] Numbers are weeks to excision or sacrifice
[c] Number of animals are indicated in parentheses
[d] Exercised groups vs. Control groups [P < 0.05] or less

weight at the initiation of the study. Trained animals after sixteen weeks of exercise with or without lipidectomy were of the same relative weight. The control groups were significantly heavier than the exercise groups ( P < 0.05 or less) at this time.

The epididymal fat pad weights at excision and at the time of sacrifice are found in Table 2-III. Regeneration of the epididymal fat is evident from the increases in pad weights after lipidectomy. All exercising groups had similar epididymal fat pad total weight after sixteen weeks of training. Those groups exercising, but with no lipidectomy, had similar weights approximately twice the size of the other exercise groups. The control animals demonstrated enormous fat pad weights when compared with all other groups.

TABLE 2-III
TOTAL EPIDIDYMAL FAT PAD WEIGHTS AT EXCISION AND
SACRIFICE AFTER BILATERAL LIPIDECTOMY

| Group[a] | 0[b] | 4 | 8 | 12 | 16 |
|---|---|---|---|---|---|
| FRIT (10) | 1295.1 | 762.8 | 860.0 | 1264.0 | 1826.2 |
| FRLT (10) | — | 2232.9 | 316.8 | 757.2 | 1891.4 |
| TC (18) | — | 2882.7 | 3183.7 | 4280.6 | 4021.0[e] |
| FRIF (8) | 1248.3 | 334.6 | 767.2 | 1232.6 | 1891.0 |
| FRLF (8) | — | 2012.3 | 297.0 | 1307.0 | 1820.0 |
| TF (18) | — | 3007.9 | 2823.0 | 4490.9 | 4020.0[e] |
| FRIC (16) | 1216.9 | 1837.6 | 2499.0 | 3871.4 | 5043.9[d] |
| C (16) | — | 4355.3 | 6109.6 | 7845.5 | 9007.3[d] |

[a] Values are group means in milligrams
[b] Numbers are weeks to excision or sacrifice
[c] Number of animals are indicated in parentheses
[d] Exercised groups vs. control groups [P < 0.05] or less
[e] Exercised lipidectomized groups vs. exercised nonlipidectomized groups[P < 0.05 or less

TABLE 2-IV

EFFECTS OF EXERCISE ON PLASMA AND ADIPOSE TISSUE FFA AND *IN VITRO* OF LIPID TISSUE FFA IN EPIDIDYMAL UNILATERAL LIPIDECTOMIZED AND CONTROL RATS

| Group[a] | Plasma FFA ueq/ml | Adipose Tissue FFA ueq/gm | | | Adipose Tissue FFA Release ueq/gm/3 hr. | | |
|---|---|---|---|---|---|---|---|
| | | Regenerating Pad at Lipidectomy | Regenerating Pad at Sacrifice | Pad Intact at Sacrifice | Regenerating Pad at Lipidectomy | Regenerating Pad at Sacrifice | Pad Intact at Sacrifice |
| FRIT (6)[b] | .333 ± .018 | —[d] | 4.94 ± .431 | 3.05 ± .583 | 4.98 ± .632 | 3.41 ± .413 | 4.49 ± .016 |
| FRIF (3) | .967 ± .141[c] | —[d] | 4.58 ± .582 | 9.05 ± 1.212 | 3.52 ± .111 | 4.55 ± .127 | 8.71 ± .136[c] |
| FRLT (4) | .412 ± .101 | 4.55 ± .841 | 4.50 ± .610 | 4.80 ± .137 | 3.85 ± .131 | 4.32 ± .202 | 4.51 ± .041 |
| FRLF (2) | .750 ± .013[c] | 4.00 ± .763 | 4.12 ± .126 | 10.75 ± 1.432[c] | 4.68 ± .411 | 3.14 ± .043 | 10.75 ± 1.362[c] |
| FRLLT (3) | .381 ± .042 | —[d] | 3.71 ± .134 | 3.12 ± .063 | 4.25 ± .382 | 4.50 ± .091 | 3.31 ± .073 |
| FRIC (8) | .357 ± .026 | | 3.65 ± .422 | 4.42 ± .137 | 3.53 ± .413 | 4.12 ± .212 | 4.34 ± .015 |
| FRLC (6) | .318 ± .013 | 3.12 ± .132 | 4.34 ± .328 | 3.31 ± .216 | 4.46 ± .683 | 4.11 ± .314 | 3.01 ± .058 |
| FRLLC (3) | .326 ± .021 | 3.45 ± .064 | 4.35 ± .531 | 4.61 ± .433 | 3.75 ± .126 | 3.95 ± .058 | 3.51 ± .037 |

a Values are group means ± SEM
b Numbers of animals per group are in parentheses
c Groups exercised to fatigue vs. rest and control groups [P < 0.05] or less
d Samples too small to analyse for both FFA release and mobilization

## Unilateral Epididymal Lipidectomy

Plasma FFA levels were once again elevated in all groups exercised to fatigue (Table 2-IV). No differences in plasma FFA values were noted between trained rested animals and control groups. Adipose tissue FFA values for regenerating fat pads were not elevated under conditions of exercise to fatigue. The intact pads did, however, demonstrate increased adipose tissue FFA levels after exercise (Fig. 2–4). The *in vitro* release of

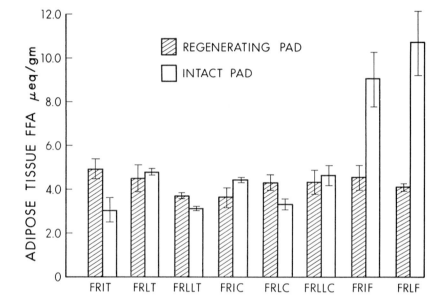

Figure 2–4. Effects of exercise on adipose tissue FFA in epididymal unilaterally lipidectomized and control rats.

FFA from adipose tissue followed a trend similar to the mobilization of FFA from regenerating and intact fat pads with the only significant release increase being found for intact pads in animals run to complete exhaustion (Fig. 2–5).

Animal body weights and epididymal fat pad regenerating and intact weights are found in Table 2-V. After twenty-four weeks of running the total fat pad weight is slightly greater than found after sixteen weeks of training for the bilateral lipidectomy study. Fat pad regeneration as indicated by increased fat pad

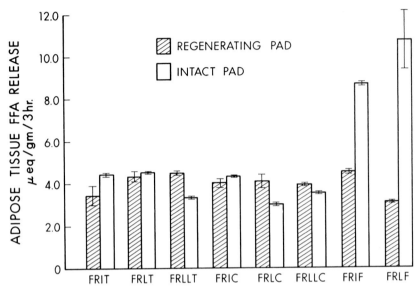

Figure 2–5. Effects of exercise on *in vitro* release of FFA from adipose tissue in unilaterally lipidectomized and control rats.

size and weight after lipidectomy is again obvious. The intact and regenerating fat pads of the control animals are greater in size and weight in all cases than the weights of the groups trained to run.

TABLE 2-V

ANIMAL BODY AND EPIDIDYMAL FAT PAD WEIGHTS INITIALLY AND AT SACRIFICE AFTER UNILATERAL LIPIDECTOMY

| Group[a] | Body Weights (gr) At Lipidectomy | Body Weights (gr) At Sacrifice | Regenerating Fat Pad (mg) At Lipidectomy | Regenerating Fat Pad (mg) At Sacrifice | Intact Fat Pad (mg) At Sacrifice |
|---|---|---|---|---|---|
| FRIT  (6)[b] | 122.67 | 397.67 | 206.56 | 487.60 | 2129.67 |
| FRIF  (3) | 139.00 | 345.67 | 212.07 | 370.67 | 1909.27 |
| FRLT  (4) | 261.25 | 381.75 | 813.80 | 381.35 | 2213.90 |
| FRLF  (2) | 272.50 | 376.00 | 720.70 | 293.90 | 1426.80 |
| FRLLT (3) | 363.33 | 404.67 | 1812.33 | 429.67 | 1885.33 |
| FRIC  (8) | 128.38 | 413.13 | 217.20 | 582.03[c] | 3052.06[c] |
| FRLC  (6) | 271.17 | 457.50[c] | 912.97[c] | 535.88[c] | 3586.60[c] |
| FRLLC (3) | 409.33[c] | 452.00[c] | 3008.13[c] | 535.50[c] | 4216.70[c] |

[a] Values are group means
[b] Numbers of animals per group are in parentheses
[c] Exercised groups vs. own control groups [P < 0.05] or less

## DNA Content

The DNA content of the epididymal fat pads for the trained and control groups which were bilaterally lipidectomized were similar for both the left and right pad. The DNA content of the regenerating and intact fat pads of the exercise group which were unilaterally lipidectomized was greater than that of the unilaterally lipidectomized control group ($P < 0.05$). The regenerating fat pad always demonstrated a higher DNA content than the intact pad in all animals from both the exercise and control groups. The control animals demonstrated less DNA content than any of the groups surgically operated upon ($P < 0.05$) (Table 2-VI).

TABLE 2-VI

DNA CONTENT (mg/gm FRESH TISSUE) OF REGENERATING AND INTACT EPIDIDYMAL FAT PADS IN RATS FOUR WEEKS OF TRAINING AFTER LIDIDECTOMY

| Group[a] | Animals Per Group | Left Pad | Right Pad |
|---|---|---|---|
| Bilaterally Lipidectomized Trained | 13 | .344 ± .018[c] | .337 ± .026[c] |
| Unilaterally (left) Lipidectomized Trained | 12 | .246 ± .013[c] | .154 ± .031[bc] |
| Bilaterally Lipidectomized Control | 4 | .329 ± .021 | .439 ± .084 |
| Unilaterally (left) Lipidectomized Control | 3 | .139 ± .023[d] | .060 ± .013[bd] |
| Control | 8 | .090 ± .011[c] | .099 ± .012[c] |

[a] Values are means ± S.E.M.
[b] Regenerating lipidectomized DNA content vs. intact lipidectomized content [$P < 0.05$] or less
[c] DNA content of lipid of trained animals vs. control animals $P < 0.05$ or less
[d] DNA content of lipid of trained unilaterally lipidectomized animals vs. control lipidectomized animals [$P < 0.05$] or less

Figure 2–6 contains the curves of DNA content for lipidectomized and control animals at four week intervals after bilateral and unilateral lipidectomy. All DNA content curves appear to converge with the line representing the DNA content of the control animals. It is interesting to note that the DNA content of the intact as well as the regenerating fat pads of the lipidectomized animals appears to approach the DNA content or perhaps cellularization of the nonlipidectomized animals in a decreasing fashion, suggesting that although the adipose tissue size and weight is increasing, the cellularity per gram of fresh tissue is gradually decreasing.

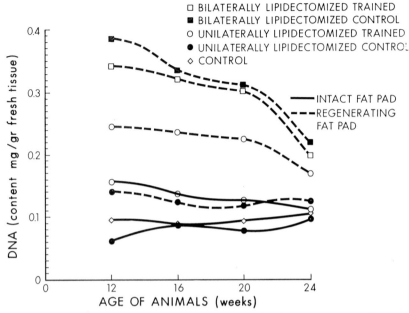

Figure 2–6. DNA content (mg/gm fresh tissue) of regenerating and intact epididymal fat pads of rats sacrificed at four week intervals after lipidectomy (at 8 weeks of age).

## Discussion

The elevated plasma FFA and adipose tissue FFA levels and the increase in *in vitro* release of FFA from the adipose tissue after exhaustive exercise in nonlipidectomized rats as well as the increased tissue FFA and *in vitro* release of FFA levels in the intact fat pads of unilaterally lipidectomized exercised animals indicates that lipid mobilization in plasma and the fat depots is stimulated by muscular work.[21,22] Similar postexercise increases have previously been found for plasma FFA levels in humans,[5,13,18] dogs[7] and rats,[60] for adipose FFA levels in rats[21,22] and for the *in vitro* release of FFA from adipose tissue.[22]

Bilateral epididymal lipidectomy altered the adipokinetic response to exercise. The lipidectomized animals were still able to run equally as long as the control exercised rats. The increased plasma FFA levels, yet complete failure of the adipose tissue to mobilize FFA or demonstrate *in vitro* release of FFA, indicate that auxiliary white adipose tissue mobilized and released adequate FFA as energy sources for the training program and the exhaustive run. Since the epididymal fat pad contains only about 15 percent of the body lipid store[51] and the metabolism of the other depots is similar to that of the epididymal fat pads, this inability of the regenerating fat pads to mobilize or release FFA is probably the result of incomplete nervous regeneration or inadequate circulation to the reforming fat pads. Wirsen[59] has shown that white adipose tissue is not directly innervated by the sympathetic nervous system as no synaptic formations are seen in the adipose cells, but terminals innervating precapillary vessels are quite evident. The possibilities exist that the norepinephrine is not released at the fat pad or that the norepinephrine, if released, cannot reach the adipose cells by way of the circulatory system and thus exert an adipokinetic effect. The lack of mobilization of FFA under exercise conditions suggests that these organs have been relegated to a relatively greater depot function and perhaps this is a reflection of decreasing metabolic activity.[56] Other hormonal systems activate lipolysis in the rat[22] and humans[5] thus liberating FFA from fat pads other than those removed.

The time of lipidectomy apparently had little effect upon the physical regeneration of the fat pads or upon the inability of the fat pads to mobilize FFA. Regeneration and a lack of increased FFA mobilization after exercise were apparent in fat pads before training, after attaining the desired level of training, and after four weeks in the trained state.

The animals used in this study were not mature and therefore possessed few if any nonmitotic cells. Since there is one nucleus per cell in most structures the number of cells is usually equal to the number of nuclei e.g. Total DNA content/DNA amount per nuclei = number of nuclei. Enesco and Leblond[17] have shown that the number of nuclei increased with age to one-hundred fifty days which is approximately the age of the animals sacrificed at the completion of the training regimen in this study. Whether the increase in cell number was due to multiplication of local fat cells or to migration of cells destined to become fat cells is unknown. Recently Rodbell[49] has demonstrated that better than 50 percent of the DNA in a portion of epididymal fat pad tissue is from the stromovascular cells. DNA content may, therefore, reflect an altered number of fat cells and/or other cells. Even though a great deal of the adipose tissue DNA is found in supportive tissue matrix and not in the adipocyte, the total DNA content is utilized in this study as we were interested in total regeneration as measured by DNA content and not simply in adipocyte regeneration.

Treadmill training programs have been shown to increase the DNA content of rat adipose tissue.[6,35,45] The abundance of DNA may indicate a change in adipose tissue metabolic activity,[45] a change in cell proliferation,[35] or both.[6] As well, training causes an increased muscle mass at the expense of fat deposition.[46] Physical activity inhibits the hypertrophy of fat cells which occurs regularly with aging and *ad libitum* feeding.[45] The animals in this study had *ad libitum* feeding. Refeeding after a previous fast[2,54] and limiting food intake to one to two hours per day[32,38] produces adipose tissue growth by enhanced cell proliferation.[6] The findings that the fat pads were relatively the same size after sixteen weeks of regeneration in all lipidectomized animals whether trained or control and that the fat pads of the trained animals had higher DNA content suggests greater cellularization in the trained animals and greater hypertrophy in the control animal fat cell size.

The finding that the DNA content of regenerating fat cells is greater than the content of intact cells in unilaterally lipidectomized animals does not favor the idea that adipocytes or their precursor cells are only formed early in life as suggested by Hirsch and Han.[31] The data in this study clearly demonstrate that adipocytes can change in size and number, although proliferation appears dominant in the bilaterally lipidectomized animals. The monthly analysis of DNA content after lipidectomy indicates that the cellularization per gram of fresh tissue gradually approaches that of the control nonlipidectomized animals. It therefore appears that cellularization or cell proliferation does occur up to twenty weeks after lipidectomy.

It would be interesting to postulate a relationship between regenerating fat pads and fat pads reduced in size by exercise, however no research indicates that the metabolism of the two tissues is similar. Plasma FFA levels, however are known to be elevated in obese subjects,[15,24] although these levels fail to rise after fasting, suggesting retarded FFA mobilization with obesity.[44] It has further been demonstrated that after brief exercise plasma FFA levels are higher or more variable in lean subjects than in obese subjects[14,36,44] indicating that lipid mobilizing processes are less active in the obese subjects. The implication for training and a cessation of training are provocative. Studies are currently being carried out in this laboratory on the effects of detraining upon cell size, number, and ability to mobilize FFA with exercise.

## References

1. Allison, J.B., Wannemacher, R.W., Hilf, R., Migliarese, J.F., and Crossley, M.L. *J Nut.* 54: 539, 1954.
2. Allman, D.W., Hubbard, D.D., Gibson, D.M.: *J. Lipid Res.* 6: 63, 1965.
3. Andres, R., Cader, G., and Zierler, K.L.: *J Clin. Invest.* 35: 671, 1956.
4. Armstrong, P.T., Steele, R., Altzuler, N., Dunn, A., Bishop, J.S., and DeBodo, R.C.: *Am. J. Physiol.* 201: 9, 1961.
5. Basu, A., Passmore, R., and Strong, J.A.: *Quart. J. Exp. Physiol.* 45: 312, 1960.
6. Braun, T., Kozdova, L., Fabry, P., Lojda, Z., and Hromadicova, V.: *Metabolism* 17: 825, 1968.
7. Cahn, T., and Bouget, J.: *Arch. Sci. Physiol.* 2: 105, 1948.
8. Cameron, G.R., Seneviratne, R.D.: *J. Path. Bact.* 59: 665, 1947.
9. Carlson, L.A., Ekelund, L.G., and Oro, L.: *J. Lab. Clin. Med.* 61: 724, 1963.
10. Carlson, L.A., Froberg, S., and Persson, S.: *Acta Physiol. Scand.* 63: 434, 1965.
11. Carlson, L.A., and Pernow, B.: *J. Lab. Clin. Med.* 53: 833, 1959.
12. Carlson, L.A., and Pernow, B.: *J. Lab. Clin. Med.* 58: 673, 1961.
13. Cobb, L.A. and Johnson, W.P.: *J. Clin. Invest.* 42: 800, 1963.
14. Dempsey, J.A. and Gordon, S.G.: *R.Q.* 36: 96, 1965.
15. Dole, V.P.: *J. Clin. Invest.* 35: 510, 1956.
16. Dole, V.P., and Meinertz, H.: *J. Biol. Chem.* 235: 2595, 1960.
17. Enesco, M., and Leblond, C.P.: *J. Embryol. and Exp. Morph.* 10: 530, 1962.
18. Friedberg, S.J., Harlan, W.R., Trout, D.L., and Estes, Jr. E.M.: *J. Clin. Invest.* 39: 215, 1960.

19. Friedberg, S.J., Sher, P.B., Bogdonoff, M.D. and Estes, Jr., E.H.: *J. Lipid Res.* 4: 34, 1963.
20. Fritz, I.B., Davis, D.C., Holtrop, R.H. and Dundee, H.: *Amer. J. Physiol,* 194: 379, 1958.
21. Gollnick, P.D.: *Amer. J. Physiol.* 213: 734, 1967.
22. Gollnick, P.D., Soule, R.G., Taylor, A.W., Williams, C., Ianuzzo, C.D. *Amer. J. Physiol.* 219: 729, 1970.
23. Gollnick, P.D. and Taylor, A.W.: *Int. Z. Angew. Physiol.* 27: 144, 1969.
24. Gordon, E.S.: *Amer. J. Clin. Nut.* 8: 740, 1960.
25. Goss, R.J.: *Science* 153: 1615, 1966.
26. Hausberger, F.X.: *Anat. Rec.* 122: 507, 1955.
27. Hausberger, F.X.: *Diabetes* 7: 211, 1958.
28. Havel, R.J., Carlson, L.A., Ekelund, L.G. and Holmgren, A. *J. Appl. Physiol.* 19: 613, 1964.
29. Havel, R.J., Naimark, A. and Borchgrevink, C.R.: *J. Clin. Invest.* 42: 1057, 1963.
30. Hellman, B. and Hellerstrom, C.: *Acta. Pathol. Microbiol. Scand.* 51: 347, 1961.
31. Hirsch, J., and Han, P.W.: *J. Lipid Research.* 10: 77, 1969.
32. Hollifield, G. and Parson, W.: *J. Clin. Invest.* 41: 245, 1962.
33. Issekutz, B. Jr., Miller, H.L., Paul, P. and Rodahl, K.: *J. Appl. Physiol.* 20: 293, 1965.
34. Issekutz, B. Jr., and Paul, P.: *Fed. Proc.* 25: 334, 1966.
35. Kazdova, L., Braun, T. and Fabry, P.: *Metabolism.* 16: 1174, 1967.
36. Klein, R.F., Troyer, W.G., Back, K.W.: *Annals. N.Y.A.S.* 131: 662, 1965.
37. Knittle, J.L., and Hirsch, J.: *J. Clin. Invest.* 47: 2091, 1968.
38. Leveille, G.A., Hanson, R.W.: *Canad. J. Physiol. Pharmacol.* 43: 857, 1965.
39. Liebelt, R.A.: *New York Acad. Sci.* 110: 723, 1963.
40. Makkas, M.: *Beitr. Klin. Chir.* 77: 523, 1912.
41. Marx, G.: *Z. Ohrenheilk* 61: 7, 1910.
42. Masoro, E.J., Rowell, L.B. and McDonald, R.M.: *Fed. Proc.* 25: 1421, 1966.
43. Maximow, A.: *Beitr. Path Anat.* 35: 93, 1903.
44. Opie, L.H., and Walfish, P.G.: *N.E.J. Med.* 268: 757, 1963.
45. Parizkova, J.: *Nutr. Soc. Proc.* 25: 93, 1966.
46. Parizkova, J. and Stanova, L.: *Brit. J. Nutr.* 18: 325, 1964.
47. Robinson, D.W. *Growth* 33: 231, 1969.
48. Robinson, D.W., Bradford, G.E.: *Growth* 33: 221, 1969.
49. Rodbell, M.: *J. Biol. Chem.* 239: 375, 1964.
50. Schotz, M.C. and Page, I.M.: *J. Lipid Res.* 1: 466, 1959.

51. Smith, T.C., Will, L., Oleson, J., Benitz, K.F., Perrine, J. and Ringler, I.: *Amer. J. Phys.* 200: 1277, 1965.
52. Steiner, G. and Cahill, Jr., G.F.: *New York Acad. Sci.* 110: 749, 1963.
53. Taylor, A.W.: *Diss. Abstracts* 28: 8, 1968.
54. Tepperman, H.M., Tepperman, J.: *Fed. Proc.* 23: 73, 1964.
55. Wannemacher, Jr. R.W., Banks, Jr. W.C. and Wunner, W.H.: *Anal. Biochem.* 11: 320, 1965.
56. Wasserman, F.: *Handbook of Physiology. Adipose Tissue.* 87, 1965.
57. Wertheimer, E., Hamosh, M., and Shafrir, E.: *Amer. J. Clin. Nutr.* 8: 705, 1960.
58. Wertheimer, E., and Shapiro, B.: *Physiol. Rev.* 28: 451, 1948.
59. Wirsen, C.: *Acta. Physiol. Scand.* 65: Supp. 252, 1965.
60. Yakovlev, N.N.: *Fiziol. Zhur.* S.S.R. 38: 332, 1952.
61. Ziegler, K.: *Beitr. Path. Anat.* 36: 435, 1904.

# Chapter 3

# The Frequency and Possible Significance of Ischemic S-T Changes in the Exercise Electrocardiogram

G.R. Cumming

Fiel and Siegel first reported the electrocardiographic changes that occurred during exercise-induced attacks of angina in 1928.[31] Earlier, in 1918, Bousfield had reported on the variations in electrocardiograms during a paroxysm of angina.[20] In 1931, Wood et al.[64] further defined the electrocardiographic phenomena during attacks of angina pectoris in patients, and supported the clinical information with studies on the effects of temporary coronary artery occlusion in animals. Goldhammer and Scherf[35] were the first in Europe (1932) to report on electrocardiogram studies in angina pectoris. Master and Openheimer devised the simple two-step exercise test with standard tables in 1929,[45] and amplified this functional test to include electrocardiographic changes in 1941 and 1942.[46,47] For the next twenty years the Master's two-step test was virtually the only exercise test used in North America. This test had the advantage of simplicity but the disadvantage of only measuring the ECG changes after the exercise was completed. In addition, the Master's test was not a good test of functional capacity, for the work done was related to age and weight of the patient, and was close to a maximal effort for some and a light effort for others. In 1950 in Sweden, some of the knowledge from exercise physiology was applied to exercise testing of patients by Sjostrand.[59] In the past ten years exercise electrocardiography has become a large and complex subject. In 1968 the Ernst Simonson conference was held in Minneapolis, and the result was a monograph of 479 pages entitled, "Measurement in Exercise Electrocardiography, edited by H. Blackburn.[14]

## Reasons for Recording Exercise Electrocardiograms

Exercise electrocardiograms are recorded in patients when there is uncertainty about the diagnosis of chest pain. They are of use in objectively following the progress of the patient, and evaluating the results of surgical or medical therapy, and of exercise rehabilitation programs. It is necessary when testing the functional capacity of patients to follow the exercise electrocardiogram for safety reasons. In some patients, symptoms are due to rhythm disturbances which come on only with exercise, and monitoring of the cardiac rhythm during exercise is the only method available for diagnosis.

Electrocardiograms during exercise are useful in screening and evaluation of cardiovascular disease in a population, and are the basis of this report. Monitoring of electrocardiogram is necessary for safety purposes, if nothing else, when testing patients in the coronary age group. The detection of S-T segment depression during exercise in a normal subject should be considered one of the risk factors for the development of coronary heart disease in the same manner as an elevation in blood cholesterol. The development of S-T segment depression, plus the appearance of chest pain, is taken as firm evidence of myocardial ischemia and coronary heart disease. The appearance of ventricular arrhythmias during exercise is also of possible prognostic import.

## Recording of the Exercise Electrocardiogram

The desirable goal is to obtain a positive test in all subjects who have abnormalities or disease, and to have a negative test in all subjects who are normal and free from disease, while, at the same time, having the test simple, painless, easy to interpret and record. In clinical practice the twelve-lead electrocardiogram has gained wide acceptance and has the background of years of empiric interpretation. The entire twelve leads may be obtained during and following exercise, but this results in a large amount of data, some of which is superfluous. The vectorcardiogram can be recorded during exercise although there is certain difficulty with the placement of inferior leads.[15] Vector analysis with computer techniques can circumvent the difficulties in routine interpretation, but these facilities are available to very few. The vector method may not be quite as sensitive to changes as those found in certain precordial leads. A bipolar lead using the manubrium, or the forehead or right side of the chest as the indifferent point, and a single exploring lead in the $V_5$ position, is the simplest approach of all, and there is evidence to suggest that if changes are to be found, the single electrode approach will record the changes in over 85 percent of subjects.[11] In our studies we have used this simple approach with the exploring electrode at the $V_5$ position, and the indifferent electrode at the manubrium or just under the medial end of the right clavicle. Skin preparation is important, and the skin should be cleansed and rubbed with alcohol until it is reddened. Recordings can be improved beyond this by scraping the outer surfaces of dermis off with a knife, or drilling a small 1 mm hole with a dental burr. Motion artifacts are reduced when the contact between the electrode and skin is by way of a thin layer of electrode jelly. The wires attached to the electrodes should be light and taped to prevent excess motion. A modern direct-writing electrocardiographic apparatus is usually satisfactory. The response of the instrument should be flat up to one hundred cycles per second, and there is now wider recognition of the importance of acurate recording at the lower end of the ECG frequency range (down to .05 HZ). Berson[19] estimates that up to 3 percent of subjects will show S-T segment displacement errors of 1 mm or more from instruments built according to American Heart Association specifications up until 1967.[1] There are many possible refinements in the design of electrocardiographic amplifiers and recorders that are not present in the commercial service machines. Tape recording systems, computer elimination of noise,[38,63] and various computer analyses[32,50,58] are available to the researcher in exercise electrocardiography.

## The Mechanism of S-T Changes With Exercise

In 1941, Barach and Steiner gave 12 percent oxygen mixtures to patients for twenty minutes and produced more S-T changes in subjects with coronary disease than in normals.[8] In experimentally produced ischemia, Case *et al.*[22] found that the depression of the S-T segment began with a rise in left atrial pressure, and a fall in myocardial extraction of lactate. When coronary obstruction was released, there was a rapid return to normal in the pressure and metabolic abnormalities while the S-T depression persisted for several minutes. In addition to lactate excretion during impaired coronary flow, myocardial cells give off potassium. These changes in potassium movement across the cell membrane may be the explanation for the S-T changes.[33] Theoretically, the electrocardiogram monitors some functional changes occurring at the myocardial cell membrane, and, while these changes may be due to relative oxygen lack in the myocardial cell, they are not specific for oxygen lack. Changes are not only found in patients with coronary artery narrowing, but also in patients receiving digitalis, patients with low blood potassium, in rheumatic and congenital heart disease, and in various myocardial disorders.

### Criteria and Coding of Interpretation

At the present time a positive test is said to be present when there is a depression in the S-T segment of 1 mm or more with a horizontal or downsloping S-T segment.[12] Some include a 0.5 to 1.0 mm S-T depression, as long as the S-T segment is horizontal or down-sloping, as a positive change.[16] Others add a slope criteria to electrocardiograms showing 1 mm S-T depression and an upsloping S-T segment (rate of rise less than 1 mv/ sec), but the significance of this change requires further study.[41] Usually the S-T segment depression occurs during the exertion, and persists for a few seconds to a few minutes after the exertion. In some subjects, the S-T change may not occur for three to four minutes after the exercise, and Bruce has reported that this occurs more frequently in the Oriental population.[23]

False positive S-T depressions apparently may occur when the T wave is superimposed on the J and early S-T segment, and Lepeshkin[40] has suggested a means of allowing for this that seems somewhat arbitrary. Whether there is any prognostic import to J depressions alone, which are observed with greater frequency in the older subjects, requires long-term evaluation.

McHenry *et al.*[51] report that hyperventilation may produce a false positive ECG exercise test, but there was no data concerning ventilation or $pCO_2$ to back up the claim, and the exercise changes were more marked than those produced by hyperventilation in the one patient reported.

## Merits of Various Types of Exercise Tests

The merits of the various types of exercise tests have been fully discussed by others.[60] We have used the bicycle ergometer rather than the treadmill in our studies of an adult population, because the work is easily quantitated, artifact-free electrocardiograms are more easily obtained, there is less patient fear, and less need to practice than with the treadmill. The main advantage of the bicycle would seem to be the quality of electrocardiographic tracings that may be obtained for monitoring and recording purposes. It is important to utilize the exercise test to assess the patient's functional capacity, as well as to record any electrocardiographic changes, and for this reason each exercise load should be at least six minutes in length to allow the attainment of a "steady state." This permits determination of submaximal functional capacity. For the attainment of maximal effort, the bicycle ergometer seems to be clearly inferior in our population because fatigue occurs in the leg muscles before the cardiorespiratory apparatus is fully taxed. Even so, most subjects can be persuaded to persist long enough to obtain values very close to maximum oxygen uptake that would be obtained on the treadmill.

## Methods and Materials

Volunteers were obtained from the employees of the city of Winnipeg. All individuals over forty years of age on the city payroll were asked, and, of some seven hundred volunteers, 475 have been tested to date.

No attempt was made to have the subjects fasting. The exercise was carried out in an air-conditioned room at 20°C using an Elema electrically braked ergometer which has been calibrated by method previously reported.[24] To compare exercise loads with those of other studies, it is absolutely imperative that this calibration be carried out. All subjects completed two submaximal loads. The first load varied from 300 to 600 kpm, the second load from 600 to 1050 kpm, depending on the age, weight, and apparent fitness of the subject. In 380 subjects, a third load of three to five mintues duration was added. This was a supermaximal load that could not be sustained in a steady state, and it was chosen according to the response to the previous two loads. The electrocardiogram was monitored by oscilloscope throughout the exercise, and recordings obtained every two minutes during the submaximal loads, and continuously during the maximal load. Oxygen uptake was measured during the last two minutes of each submaximal load, and continuously during the maximal load. Electrocardiograms were also obtained two minutes and five minutes after completion of the exercise with the subject sitting relaxed in a chair beside the bicycle. Subjects were asked to terminate the exercise with the appearance of any chest discomfort, with the appearance of more than a 2 mm S-T depression on the monitored electrocardiographic lead, or with the appearance of frequent ventricular extrasystoles. According to these criteria, the exercise was terminated in twenty subjects.

Prior to the performance of the test, all subjects were examined medically, all had a resting electrocardiogram. All subjects with known abnormalities were included in the study, but maximal exercise testing was not carried out on those who had a previous myocardial infarction, resting blood pressure of greater than 180/120, a history of angina, or musculoskeletal problems. Maximal testing was also omitted if a physician was not nearby.

The electrocardiograms were analyzed and the electrocardiographic changes were recorded according to the code devised by Blackburn *et al.*[10] as modified by Astrand[4] for electrocardiographic monitoring during exercise.

The code categories IV-1 to IV-3 were considered to be positive, raising the suspicion of subclinical coronary disease. Only one patient in this series developed angina during the exercise test.

## Results

Table 3-I shows the age incidence of positive tests—increasing from 4.3 percent at forty to forty-five years, to 30 percent at sixty-one to sixty-five years. We have no explanation why the incidence was similar in the first and second halves of the sixth decade, then doubles at age sixty-one to sixty-five, other than the small numbers involved.

TABLE 3-I
AGE INCIDENCE OF POSITIVE EXERCISE ECG TESTS

| Age Group | No. of Subjects | No. of Positive Tests | Percent |
|---|---|---|---|
| 40–45 | 140 | 6 | 4.3 |
| 46–50 | 145 | 14 | 9.7 |
| 51–55 | 101 | 18 | 17.8 |
| 56–60 | 59 | 10 | 17.0 |
| 61–65 | 30 | 9 | 30.0 |

An attempt has been made to document the frequency of risk factors in subjects with positive responses. Risk factors are defined in Table 3-II.

Obesity was present in over 70 percent of those examined using two criteria—a weight 15 percent above ideal based on the actuarial studies, assuming medium frame for all, and body fat content of greater than 18 percent of body weight determined from four skinfolds as presented by Durnin.[30]

TABLE 3-II
DEFINITION OF RISK FACTORS

| | |
|---|---|
| Obesity | —1.15 ideal weight or >18% fat |
| Cholesterol | —above 210 mg% |
| Fitness | —PWC$_{150}$ <7.5 kpm/min/kg |
| Activity | —no sports, sedentary work |
| Family History | —parent or sibling <60 with fatal coronary |
| Vital Capacity | —<4.0 L |
| Smoking | —>5/day |
| Blood Pressure | —> 140/90 |
| Resting ECG | —L. axis, LVH, T wave, S-T, codable Q |

The autoanalyzer method used for cholesterol determination gave values up to 30 mg percent lower than those generally found in the Canadian population. Test retest reliability values were within 5 percent. Fifteen percent of the population were above 210 mg percent, and we arbitrarily selected this value as abnormal.

Fitness declines with age as measured by maximum oxygen uptake. As all subjects did not have maximal oxygen uptake determinations, we used the $PWC_{150}$ value as a criteria of fitness. This value is relatively stationary with age, because maximum heart rate decreases, the $PWC_{150}$ becomes a greater percentage of maximum as age increases, and therefore the value is relatively the same in different ages. We arbitrarily chose values under 7.5 kpm/min/kg as indicating low fitness.

Activity—a brief questionnaire was sent ou. Those who took part in no regular sporting activity, and those whose occupation involved primarily desk work, were labelled as at risk for having no physical activity.

Family history was briefly recorded, particularly as to whether a parent or sibling died under the age of sixty with a fatal coronary attack. A positive risk factor was recorded with this occurrence.

A positive risk factor for vital capacity was recorded when this value was under 4 liters. No correction was made for body size in this prediction.

Regular cigarette intake in excess of five per day was considered a positive risk factor.

A lying blood pressure of greater than 140/90 was considered a positive risk factor regardless of age.

In the resting electrocardiogram, left axis deviation in excess of $-30°$, definite left ventricular hypertrophy by the accepted criteria, T wave flattening or inversion, S-T changes coded IV-1 to IV-3, and codable Q waves were all considered risk factors. Right bundle branch block was not considered a risk factor, nor were minor decreases in T wave voltage.

Table 3-III lists the number of subjects with positive exercise tests who had positive risk factors. Obesity was present in 89.5 percent of the subjects, and possibly the definition for this was

TABLE 3-III
FREQUENCY OF POSSIBLE RISK FACTORS IN FIFTY-SEVEN
SUBJECTS WITH POSITIVE EXERCISE TESTS

| Risk Factor | Number | Percent |
|---|---|---|
| Obesity | 51 | 89.5 |
| Cholesterol | 12 | 21.1 |
| Fitness | 16 | 28.1 |
| Activity | 31 | 54.5 |
| Family History | 25 | 43.8 |
| Vital Capacity | 35 | 61.5 |
| Smoking | 21 | 36.9 |
| Blood Pressure | 28 | 49.2 |
| Resting ECG | 20 | 35.1 |

too strict. The most frequent positive risk factor was a low vital capacity, and this data will be reanalyzed using predicted values based on surface area. This was followed by a low activity pattern and an elevation in blood pressure. Resting ECG abnormalities were present in one-third of those with positive exercise tests, a similar incidence to that of smoking. Low fitness and elevated cholesterol were found in about one-fourth of the subjects. The question is raised as to whether the exercise ECG selects out those at risk for coronary heart disease and provides information in addition to what can be provided by resting data.

In Table 3-IV the major risk factors, elevated cholesterol, smoking, blood pressure elevation, and resting ECG abnormalities only are considered. One-fourth of those with abnormal exercise ECGs had none of these risk factors positive, while one-fifth of the subjects had three or four of these risk factors positive. The exercise ECG, therefore, appeared to offer information not provided by the other factors in at least one-fourth of the cases with positive tests.

Another point of contention is whether the exercise used for the detection of occult coronary disease needs to be a maximum

TABLE 3-IV
INCIDENCE OF NUMBER OF MAJOR RISK FACTORS
CHOLESTEROL, SMOKING, BLOOD PRESSURE, RESTING ECG

| | Number | Percent |
|---|---|---|
| Zero Factors | 14 | 24.6 |
| One Factor | 19 | 33.4 |
| Two Factors | 13 | 22.8 |
| Three Factors | 8 | 14.0 |
| Four Factors | 3 | 5.3 |

effort or whether submaximal tests suffice. Another contention is whether it is necessary to record the electrocardiogram during the exercise, or whether it is satisfactory to obtain a record immediately after. Table 3-V shows an enquiry into these points on those with the positive execise test in this series. The abnormality appeared during recovery in over 50 percent of the cases, but, on the other hand, if recovery records alone had been used over 40 percent of the abnormalities would have been missed. Three-fourths of the abnormalities showed up without resorting

TABLE 3-V

OCCURRENCE OF S-T DEPRESSION—%

| | |
|---|---|
| Submax Exercise Only (No Max Done) | 26 |
| Max Only | 12 |
| Recovery Only | 5 |
| Submax and Recovery (No Max Done) | 33 |
| Submax and Max | 5 |
| Max and Recovery | 7 |
| Submax, Max and Recovery | 12 |
| | 100 |
| *Total Recovery* | 57 |
| *Without Max* | 74 |

to maximum exercise. In many of the subjects who exercised at submaximal loads only, maximum exercise was not carried out as the appearance of S-T changes lead us to terminate the test.

## Discussion

Table 3-VI lists the frequency of ischemic S-T changes found in the so-called asymptomatic healthy population. The values found in our city of Winnipeg workers were in agreement with the result of Astrand[6] and Bruce.[26] The results were at variance with those of Lester[42] who found very few changes in the forty to sixty year age group. Some of the discrepancy between various studies depends on whether the asymptomatic patient who shows up in the population survey but who has such diseases as aortic stenosis, idiopathic atrial fibrillation, angina, hypertension, ECG evidence of LVH, or a previous healed myocardial infarction, is excluded from the survey or not. If these subjects with abnormalities found on the screening tests are completely excluded, the incidence of ischemic S-T changes is likely to be somewhat less.

TABLE 3-VI
REPORTED FREQUENCY "ISCHEMIC" S-T CHANGES

| Age | I. Astrand[5] Men | I. Astrand[6] Women | Bruce[29] Seattle | Li[43] Taiwan | Railway[61] U.S.A. | Farm[21] Yugoslav | Lester[41] Alabama | Chicago[34] Executives | Winnipeg All Workers |
|---|---|---|---|---|---|---|---|---|---|
| <40 | <10 | — | 2 | 2 | — | — | — | 0 | 2.0 |
| 40–50 | 15 | 20 | 9 | 4 | 5.9 | 2.9 | 3.6 | 6.8 | 7.0 |
| 51–60 | 20 | 30 | 25 | 12 | 12.0 | 4.3 | 2.4 | 27.0 | 17.4 |
| 61–65 | 35 | 55 | 46 | 14 | — | — | 17.6 | — | 30.0 |

The values of physical fitness and the protective effects of physical activity, either as recreation in play, or as occupation, in preventing coronary heart disease, is unsettled.[34] Grimby and Saltin[36] studied well-conditioned middle-aged and old athletes in Sweden and found just as many S-T changes of an ischemic type in these subjects as was present in the normal nonathletic population in Sweden.

There is an indication that physical training will decrease or eliminate positive S-T changes in the exercise electrocardiogram. In some instances, the S-T changes will appear after training when the exercise is continued to the same heart rate, but, as

TABLE 3-VII

FREQUENCY OF "ISCHEMIC" S-T CHANGES IN WELL-TRAINED MIDDLE-AGED AND OLD ATHLETES IN SWEDEN

| Age | Average Population I. Astrand[5] | Athletes Grimby and Saltin[36] |
|---|---|---|
| 40–50 | 15 | 14 |
| 50–59 | 20 | 27 |
| 60–70 | 35 | 50 |

the heart rate for a given load declines, the subject is able to do more work without showing S-T changes. This relationship between S-T changes and physical training has not been studied completely, nor are full reports documenting these changes available.[39,56]

A problem in exercise testing is at what intensity of exercise to stop the test. True maximal testing involves the attainment of a plateau in oxygen uptake which may require two or three days of separate testing and is not applicable to population studies. It also means pushing patients close to the point of exhaustion which may carry a slight but definite risk. Ideally, it also involves determination of blood lactic acid. In some of the tests, such as the multistage test used extensively by Bruce,[19] the patient determines his own end-point by stopping voluntarily when fatigued. This is usually a near maximal rather than maximal test, and the degree to which maximum is approached must vary from patient to patient. Some authors advocate having the patients stop at a defined heart rate, and this rate is usually decreased with age to take into consideration the change in maximum heart rate with age. Table 3-VIII lists

TABLE 3-VIII
MAXIMUM HEART RATES IN VARIOUS STUDIES

| Age | Robinson[54] (1938) Treadmill | Bruce[17] (1965) Treadmill | Lester[42] (1968) Treadmill | Astrand[3] (1960) Bicycle | Anderson[2] (1964) Bicycle | Cumming[26] (1967) Bicycle |
|---|---|---|---|---|---|---|
| 20–29 | 194 ± 8 | 190 ± 10 | 195 | 195 ± 11 | — | 195 ± 8 |
| 30–39 | 187 ± 7 | 180 ± 10 | 191 | 181 ± 12 | 180 | 184 ± 10 |
| 40–49 | 177 ± 8 | 174 ± 11 | 187 | 173 ± 9 | 173 ± 11 | 178 ± 12 |
| 50–59 | 170 ± 9 | 170 ± 14 | 183 | 161 ± 11 | 165 ± 14 | 168 ± 15 |
| 60–69 | 160 ± 7 | 146 ± 25 | 179 | 159 ± 9 | 150 ± 12 | 160 ± 15 |

some of the maximum heart rates found at various age groups in several different studies, including one from this center. If one is to use ±2 standard deviations as the normal range, then the maximum heart rate at aged fifty to fifty-nine varies from 138 to 198, and a rate of 150 may be more than the maximum for one subject and less than 70 percent of maximum for another. The limitation of arbitrary pulse rate end-points is obvious. Despite this, some authors advise stopping the exercise when 75% or 85% of the maximum predicted heart rate is reached.

## The Prognostic Value of Ischemic S-T Response in the Exercise Electrocardiogram in Normal Subjects

Some information is available on this point and summarized in Table 3-IX. The important column is the last which is the risk ratio, defined as the incidence of coronary heart disease developing in those who have a positive exercise response compared with the incidence of coronary disease developing in those who have a negative response. This risk ratio varied from 3.6 in a study of Robb and Marks, to 48.5 in the study of Mattingly. If subjects who show S-T changes in the exercise electrocardiogram are more than three times likely than subjects without exercise S-T changes to develop coronary heart disease in a ten-year period, this is a risk factor worthy of note, particularly as the highly popularized risk factors found in the Framingham study, such as elevated cholesterol and blood pressure, and resting ECG abnormalities, have risk ratios in the range of 2:1 to 4:1. It should be noted that the combination of several

TABLE 3-IX
PROGNOSTIC VALUE OF ISCHEMIC S-T RESPONSE
IN NORMAL SUBJECTS

| Source | Positive Tests | Subjects | Age | Follow-up | % Developing CHD | Risk Ratio |
|---|---|---|---|---|---|---|
| Rumball and Acheson[55] | 37 | Service | 40–54 | 7 | 29.8 | 11.8 |
| Robb and Marks[53] | 201 | Insurance | >40 | 5.6 | 5.0* | 3.6 |
| Mattingly[49] | 6 | Service | 25–60 | 10 | 50 | 48.5 |
| Most et al.[52] | 22 | YMCA | 34–67 | 5 | 13.6 | 13.6 |

* Fatalities only

risk factors in the Framingham study raises the risk ratio as high as 40:1.[28] The lack of a large number of subjects with ischemic S-T changes, as indicated in Table 3-IX permits but tentative conclusions as to the validity of ECG changes in normal subjects.

### Some Questions About the Ischemic S-T Change

There are several observations which require explanation before the ischemic response on the exercise ECG in the otherwise normal population may be considered definite evidence of ischemia. Women have a 50 percent higher incidence of exercise S-T changes than men, and yet far fewer myocardial infarctions.[6] Trained middle-aged athletes show as many S-T changes on exercise as the normal population, and yet are said to be protected from ischemic heart disease.[36] Exercise ECG changes occur as frequently in the normal population in Sweden as they do in the United States, yet there is less coronary heart disease in Sweden.[5,52] In the United States the incidence of ischemic S-T changes with maximum exercise varies from 3 percent in one population study to 10 percent or more in another population study. [41,52] There is only one available maximum study with a follow-up of eight years. There was but one case of myocardial infarction in the eight years of follow-up, and this subject had a normal ECG response to exercise.[5] In the Seattle study[18] (follow-up of five years), there has been but one myocardial infarction, this being silent, and one sudden death, the cause unconfirmed with autopsy. Both these subjects had an abnormal ECG response to near-maximal exercise. One or two cases are hardly sufficient evidence on which to base the validity of the maximum exercise ECG, and considerably larger numbers of subjects need to be studied for longer periods of time. It may be that maximal tests with ECG monitoring during exercise is too sensitive a test, and that there are too many false positives. The Master's test has had a considerably longer period for evaluation, and there is little doubt of the prognostic power of the Master's test. However, subjects with extensive coronary disease may not show an ischemic response to the two-step test, and hence the current interest in multistage near-maximal tests with ECG monitoring during the test.

Master claims that his test procedure will identify 93 percent of typcial coronary cases with a false positive rate of only 2 percent.[18] The statement, "It is clear that in patients with normal resting ECGs a negative double two-step test practically excludes ischemic heart disease," would find strong argument from almost every center. Master followed eight hundred patients for an average of 8.6 years to reach this conclusion. Master and Rosenfeld also concluded that monitoring the patient during the exercise test did not alter the diagnostic yield. They placed faith in the QX/QT ratio, which others have discounted as being of diagnostic value.

Robb and Marks[53] followed 2,224 insurance applicants, of whom 299 had an abnormal or ischemic response to the Master's test. Of these 299, twenty-eight had angina, twenty-six had a healed infarct, thirty-three had suspected coronary occlusion, one hundred two had an ECG anomaly at rest, and eighty-five had atypical chest pains. In other words, over 90 percent of the subjects had symptoms suggestive, or highly suggestive, of cardiac disease, and the subjects were, therefore, not asymptomatic. Nonetheless, of those subjects having these symptoms, there were five times as many deaths in those with the ischemic exercise test compared to those without. A similar mortality ratio (5:1) was found for those without these symptoms, confirming the prognostic value of exercise response in the asymptomatic as well as the symptomatic subject.

In the large international study under the direction of Keys, electrocardiograms were recorded after a three minute step test (a standardized rate of 20 steps per minute). Those with ischemic responses had twice the incidence rate of clinical coronary heart disease as those with a normal response after five years had elapsed. This bad outlook persisted after matching the subjects for age, blood pressure, weight, cholesterol, physical activity, and smoking. There were some differences from country to country in this study of Keys in that the ischemic S-T change was highly predictive in the United States with a mortality ratio of 3:1, but barely significant in the countries outside of the United States.

Mattingly administered the Master's test to three hundred officers in 1951, with an ischemic response in only 2 percent. However, in a ten year follow-up, three of the six with the ischemic response had infarctions (i.e. 50%) whereas only two occlusions occurred in the 294 subjects with a normal response (0.7%).[49] In a larger series of serve personnel given the test for clinical indications, 145 subjects had positive tests, and 31.7 percent developed coronary occlusions within seven years. Of the 726 with a normal response, coronary occlusions occurred in only 3.6 percent. A positive response to the Master's test is thus of considerable prognostic value. A positive response to more severe stress testing with any type of lead system requires further evaluation in number of subjects tested and in years of follow-up. Compounding the difficulties of evaluation are the multitude of other variables including technical details of recording and interpreting the exercise ECG, including observer error, and the many factors casually or incidentally related to coronary heart disease. These problems have been well reviewed by Blackburn.[13]

### Coronary Arteriography vs. Exercise Tests

Several correlative studies are available comparing the results of exercise tests and coronary angiography in the same patients. These studies have the drawback that there are limitations to both procedures. The arteriography is an anatomic study, and does not directly assess blood flow or tissue perfusion. Arteriography may not assess small vessel disease, and, in particular, may miss small localized areas of ischemia or deficiencies in the microcirculation. On the other hand, the ECG changes are not specific for ischemia with changes being seen in the hypertensive and digitalis treated patients, and others without ischemia. Exercise may not be sufficiently intense to provoke ischemia or indeed the patient's ischemia may be precipitated only by emotional factors. A patient with a healed infarction may have a normal perfusion of functioning muscle and show no ECG changes with exercise, yet have a complete occlusion of one of the major coronary vessels. There are rare syndromes, such as changes in hemoglobin affinity with oxygen, that are associated with myocardial ischemia in the absence of anatomic coronary artery disease. Mason *et al.*[44] found that of those subjects with significant coronary disease as revealed by coronary angiography, 74 percent had positive ECG changes, 26 percent had normal exercise tests. Of those with abnormal exercise tests, 81 percent had significant anatomic coronary artery disease, 19 percent false positives. In the investigation of Selzer *et al.*,[57] the exercise test was positive in nearly all patients with involvement of two or three of the major coronary arteries in the angiograms, but in patients with single vessel disease, the hemodynamic response to exercise was normal, and the multistage treadmill test was negative in all.

### Exercise Tests in Patients with Previous Myocardial Infarction

Weeda performed maximal ergometer tests in sixty-three subjects who had previous myocardial infarctions.[62] The test was negative in 43 percent of those with previous anterior infarction, and in 53 percent of those with previous inferior infarction. Hellerstein *et al.* have reported a similar incidence of negative tests from those with previous infarction.[37] Both Hellerstein *et al.* and Areskog *et al.*[7] found a higher frequency of negative tests in those with previous inferior infarctions. Either the ECG lead system is not monitoring an ischemic zone, or there is a healed scar and no ischemia, but the failure of exercise tests to reveal an abnormality in half of all patients with old infarctions is diconcerting.

When the resting ECG is abnormal, the criteria for judging the abnormal response are not as well-defined as when the resting ECG is normal. The large series of Robb and Marks[53] suggest that the further changes produced by exercise (Master's test) in patients with an abnormal resting ECG carry the same prognostic significance as those with normal resting ECGs, but there has been no evaluation of this problem with maximal or near-maximal exercise tests.

# References

1. American Heart Association Committee on Electrocardiography: *Circulation*, 35:583, 1967.
2. Anderson, K.L.: Interaction of chronic cold exposure and physical training upon human body tolerance to cold. Report AF61 (052758) Institute of Work Physiology, Oslo, 1964.
3. Astrand, I.: *Acta Physiol. Scand.* 49:1 (Suppl 169), 1960.
4. Astrand, I.: *Acta Med. Scand.*, 173:257, 1963.
5. Astrand, I.: *Acta Med. Scand.*, 178:27, 1965.
6. Astrand, I.: Electrocardiographic changes in relation to type of exercise, the work load, age and sex. In *Measurement in Exercise Electrocardiography*, H. Blackburn, Ed. Springfield, Thomas, 1969 (page 309)
7. Areskog, N.H., L. Bjork, V.C. Bjork, A. Hallen, and G. Strom. *Acta Med. Scand.*, *Suppl.* 472:9, 1967.
8. Barach, A.L., and A. Steiner: *Amer. Heart J.*, 22:13, 1941.
9. Berson, A.: In *Measurement in Exercise Electrocardiography*, H. Blackburn, Ed. Springfield, Thomas, 1969 page 181.
10. Blackburn, H., A. Keys, E. Simonson, P. Rautaharju, and S. Punsar: *Circulation*, 21:1160, 1960.
11. Blackburn, H.: *Ann. NY Acad. Sci.*, 126:882, 1965.
12. Blackburn, H., I. Astrand, G. Blomqvist, and P. Rautaharju: Standardization of the electrocardiogram for exercise tests. In *Physical Activity and the Heart*, M.J. Karvonen and A.J. Barry, Eds. Springfield, Thomas, 1967.
13. Blackburn, H.: The exercise electrocardiogram. Technological, procedural and conceptual developments. In *The Ernst Simonson Conference, Measurement in Exercise Electrocardiography*, H. Blackburn, Ed. Springfield, Thomas, 1969 (page 220).
14. Blackburn, H.: *Measurement in Exercise Electrocardiography*. Springfield, Thomas, 1969.
15. Blomqvist, G.: *Acta Med. Scand.*, 178:1, 1965.
16. Brody, A.J.: *JAMA*, 21:495, 1959.
17. Bruce, R.A., J.R. Blackman, J.W. Jones, and G. Strait: *Pediatrics*, 32 (Suppl 742), 1963.
18. Bruce, R.A., and J.R. McDonough: *Bull NY Acad. Med.*, 45:1288, 1969.
19. Bruce, R.A., and T.R. Hornsten: *Progr. Cardiov. Dis.*, 11:371, 1969.
20. Bousfield, G.: *Lancet*, 2:457, 1918.
21. Buzina, R., A. Keys, I. Mohacek, M. Marinkovic, A. Hahn, and H. Blackburn: *Circulation*, 41 (Suppl.I):40, 1970.
22. Case, R.A., H.A. Roselle, and R.S. Crampton: *Cardiologia*, 48: 32, 1966.

23. Chiang, B.N. *et al.: China Med.*, 14:239, 1967.
24. Cumming, G.R., and W.D. Alexander: *Canad. J. Physiol. Pharmacol.*, 46:917, 1968.
25. Cumming, G.R.: Editorial—Physical fitness and cardiovascular health. *Circulation*, 37:4, 1968.
26. Cumming, G.R.: Unpublished data.
27. Cumming, G.R.: Use of S-T changes after maximal exercise in a population survey for coronary heart disease. (In preparation)
28. Dawber, T.R., and W.B. Kannel: *Mod. Conc. Cardiov. Dis.*, 30:671 1961.
29. Doan, A.E., D.R. Petersen, J.R. Blackman, and R.A. Bruce: *Amer. Heart J.*, 69:11, 1965.
30. Durnin, J.V.G.A., and M.M. Rahaman: *Brit. J. Nutr.*, 21:681, 1967.
31. Fiel, H., and M.L. Siegel: *Amer. J. Med. Sci.*, 175:255, 1928.
32. Freiman, A.H.: Arrhythmia and wave form analysis program. In *Measurement in Exercise Electrocardiography*, H. Blackburn, Ed. Springfield, Thomas, 1969 page 118.
33. Friesen, W.J., and G.R. Cumming: *Canad. Med. Ass. J.*, 97:960, 1967.
34. Goldberg, A.M., J.F. Moran, R.W. Childers, and H.T. Richets: *Amer. Heart J.*, 79:194, 1970.
35. Goldhammer, S., and D. Scherf: *Z. Klin. Med.*, 122:134, 1932.
36. Grimby, G., and B. Saltin, *Acta Med. Scand.*, 179:513, 1966.
37. Hellerstein, H.K., G.B. Prozan, I.M. Liebow, A.E. Doan, and J.A. Henderson: *Amer. J. Cardiol.*, 7:234, 1961.
38. Jakson, L.K. *et al.*: Noise reduction and representative complex selection in the computer analyzed exercise electrocardiogram. In *Measurement in Exercise Electrocardiography*, H. Blackburn, Ed. Springfield, Thomas, 1969 page 73.
39. Kilbom, A., L.H. Hartley, B. Saltin, J. Bjure, G. Grimby, and I. Astrand: *Scand. J. Clin. Lab. Invest.*, 24: 315, 1969.
40. Lepeshkin, E., and B. Surawicz: *New Eng. J Med*, 258:511, 1958.
41. Lester, F.M., L.T. Sheffield, and J.T. Reeves: *Circulation*, 26:5, 1967.
42. Lester, M., L.T. Sheffield, P. Trammell, and T.J. Reeves: *Amer. Heart J.*, 76:370, 1968.
43. Li, Y.B., N. Ting, B.N. Chiang, *et al.: Amer. J. Cardiol.*, 20:541, 1967.
44. Mason, R.E., J. Litar, R.O. Biern, and R.S. Ross: *Circulation*, 36:517, 1967.
45. Master, A.M., and E. Openheimer: *Amer. J. Med. Sci.*, 177:223, 1929.
46. Master, A.M., and H.L. Jaffe: *Mount Sinai J. Med. NY*, 7:629, 1941.
47. Master, A.M., R. Friedman, and S. Dack: *Amer. Heart J*, 24:777, 1942.

The Frequency and Possible Significance of Ischemia    59

48. Master, A.M., and I. Rosenfeld: *JAMA, 190*:102, 1964.
49. Mattingly, T.: *Amer. J. Cardiol., 9*:393, 1962.
50. McHenry, P.L.: Computer quantitation of the S-T segment response to maximal treadmill exercise. In *Measurement in Exercise Electrocardiography*, H. Blackburn, Ed. Springfield, Thomas, 1969. (page 61).
51. McHenry, P.L., O.J. Cogan, W.C. Elliott, and S.B. Knoebel: *Amer. Heart. J., 79*:683, 1970.
52. Most, A.S., T.R. Hornstein, V. Hofer, and R.A. Bruce: *Arch Intern. Med., 121*:225, 1968.
53. Robb, G.P., and H.H. Marks: *JAMA*, 200:918, 1967.
54. Robinson, S.: *Arb. Physiol., 10*:251, 1938.
55. Rumball, C.A., and E.C. Acheson: *Brit. Med. J.*, 1:423, 1963.
56. Salzman, S.H., H.K. Hellerstein, J.D. Radke, H.W. Maistelman, and R. Ricklen: Quantitative effects of physical conditioning on the exercise electrocardiogram of middle-aged subjects with arteriosclerotic heart disease. In *The Ernst Simonson Conference, Measurement in Exercise Electrocardiography*, H. Blackburn, Ed. Springfield, Thomas, 1969, page 388.
57. Selzer, A., F.J. Sakai, K. Cohn, and W.L. Anderson: *Israel J. Med. Sci., 5*:715, 1969.
58. Sheffield, L.T., M.D. Perry, L.N. Larkin, J.A. Burdenshaw, D.V. Conray, and J.T. Reeves: Electrocardiographic signal analysis without averaging of complexes. In *Measurement in Exercise Electrocardiography*, H. Blackburn, Ed. Springfield, Thomas, 1969, page 108.
59. Sjostrand, T.: *Acta Med. Scand., 138*:201, 1950.
60. Taylor, H.L., W. Haskell, S.M. Fox, and H. Blackburn: Exercise tests: A summary of procedures and concepts of stress testing for cardiovascular diagnosis and function evaluation. In *The Ernst Simonson Conference, Measurement in Exercise Electrocardiography*, H. Blackburn, Ed. Springfield, Thomas, 1969, page 259.
61. Taylor, H.L., H. Blackburn, A. Keys, R.W. Parlin, C. Vasquez, and T. Puchner: *Circulation*, 41:20 (Suppl. I), 1970.
62. Weeda, H.W.H.: *Mal Cardiov* 10:61, 1969.
63. Winter, D.A.: Noise measurement and quality control techniques in recording and processing of exercise electrocardiograms. In *Measurement in Exercise Electrocardiography*, H. Blackburn, Ed. Springfield, Thomas, 1969, page 159.
64. Wood, F.C., C.C. Wolferth, and M.M. Livezey: *Arch. Intern. Med., 47*:339, 1931.

# Chapter 4

# Metabolic Acidosis During Muscular Exercise, Its Repercussions on Ventilation

R. Vanroux

Metabolic acidosis normally occurs in muscular exercise of a certain intensity. It is usually attributed to lactic acid formation at the level of the muscular cell placed in anaerobic conditions when an insufficient blood flow creates an oxygen-lack.

Cell and extracellular liquid chemical buffers make up the first protection line: important lactic acid quantities liberated in the circulation are neutralized by standard blood bases.

Most of the time, however, the amount of bicarbonate decrease exceeds the amount of lactate increase in a proportion of two to one according to our experiments (Fig. 4–1). It is only in hypoxic exercise or more rarely in exhaustive efforts that this repartition is equimolar.

The preservation of the pH homeostasis of which the drop is undoubtedly limited by the buffer effect is guaranteed by the hyperventilation provoked by this pH drop. As a matter of fact in the Henderson-Hasselback equation

$$pH = pK + \log \frac{base}{acid}$$

the base/acid ratio is approximately equal to twenty, the bases being equal to sixty volumes, the free acid to three.

If the pouring of a certain quantity of metabolic acids causes a bicarbonate drop of twenty volumes, for example, and at the same time a drop in pH, it will suffice that the denominator drops from three to two volumes following the hyperventilation

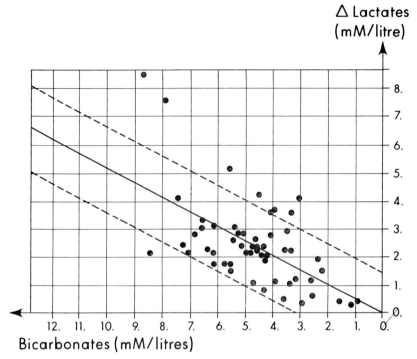

Figure 4–1. Relation between lactic acid/bicarbonates in arterial blood collected during exercises of various intensities from subjects of different aptitudes.

X : Δ bicarbonates (mM/lit.);        Y : 0,5166 x + 0,0477
Y : Δ lactates (mM/lit.);            r : 0,5898

provoked by this acidosis to reestablish the normal pH values.

From arterial blood collected in these conditions, we can easily dissociate the metabolic and ventilatory elements by inversing the reasoning, that is, recalculating pH $paCO_2$ supposedly equal to 40 mm Hg, or better yet, by using Davenport's chart: from the intersection point defining the arterial blood a line is drawn parallel to the blood base buffer line: from the intersection of this straight line with the $paCO_2$ 40 mm Hg iso-bar line, a perpendicular is dropped on the abscissa. This point defines the metabolic pH (Fig. 4–2, 4–3).

## CO₂ total plasma (Vol. p.100)

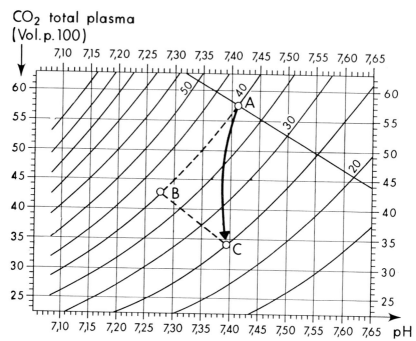

Figure 4–2. Utilization of Davenport's chart during acid-base equilibrium modifications in the course of muscular exercise. Arterial blood collected at rest is defined by Point A. During exercise it is defined by point C, resultant of a metabolic acidosis (AB) and of a compensating respiratory alkalosis BC.

### Study of Ventilatory Parameters Relative to Metabolic Acidosis

As expected a correlation is found between respiratory equivalent and metabolic pH. In normal subjects, in pathological subjects and in athletes this measure shows a dispersion which is a function of the individual mechanical qualities of the thoraco-pulmonary system. This is why for an equal pH of 7.37 the respiratory equivalent lies between twenty-five and thirty-five. It is important to note however that the respiratory equivalent is always above thirty, a value considered as a lyspnea index, when metabolic pH is below 7.30 (Fig. 4–4).

Alveolar ventilation calculated with Enghoff Rossier's equa-

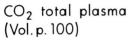

CO₂ total plasma
(Vol. p. 100)

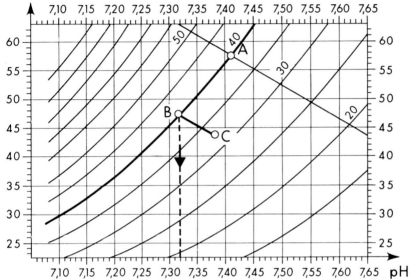

Figure 4–3. Metabolic acidosis degree expressed in pH.

tion increases as metabolic pH decreases which also automatically means that $paCO_2$ decreases (Fig. 4–5).

This result could be foreseen because it is the sole factor that will allow a reduction of the acidosis degree. The respiratory quotient (R) values are in turn influenced by this excess $CO_2$ rejection. As the load increases the respiratory quotient tends toward unity, it even exceeds this number at times (Fig. 4–6). It is accepted that during exercise glucides are the fuel of choice, but this reasoning seems to be erroneous because as the effort increases $paCO_2$ decreases following metabolic acidosis which appears at a certain threshold.

In evaluating energy cost from respiratory quotient values it is therefore important to recalculate the respiratory quotient with a pa $CO_2$ of 40 mm Hg. In doing so, we see that the respiratory quotient, which we shall call metabolic, decreases and tends toward 0.7. One would be inclined to conclude in first approximation that the glucide metabolism is set aside in

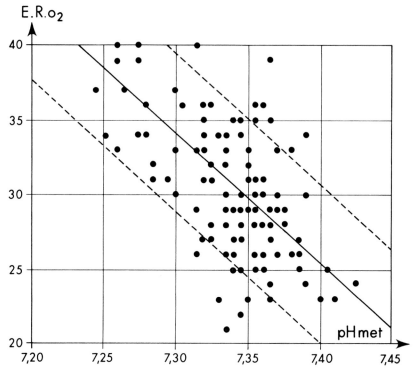

Figure 4–4. Correlation between respiratory equivalent and metabolic pH in arterial blood during muscular exercise.

    X : metabolic pH
    Y : respiratory equivalent (ERO2)
    $\sigma Y$ : 5,337 2
    Y : −87,475 5x + 672,653 5
    r : 0,612 9

favor of lipid metabolism from which a share of the energy is derived.

## Ventilation Evolution During Increasing Load Efforts and Constant Load Efforts

Whether the effort is done on a cycle ergometer or a treadmill with increasing work loads as it is usually the case in oxygen consumption determinations, ventilation increase is asymptotic

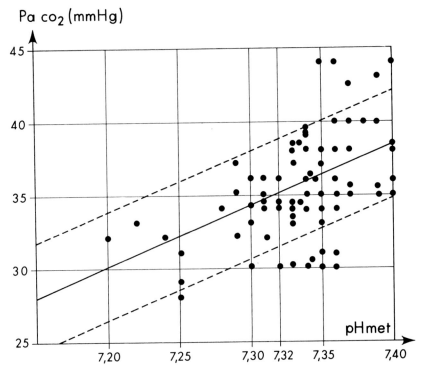

Figure 4–5. Correlation between $PaCO_2$ and metabolic pH in arterial blood during muscular exercise.

X : metabolic pH
Y : PaCO2
$\sigma Y = 3,668$  I
$Y = 42,544\ 2x - 276,431\ 3$
$r = 0,501\ 2$

while oxygen consumption is a linear function of the work load. The ventilation slope flattening coincides with the appearance of metabolic acidosis.

The ventilation study techniques during constant load efforts intend to determine the maximum effort sustained in ventilatory steady state conditions which, of general agreement, corresponds to two-thirds of maximal $Vo_2$.

An analysis of the intersection points which define arterial blood on Davenport's chart and the metabolic pH deter-

**Respiratory Quotient**

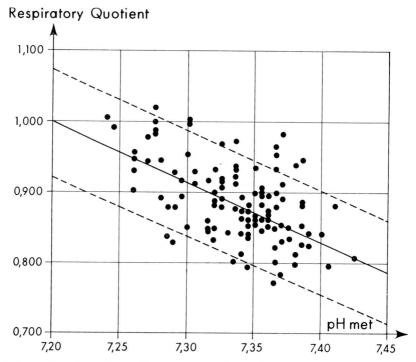

Figure 4–6. Correlation between R and metabolic pH in arterial blood during muscular exercise.

X : metabolic pH
Y : RQ
$\sigma Y = 0{,}074\ 8$
$Y = -816\ 2x + 6{,}871\ 7$
$R = 0{,}406\ 6$

mined for each of them by this method enables us to set at 7.32 ± 0.02 the maximum degree of metabolic acidosis compatible with a well-supported exercise. (Fig. 4–7 and 4–8).

The metabolic acidosis study during exercise brings in a determinant element in defining a more or less well-supported effort that is made or not in ventilatory steady state.

Surprisingly repeatable, this measure can be considered as the most reliable of all ventilatory and hemo-respiratory parameters used during a muscular effort.

One cannot doubt moreover of the metabolic acidosis im-

## CO₂ total plasma (Vol. %)

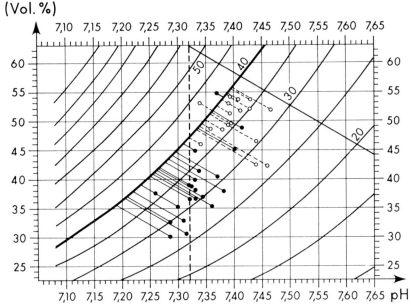

Figure 4–7. Metabolic acidosis variation during more or less well-supported muscular effort according to ventilatory criterions.
Broken Lines: well-supported efforts where ventilatory steady state is held.
Solid Lines: less well-supported efforts, where ventilation increases by more than 5% between the tenth and twentieth minutes of exercise.

portance in the ventilation evolution as shown by the following experiment: a predetermined work load is successively carried on the bicycle ergometer during ten minutes with both legs and then with a single leg. In the first part of the experiment the ventilatory flow is stable while it is progressively increasing in the second part (Fig. 4–9).

It can be noted during these two tests that Vo₂ is strictly the same. Only metabolic acidosis is different since in the first case metabolic pH is equal to 7.38 while it is 7.32 in the second.

The following interpretation of the results can be given: when cycling with one leg the muscular group involved must double the load supported by both legs in an identical exercise. This

CO$_2$total plasma
(Vol. %)

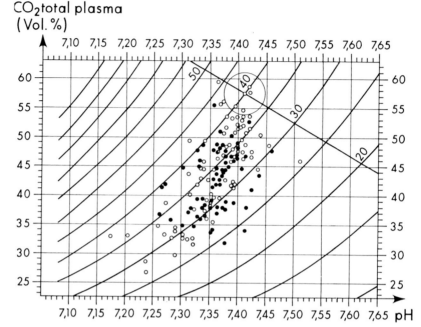

Figure 4–8. Acid-Base equilibrium evolution during a 120-watt muscular exercise. Arterial blood is collected between the nineteenth and twentieth minutes of effort. Subjects are separated in two groups according to their P.M.S.:

*First group,* forty-five cases (open circles): P.M.S. equal or superior at 120 watts (mean pH: 7,365, $\sigma = 0.026$).

*Second group,* seventy-two cases (closed circles): P.M.S. falls between 100 and 120 watts (mean pH: 7,303, $\sigma = 0.039$).

implies that the local blood flow increases proportionately. The metabolic acidosis increase indicates that the blood flow increase is insufficient to maintain the muscle fiber metabolism in aerobic conditions; this acidosis is responsible for the hyperpnea unlatching to maintain pH homeostasis.

## Conclusions

Many authors attempted to explain ventilatory parameter evolution and appearance of metabolic acidosis during muscular

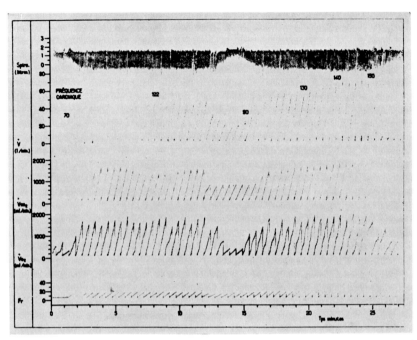

Figure 4–9. Ventilatory parameter variations during a muscular exercise of the same type and load, where various muscular groups come into action. Registration of $\dot{V}$ (vertical coordinate, in liters), $\dot{V}CO_2$ (vertical coordinate in ml), $\dot{V}O_2$ (vertical coordinate, in ml) and respiratory frequency (vertical coordinate, in numbers of pulsations). On the left side of the graph are the results of a 100 watt effort made in normal pedalling conditions, that is with both legs. On the right side are the results of the same work load done with a single leg. In the latter case ventilation increases progressively.

effort by quantifying blood lactate amounts. However it does not seem that an explicit correlation was ever established between the value of this amount and exercise hyperpnea. An explanation of the impossibility of this correlation is given by our experiments which have shown the differential evolution of lactates and bicarbonates during effort metabolic acidosis.

On the other hand, the only control criterion for this metabolic acidosis lies in the expression of the metabolic pH value. This parameter alone enables one to define a tested subject's aptitude for exercise as well as the efficiency of the training he underwent.

# Chapter 5

# The Effects of Three Types of Warm-up on the Total Oxygen Cost of a Short Treadmill Run

R.T. HERMISTON

M.E. O'BRIEN

Warm-up, as a preparation prior to physical work, attempts to produce optimum performance by increasing one or more of the following readiness factors: muscle temperature, circulation and/or joint mobility. Previous studies have utilized massage, light exercise, calisthenics, diathermy and shower techniques to produce these conditions of readiness. Numerous studies[3,6,10,11,12] have investigated the effects of various warm-up techniques on athletic performance and physical work. Actual performance or certain physiological change, such as oxygen uptake ($VO_2$) and heart rate, have been utilized to assess the effects of warm-up,[5] but physiological phenomena are not generally reported as measures of the intensity of the warm-up.

Metabolic energy sources are derived from the aerobic and the anaerobic systems. Not all of the energy cost of work can be paid for by aerobic processes during the actual work period. Hermansen[8] has reported that in hard work tasks $VO_2$ increases during the first minutes of exercise until it reaches maximum oxygen uptake (Max. $VO_2$). The lack of oxygen in the initial period is referred to as oxygen deficit (an anaerobic process). If an individual can raise his $VO_2$ quickly, accumulating a small oxygen deficit, he may pay for the initial stages of the work aerobically and thus will conserve his internal anaerobic processes for utilization during a different time period in the work task. Specifically, in track and field, if by warming up an athlete can raise his $VO_2$ near maximum, he can perform aerobically for a major portion of the race. Thus he will incur

70

a smaller oxygen deficit at the beginning of the race, conserving his alactic energy reserves for the final sprint to the finish.

The purpose of this study was to investigate the effects of three types of warm-up on the oxygen cost of a short treadmill run. Warm-up was defined as a percentage of each individual's maximum oxygen uptake.

## Methods and Materials

Six well-trained subjects participated in this study. Their physical characteristics are presented in Table 5-I.

TABLE 5-I

ANTHROPOMETRIC, PHYSIOLOGIC, AND TIME DATA
DESCRIBING CHARACTERISTICS OF THE SUBJECTS

| Subject | Age (Yr) | Weight (lb.) | Max $VO_2$ (liter/min) | $VO_2$ (ml/kg/min) | 220 Yd Time (sec.) | Calculated Treadmill Speed (mph) |
|---|---|---|---|---|---|---|
| RH | 33 | 180 | 4.52 | 55 | 28.6 | 15 |
| JC | 22 | 150 | 4.40 | 75.6 | 25.0 | 18 |
| PR | 23 | 141 | 4.10 | 63.6 | 27.9 | 16 |
| GS | 29 | 185 | 5.04 | 60 | 26.5 | 17 |
| MO | 23 | 155 | 3.30 | 48 | 29.7 | 15 |
| BW | 24 | 142 | 4.52 | 70.6 | 27.5 | 16.3 |

Best consistent running times for a 220-yard run were established on a Grasstex track. All subjects ran the 220 yards from a running start. Three trials were given with a ten-minute rest between trials. The median of the three trials was accepted as the best consistent time.

A 2 percent grade was arbitrarily chosen on the treadmill and the speed was set at a rate equivalent to each individual's prescribed time (unpublished data from the University of Windsor, 1969).

To establish consistency for each individual's maximum oxygen uptake, all subjects ran both the Cureton[2] and the Taylor[14] treadmill tests to volitional fatigue. Thirty and sixty percent of each subject's calculated maximum oxygen uptake were designated as two of the types of warm-up. The third type was preexercise $VO_2$ and called no warm-up (NW).

The length of the warm-up was arbitrarily chosen as ten minutes. A one-minute rest followed the warm-up period preceding each run.[9] The 30 percent and 60 percent levels of warm-up were calculated from the expired volume during the last thirty seconds of the one-minute rest interval, between the ten-minute warm-up and the treadmill run. By a trial and error method, ten-minute warm-up programs were developed so that each subject began the run with: (a) no warm-up (NW), (b) a 30 percent warm-up, and (c) a 60 percent warm-up. The oxygen debt of the warm-up programs was calculated for both the 30 percent warm-up and the 60 percent warm-up.

During the trial and error sessions, both warm-up programs and sampling times were established. A preexercise resting gas sample was drawn for the last minute of a two-minute rest period. Two thirty-second post warm-up gas samples were collected immediately prior to the run. Expired gas was collected in fifteen-second samples during the run. A six-minute debt was collected during the recovery period. The length of time that the recovery gas was collected was an arbitrary decision based on an analysis of the results of pilot runs which indicated that all subjects had recovered to near preexercise levels in six minutes.

The total metabolic cost was calculated by combining the net aerobic and anaerobic metabolic values. The net aerobic cost was computed from the oxygen utilized above the preexercise values for the exercise period. The net anaerobic metabolic cost was calculated by subtracting six times the preexercise $VO_2$ from the gross $VO_2$ for six minutes of recovery.

## Results

Maximum oygygen uptake values, the median of the 220-yard time, and the equivalent times in mph for each individual are presented in Table 5-I.

Figure 5–1 indicates graphically the mean values for each warm-up condition in terms of aerobic cost, anaerobic cost, and total oxygen cost. A repeated measures analysis of variance was used to evaluate the variances in these means. The mean scores

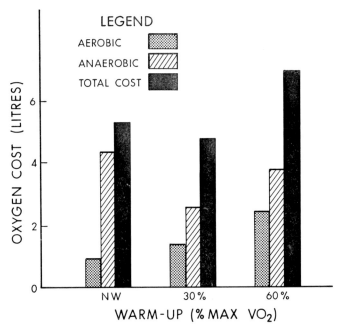

Figure 5–1. The mean values for each warm-up condition in terms of aerobic cost, anaerobic cost and total oxygen cost.

and F-ratios are presented in Table 5-II. An $F_{(.05)}$ $(2,10)$ > 4.10 was required to show significance in the aerobic and the anaerobic costs of the run, as well as in the total cost of work. A Newman-Keuls procedure indicated that the 30 percent warm-up and the 60 percent warm-up appeared to be different than no warm-up in terms of aerobic cost. By warming up at 30 percent and 60 percent of maximum oxygen uptake, the subjects were able to utilize more oxygen aerobically.

TABLE 5-II

AEROBIC, ANAEROBIC, AND TOTAL OXYGEN COST OF A SHORT TREADMILL RUN WITH 0% (NW), 30%, AND 60% (OF MAX VO₂) WARM-UP

| Oxygen Cost (Liters, STPD) | % (NW) | 30% | 60% | *F |
|---|---|---|---|---|
| Aerobic | .90 | 1.41 | 1.47 | 45.45* |
| Anaerobic | 4.42 | 2.60 | 3.83 | 10.61* |
| Total Cost | 5.32 | 4.81 | 6.88 | 10.31* |

* $F_{(.95)}(2,10)$ > 4.10.
F statistic calculated by means of Repeated Measures Analysis of Variance

Newman-Keuls procedure showed that the 30 percent warm-up was significantly different from both the 60 percent warm-up and no warm-up. As indicated in Figure 5–1, a greater anaerobic cost was accumulated with both the 60 percent warm-up and no warm-up than with the 30 percent warm-up.

In terms of the total cost of work, the Newman-Keuls procedure indicated that the 60 percent warm-up was significantly different from both the 30 percent warm-up and no warm-up. Figure 5–1 indicates that the total oxygen cost was less in the 30 percent warm-up than in the other two warm-ups; however, it was not significantly less.

### Discussion

By warming-up to 30 percent Max $VO_2$ the subjects utilized more oxygen aerobically. By utilizing more oxygen aerobically, the subjects incurred a smaller anaerobic debt during the race. Since the aerobic oxidative mechanism is delayed and takes at least one minute to reach full capacity during the run with no warm-up, the subject must be in a state of relative anoxia.[9] More energy is then drawn from anaerobic mechanisms. Since the capacity of the alactic system is limited,[9] the physiological processes rely on the lactacid mechanism to fulfill their metabolic requirements. If the rest period after a work session is greater than twenty-five seconds, the phosphagen source[9] is considered adequate to repay the incurred debt since the payment of the alactic oxygen debt takes place quickly during the initial stages of recovery.

Since the warm-up programs were neither gradual enough nor discontinuous, the subjects incurred a large debt from the warm-up sessions. This accumulated warm-up debt confounded the total cost calculations for the subjects because the warm-up as prescribed did not raise the subject's metabolic $VO_2$ slowly and thus allow him to repay the incurred deficit at each increased work level. With a proper program, a subject should be able to start the run with minimal debt from the warm-up procedure. A slower accumulation of lactic acid, and therefore the delay in the onset of fatigue, resulting from replenishment and reutilization of part of the alactacid energy reserves, should enable the athlete to handle greater quantities of work at high intensities.[4]

In addition, the length of the race may be a limitation. Perhaps a longer race, utilizing the total aerobic system more efficiently and for a greater percentage of the total time period, would add to the knowledge of physiological processes produced by oxygen utilization.

## References

1. Astrand, P., and Saltin, B.: *J. Appl. Physiol.* 16(6): 971–976, 1961.
2. Consolazio, C.F., Johnson, R. and Pecora, L.: *Physiological Measurements of Metabolic Functions in Man.* McGraw-Hill Book Company, New York, 1963.
3. Costill, D.: *J. Appl. Physiol.* 28(3): 251–255, 1970.
4. Falls, H. and Weibers, J.: *Res. Quart.* 36(3): 243–250, 1965.
5. Fox, E., Robinson, S., and Wiegman, D.: *J. Appl. Physiol.* 27(2): 174–178, 1969.
6. Grodjinovsky, A., and Magel, J.: *Res. Quart.* 41(1):116–119, 1970.
7. Grose, J.: *Res. Quart.* 29(1): 19–30, 1958.
8. Hermansen, L. *Med. Sci. Sports.* 1(1):32–38, 1969.
9. Margaria, R., Cerretelli, P., Aghemo, P. and Sassi, G.: *J. Appl. Physiol.* 18(2):367–370, 1963.
10. Margaria, R., Oliva, R.D., DiPrampiro, P., and Cerretelli, P.: *J. Appl. Physiol.* 26(6):752–756, 1969.
11. Massey, B., Johnson, W., and Kramer, G.: *Res. Quart.* 32:63–71, 1961.
12. Mathews, D., and Snyder, A.: *Res. Quart.* 30:446–451, 1959.
13. McGavin, R.: *Res. Quart.* 39(1):125–129, 1968.
14. Schneider, E.G., Robinson, S., and Newton, J.: *J. Appl. Physiol.* 25(1):58–62, 1968.
15. Taylor, H.L., Buskirk, E., and Henschel, A.: *J. Appl. Physiol.* 8: 73–80, 1955.
16. Whipp, B., Seard, C., and Wasserman, K.: *J. Appl. Physiol.* 28(4): 452–456, 1970.

# Application of a Practical Test to Predict the Maximal Oxygen Intake of High School Boys

Denis Massicotte

## Abstract

Forty (40) high school boys, aged from fourteen to seventeen years old, were evaluated during a twelve minute field performance test and retest and on a treadmill maximum-oxygen-intake test. A correlation of 0.80 (r = 0.80) was obtained between the field-test data and the laboratory oxygen consumption results. The correlation of the twelve minute test and retest results, at three days interval, was 0.93 (r = 0.93). The analysis of variance revealed no significant differences (P ≤ .05) between these three series of values (treadmill, 12 minute tests 1 and 2). The correlation of the treadmill test and retest data for nine subjects was 0.86 (r = 0.86). The significance of this relationship makes it possible to estimate with considerable accuracy the maximum oxygen intake from only the results of the twelve minute running test. Because of the high correlation with maximal oxygen intake, it can be assumed that the twelve minute field test is an adequate measure of physical fitness reflecting the cardiorespiratory status of an individual. This test is readily applicable to large groups of high school students and requires minimum equipment.

Numerous investigators[2,5,7,12,14] have indicated that maximum oxygen intake is an adequate measure of cardiorespiratory fitness. Others, among them, Hill,[10] Asmussen and Nielsen,[1] Margaria,[11] Astrand[2,4] and Wyndham[15,16] devised some direct and indirect methods of measuring and predicting individual aerobic capacity. In 1923, Hill[10] suggested a linear relationship between oxygen intake and submaximal work intensity. In 1954, Astrand[4] used this relationship to predict the maximum oxygen consumption. His nomograms were based on the interrelationship between the heart rate and the oxygen requirements at various submaximal work loads.

Many others[2,5,8,13,15] considered running as one of the most efficient methods of measuring an individual's aerobic capacity. Astrand[2] and Balke[5] revealed a linear relationship between oxygen requirements at various running speeds (5 mph to 11 mph) on a treadmill. Considering this relationship, Balke[5] developed a practical test to predict the maximal oxygen consumption from the maximal distances covered in one, five, eight, twelve, fifteen, eighteen, twenty and thirty minutes. For each period of running, individual physical condition was expressed in terms of oxygen intake. The maximal oxygen consumption values recorded during a strenuous workout on a treadmill, were quite close to the values obtained during those running periods varying from twelve to twenty minutes. Balke,[5] Cooper,[8] Doolittle and Bigbee[9] reported correlations of 1.0, 0.89 and 0.85 respectively between the maximum distances run in twelve or fifteen minutes and the maximal oxygen intakes measured on a treadmill.

## Method and Materials

Forty (40) High School boys (14 to 17 years old) acted as subjects to compare the results of a twelve minute performance field test and retest, with a treadmill maximum oxygen consumption test.

The maximum oxygen intake in the laboratory was determined through a open-circuit system. The test consisted of a series of five minute running exercises at a constant speed of 7 mph on a treadmill whose slope varied between 0 percent and 9 percent at intervals of 3 percent. A rest period of five to ten minutes between each running level was allowed each participant. The subject must complete the five minute period before a further slope increase. Heart rate (Oscillographic Recording System, model 7718A, Sanborn), oxygen intake (Beckman Model $E_2$ Oxygen Analyser), carbon dioxide (Carbon Dioxide Model LR 215 Infrared Analyser), production and ventilation (Tissot: Chain Compensated Gasometer, 150 liters) were measured between the second and third minute and between the fourth and fifth minute at each level of work. The reliability of the laboratory test had been determined beforehand with nine subjects who completed the test twice as described.

The twelve minute run test was performed on a 284 meters gymnasium track. A stopwatch was used to time the twelve minute duration, and the subjects were instructed to complete the last lap when they heard the whistle signaling the end of the twelve minute period. The exact time was recorded when the subject crossed the finish line. Subjects were notified of the remaining time at 6, 9, 11 and 11.5 minutes. They were asked to run for the entire twelve minutes and that if walking became necessary, not to walk for more than one-fifth of a lap at a time. They were also instructed to cover the longest distance possible in twelve minutes. The retest was performed under the same conditions within three days of the first test. On the basis of the average speed maintained, the maximum oxygen consumption was determined by Balke's formula:

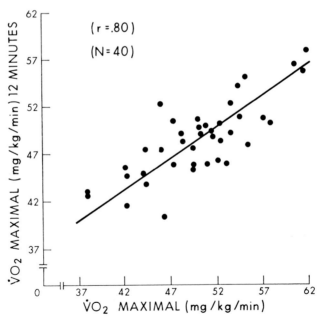

Figure 6–1. Correlation between maximal oxygen consumption on treadmill and twelve minute walk-run performance test. The regression coefficient bxy = 0.57 was calculated in function of rxy (40 subjects).

$$VO_2 \ (ml/kg/min) = 33 + .17 \ (\text{speed in meters/min} - 133)$$

in which a standard oxygen consumption of 33 ml was used for a specific speed of 133 meters/min.

## Results and Discussion

The averages and standard deviations for the maximum oxygen consumption of the forty subjects in the three tests were as follows:

50.31 ± 5.46 ml/kg/min on the treadmill
48.31 ± 3.72 ml/kg/min in the first 12 minute run test
48.41 ± 3.91 ml/kg/min in the second 12 minute run test

A correlation of 0.80 (r = 0.80) (Fig. 6–1) was obtained between the treadmill values and the twelve minute run test data. Figure 6–2 presents a correlation of 0.93 (r = 0.93) between the maximal oxygen consumption values of the first and

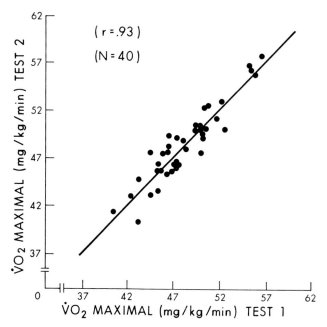

Figure 6–2. Correlation between test-retest values of maximal oxygen intake on the twelve minute performance (40 subjects).

second twelve minute test. The analysis of variance (Table 6-I) indicated no significant differences (P ≤ .05) between the treadmill and the two twelve minute run test values. Previous studies (Table 6-II) cited by Balke,[5] Cooper[8] and Doolittle[9] showed correlations higher than 0.85, using running exercises of twelve to fifteen minutes in length.

TABLE 6-I
VARIANCE ANALYSIS FOR THREE TESTS OF MAXIMUM
OXYGEN CONSUMPTION (ML/KG/MIN)

| Variance | Sum of Squares | Degrees of Freedom | Estimation of Variance | F |
|---|---|---|---|---|
| Intergroup | 99.03 | 2 | 49.52 | 2.43* |
| Intragroup | 2387.22 | 117 | 20.40 | |
| Total | 2486.25 | 119 | | |

* No significant differences at the .05 level

The averages of maximal oxygen consumption of the nine subjects in the test and retest on the treadmill were as follows:

49.02 ml/kg/min in the first treadmill test

48.61 ml/kg/min in the second treadmill test

Moreover, the "t" analysis revealed no significant differences (P ≤ .01) between these two-series of values. The correlation between these data was 0.86 (Fig. 6–3).

Figure 6–4 presents the relationship between the oxygen intake and the intensity of work on the treadmill. The subjects were divided into four different groups, relative to their tread-

TABLE 6-II
COMPARISONS WITH PREVIOUS CORRELATIONS OBTAINED
BETWEEN RUNNING TESTS AND LABORATORY TESTS
MEASURING THE MAXIMUM OXYGEN CONSUMPTION

| | Subject Number | Age Mean | (Variations) | Correlations |
|---|---|---|---|---|
| Present Study* | 40 | 16 | (14–17) | 0.80 |
| Balke[21]*** | 34 | 15.9 | (14–18) | 1.00 |
| Balke[21]** | 9 | 31.5 | (29–36) | 1.00 |
| Cooper[34]* | 115 | 22 | (17–52) | 0.897 |
| Doolittle et al.[55]* | 9 | 14 | (13–16) | 0.85 |
| Ribils et al.[101]*** | 24 | middle age | | 0.85 |

* 12-minute running test
** 15-minute running test
*** two-mile running test

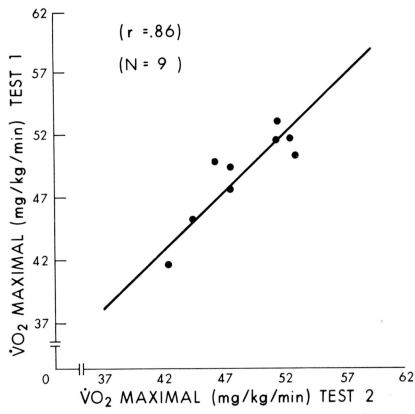

Figure 6–3. Correlation between test-retest values of maximal oxygen intake on treadmill (9 subjects).

mill performance. This performance was determined by the maximum slope on the treadmill and the maximum time up to five minutes that each subject was capable of performing.

> GROUP 1: maximum slope 6%, maximum running time = 2–3 minute
>
> GROUP 2: maximum slope 6%, maximum running time = 4–5 minute
>
> GROUP 3: maximum slope 9%, maximum running time = 2–3 minute
>
> GROUP 4: maximum slope 9%, maximum running time = 4–5 minute.

Figure 6–4 also shows that oxygen consumption curves level off for each group. Astrand[2,3] and Wyndham[15,16] considered this factor as a major criterion for indicating the maximum oxygen intake.

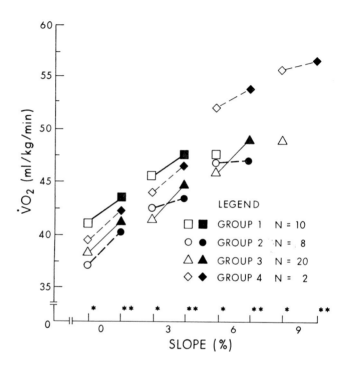

* O□△◇  MEASUREMENT BETWEEN 2nd-3rd MINUTE

** ●■▲◆  MEASUREMENT BETWEEN 4th-5th MINUTE

Figure 6–4. Relationship between maximal oxygen intake (ml/kg/min) and treadmill slope (%) (40 subjects divided into four groups relative to their performance on treadmill).

The maximum heart rates on the treadmill test varied from 180 to 190 beats/min (Fig. 6–5); these heart frequencies were considered by Balke[5] as maximum work. Most of the subjects reached the peak of their aerobic work capacity at this point. The four groups demonstrated a hyperventilation at the end of the treadmill exercise (Fig. 6–6). This reaction during a strenuous work is caused by an excessive amount of carbon dioxide in the blood; the body tries to reestablish equilibrium by increasing circulation and respiration. Figure 6–7 reports the relationship between oxygen pulse and work intensity on

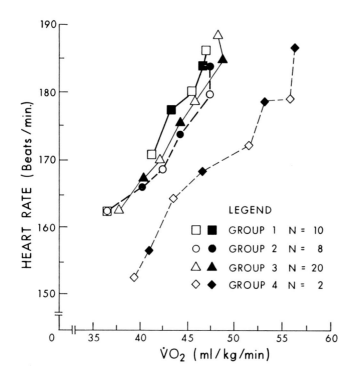

O□△◇ MEASUREMENT BETWEEN 2nd - 3rd MINUTE

●■▲◆ MEASUREMENT BETWEEN 4th - 5th MINUTE

Figure 6–5. Relationship between heart rate (beats/min) and oxygen consumption (ml/kg/min) on treadmill (40 subjects).

the treadmill. The curves levelled off (groups 1 and 4) and decreased (groups 2 and 3) at a high work intensity. This drop in oxygen pulse may be caused by a reduction of systolic volume when the heart rate reached 180 beats/min.

Table 6-III includes the relationship between the performances attained in the twelve minute run test and various

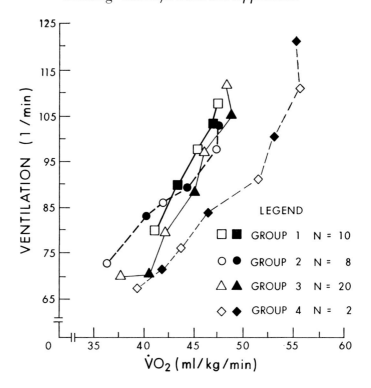

O□△◇  MEASUREMENT BETWEEN 2nd - 3rd MINUTE

●■▲◆  MEASUREMENT BETWEEN 4th - 5th MINUTE

Figure 6–6. Relationship between ventilation (liters/min) and oxygen consumption (ml/kg/min) on treadmill (40 subjects).

TABLE 6-III

RELATIONSHIP BETWEEN PERFORMANCES DURING TWELVE-MINUTE RUN TEST AND VARIOUS PHYSIOLOGICAL MEASUREMENTS REVEALING THE PHYSICAL CONDITION ON TREADMILL FOR EACH GROUP

| Group | 12-Minute Run Test | | $HR^*$ (beat/min) | $VO_2^{**}$ (ml/kg/min) STPD | $VO_2/HR^*$ (ml/beat) | $VE/VO_2^*$ STPD |
|---|---|---|---|---|---|---|
| | Distance (meters) | Speed (meter/min) | | | | |
| 1 (10 Subjects) | 2484.0 | 207.0 | 184 | 47.58 | 14.37 | 33.14 |
| 2 ( 8 Subjects) | 2646.0 | 220.5 | 174 | 47.43 | 15.01 | 28.40 |
| 3 (20 Subjects) | 2754.0 | 229.5 | 175 | 48.24 | 14.45 | 27.81 |
| 4 ( 2 Subjects) | 3387.0 | 290.5 | 168 | 56.43 | 17.41 | 23.32 |

\* Submaximal values measured between the 4th–5th at 3% slope
\*\* Maximal values (treadmill)

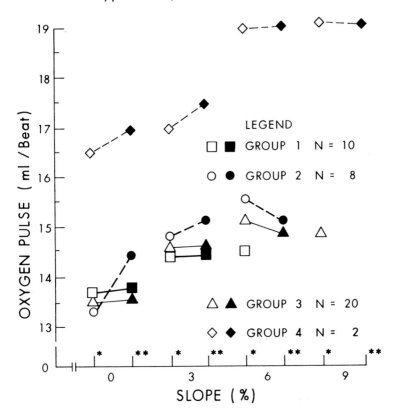

* ○□△◇  MEASUREMENT BETWEEN 2nd -3rd MINUTE
** ●■▲◆  MEASUREMENT BETWEEN 4th - 5th MINUTE

Figure 6–7. Relationship between oxygen pulse (ml/beat) and treadmill slope (%) (40 subjects).

physiological measurements studied in revealing the physical condition of the subjects on the treadmill. The better physical condition of groups three and four compared with groups one and two, was characterized by the following:

1. a longer distance run in the twelve minute test;
2. a lower heart rate at any given submaximal work load;
3. a higher maximum oxygen consumption;
4. a higher oxygen pulse at any given submaximal work load;

5. a lower respiratory equivalent at any given submaximal work load.

The twelve minute run test can be used by all physical education teachers, coaches or anyone working in sport field. It requires a minimum of equipment, and can be applied to many subjects in a short period of time. It can be also used to classify the students in a school, revealing one major aspect of their total physical fitness.

## References

1. Asmussen, E., and Nielsen, M.: *Scand. J. Clin. Lab. Invest.* 10: 67, 1958.
2. Astrand, P.O.: *Canad. Med. Ass. J.* 96: 732, 1967.
3. Astrand, P.O.: *Physiol. Rev.* 36: 307, 1956.
4. Astrand, P.O., and Rhyming, I.: *J. Appl. Physiol.* 7: 218, 1954.
5. Balke, B.: CARI Reports 63–6, Civil Aeromedical Research Institute. *Federal Aviation Agency*, 1963.
6. Benedict, F.G., and Cathcart, E.P.: *Muscular Work: A Metabolic Study with Special Reference to the Efficiency of the Human Body as a Machine.* Carnegie Institution of Washington, 1913.
7. Brouha, L., Graybiel, A., and Hearth, C.W.: *Rev. Canad. Biol.* 2: 86, 1943.
8. Cooper, K.H.: *J.A.M.A.* 203: 201, 1958.
9. Doolittle, T.L., and Bigbee, R.: *Res. Quart. Amer. Ass. Health. Phys. Educ.* 39: 491, 1968.
10. Hill, A.V.: *Proc. Roy. Soc. London.* 96: 438, 1923.
11. Margaria, R.: *J. Appl. Physiol.* 20: 1070, 1965.
12. Mitchell, H., Sproule, B.J., and Chapman, C.B.: *J. Clin. Invest.*, 37: 538, 1958.
13. Shephard, R.J.: *Int. Z. Angew. Physiol.* 23: 219, 1966.
14. Taylor, H.L., Buskiak, E., and Henschel, A., *J. Appl. Physiol.* 8: 73, 1955.
15. Wyndham, C.H.: *Int. Z. Angew. Physiol.* 22: 285, 1966.
16. Wyndham, C.H.: *Int. Z. Angew. Physiol.* 23: 354, 1967.

# Chapter 7

# Maximal Cardiac Output by "CO$_2$ Rebreathing"

R.J. Ferguson
L. Leger
M. Nadeau
P. Gauthier

Although the direct Fick and dye-dilution techniques are the methods of choice for the estimation of cardiac output ($\dot{Q}c$) in basic physiological research, indirect techniques such as "CO$_2$ rebreathing" can be useful for serial determination in patients or athletes during periods of treatment and physical training or in other situations requiring noninvasive techniques. During exercise up to 80 percent of the maximal oxygen uptake ($\dot{V}O_2$ max), performed by healthy young adult males, the "CO$_2$ rebreathing" method has been shown to be reproducible and furnish similar $\dot{Q}c$ values as the dye-dilution method.[5] The purposes of this study were (a) to determine the reproducibility of $\dot{Q}c$ max at workloads demanding the $\dot{V}O_2$ max and (b) to compare $\dot{Q}c$ max during work on a bicycle ergometer and motor-driven treadmill.

## Methods and Materials

The subjects were five normal, physically active males aged twenty to twenty three years. Oxygen consumption was measured by an open circuit technique in which one-min aliquot samples of expired gas were taken from an 8 liter mixing chamber and analyzed for oxygen and carbon dioxide fractions by means of Beckman E2 and LBI gas analyzers respectively. A three-point calibration of the CO$_2$ analyzer was performed prior to each recording of a rebreathing curve. $\dot{V}O_2$ max was determined for work on the bicycle ergometer and treadmill according to a procedure described by Hermansen and Saltin.[8] An estimate of the $\dot{V}O_2$ max was made from the submaximal heart rate and $\dot{V}O_2$. Following a warm-up the subject performed at a workload chosen to require the estimated $\dot{V}O_2$ max. On subsequent visits to the laboratory the workload was elevated by 2 km/hr for the treadmill and 200 kgm/min for the bicycle. The $\dot{V}O_2$ max was obtained when the subsequent $\dot{V}O_2$ did not increase by more than 3 percent. The pedalling rate during cycling was 50 rpm. All running was performed at a grade of 5.25 percent. During these first visits to the laboratory the subjects were given instruction and practice for the rebreathing technique.

Based on the findings of Karlsson and Astrand[10] some subjects, prior to the $\dot{Q}c$ max experiments, underwent additional tests in order to find a submaximal running speed which would demand a $\dot{V}O_2$ max and which could be maintained for six to seven min. From two to four determinations of $\dot{Q}c$ max were obtained on each subject during both bicycle and treadmill work. The subjects were accustomed to work on both ergometers. Only one maximal workload was performed per day. Cardiac output was determined by "$CO_2$ rebreathing" according to the method of Defares[4] as modified by Klausen[11] and Ferguson *et al.*[8] $PvCO_2$ was obtained from the graphical extrapolation of the exponential rise of $CO_2$ during rebreathing from a bag containing 100 percent oxygen.

Due to the high concentration of $O_2$ in the rebreathing bag it was assumed that the mixed venous blood was oxygenated. Arterial $P_{CO_2}$ was calculated using the Bohr formula and a deadspace estimate from the data of Asmussen and Nielsen.[1] All blood $P_{CO_2}$ estimates were converted to concentrations using a standard $CO_2$ dissociation curve for oxygenated blood.

Cardiac output was calculated using the Fick equation:

$$\dot{Q}c = \frac{\dot{V}_{CO_2}}{C\bar{v}_{CO_2} - Ca_{CO_2}}$$

where $\dot{Q}C$ = cardiac output in liters/min; $\dot{V}_{CO_2}$ = the expired volume of $CO_2$ (ml/min STPD); $C\bar{v}_{CO_2}$ = $CO_2$ content (ml/

liter mixed venous blood); and Ca$_{CO2}$ = CO$_2$content (ml/liter arterial blood.

The student t test for paired observations was employed in order to compare the physiologic responses to maximal treadmill and bicycle exercise. The mean of the subjects' first two determinations was used for this comparison. The calculation of the standard error of the method (SEM) was calculated by considering, as duplicates, the first two determinations of Q̇c max for each subject. The variability was expressed as a percent error.

## Results

The individual values for each subject are presented in Table 7-I. By considering the first two Q̇c max values on each ergometer and for each subject as duplicate determinations, the SEM (Table 7-II) was found to be 1.5 liters (6.6%). Although the second determination tended to be higher there was no significant difference between the means of the first and second Q̇c max. The largest difference was 3.4 liters. Using all the maximal data the intraindividual variability of Q̇c max determinations is also expressed as deviations from individual mean values (Fig. 7–1). Four of thirty-five maximal exercise tests were unsuccessful due to the poor technical quality of the rebreathing curves. Two were on subject M.N. at the beginning of bicycle ergometer testing. It was difficult for this subject to work for six minutes due to leg fatigue which distracted him from the performance of rebreathing. The remaining two occurred on subject L.L. who took an unusally long time to learn the rebreathing technique. No significant test-retest differences were found for maximal V̇O$_2$, heart rate, stroke volume or calculated arteriovenous difference.

V̇O$_2$ max (Fig. 7–2) was higher during running than during cycling (Table 7-III). The difference was 0.32 liters/min (3.89 — 3.57). This 8.2 percent higher V̇O$_2$ max was brought about by an elevated cardiac output of 8.8 percent (Fig. 7–3) with little variation in the a-vO$_2$ difference. Stroke volume and heart rate (Fig. 7–3) tended to be higher in maximal treadmill exercise.

TABLE 7-I

INDIVIDUAL VALUES FOR MAXIMAL TREADMILL (T) AND BICYCLE (B) EXERCISE

| Subject | $\dot{V}O_2$ (liter/min) | $\dot{V}O_2$ (ml/kg-min) | $\dot{Q}c$ (liter/min) | Heart Rate | Stroke Vol (ml) | $\Delta a\text{-}vO_2$ (ml/liter) | $\dot{V}e$ BTPS (liter/min) | RER | $PaCO_2$ (mmHg) | $P\bar{v}CO_2$ (mmHg) |
|---|---|---|---|---|---|---|---|---|---|---|
| **PG** | | | | | | | | | | |
| T | 3.81 | 53.2 | 24.7 | 188 | 131 | 154 | 132.0 | 1.10 | 33.7 | 76.2 |
|   | 3.79 | 52.9 | 24.6 | 187 | 132 | 154 | 127.1 | 1.03 | 32.6 | 71.3 |
|   | 3.68 | 51.4 | 22.3 | 183 | 122 | 166 | 139.9 | 1.15 | 32.2 | 80.2 |
|   | 3.74 | 51.9 | 21.2 | 181 | 117 | 176 | 151.0 | 1.13 | 29.8 | 78.6 |
| B | 3.58 | 49.5 | 23.1 | 177 | 130 | 155 | 141.5 | 1.02 | 27.8 | 62.3 |
|   | 3.53 | 49.0 | 20.4 | 181 | 113 | 172 | 142.8 | 1.08 | 28.2 | 72.9 |
|   | 3.67 | 51.4 | 26.3 | 179 | 147 | 139 | 145.8 | 1.08 | 29.0 | 62.6 |
|   | 3.25 | 45.2 | 22.3 | 176 | 131 | 145 | 136.4 | 1.11 | 28.3 | 64.5 |
| **LL** | | | | | | | | | | |
| T | 4.57 | 66.4 | 23.1 | 181 | 128 | 198 | 168.4 | 1.02 | 29.8 | 79.7 |
|   | 4.50 | 64.9 | 26.5 | 181 | 146 | 170 | 165.3 | 1.10 | 32.0 | 78.9 |
|   | 4.64 | 67.8 | 28.6 | 183 | 156 | 162 | 168.8 | 1.04 | 30.6 | 71.1 |
|   | 4.60 | 67.5 | 27.5 | 183 | 150 | 168 | 164.8 | 1.04 | 31.2 | 71.5 |
| B | 3.93 | 57.0 | 24.9 | 180 | 138 | 158 | 165.3 | 1.17 | 28.9 | 72.0 |
|   | 4.11 | 59.6 | 23.3 | 174 | 134 | 176 | 143.2 | 1.02 | 30.8 | 74.7 |
|   | 4.02 | 58.7 | 24.9 | 183 | 136 | 161 | 181.9 | 1.15 | 26.8 | 68.4 |
|   | 4.07 | 60.6 | 26.8 | 176 | 152 | 152 | 161.1 | 1.16 | 30.7 | 73.2 |
| **JL** | | | | | | | | | | |
| T | 4.49 | 60.4 | 28.2 | 192 | 147 | 160 | 159.8 | 1.12 | 33.9 | 79.9 |
|   | 4.46 | 60.0 | 28.0 | 190 | 147 | 159 | 144.5 | 1.08 | 35.6 | 80.0 |
|   | 4.19 | 56.5 | 24.0 | 190 | 126 | 175 | 151.8 | 1.11 | 32.9 | 82.2 |
| B | 4.13 | 55.5 | 23.7 | 183 | 129 | 174 | 150.3 | 1.09 | 31.7 | 79.6 |
|   | 3.96 | 53.1 | 26.4 | 183 | 144 | 150 | 142.7 | 1.15 | 34.1 | 78.0 |
|   | 3.83 | 52.6 | 19.7 | 187 | 105 | 194 | 135.1 | 1.05 | 31.7 | 83.4 |

| | | | | | | | | | | |
|---|---|---|---|---|---|---|---|---|---|---|
| MG | T | 3.43 | 59.5 | 18.0 | 195 | 93 | 190 | 128.8 | 1.14 | 33.0 | 88.9 |
| | | 3.30 | 57.3 | 19.0 | 192 | 99 | 174 | 123.0 | 1.05 | 31.0 | 76.1 |
| | B | 2.92 | 49.8 | 18.6 | 193 | 96 | 157 | 142.5 | 1.14 | 25.2 | 69.0 |
| | | 3.56 | 61.2 | 18.2 | 183 | 99 | 196 | 139.2 | .99 | 27.4 | 72.3 |
| | | 3.38 | 57.6 | 21.0 | 188 | 111 | 161 | 143.3 | 1.10 | 27.9 | 68.6 |
| MN | T | 3.20 | 55.1 | 24.0 | 184 | 130 | 133 | 107.8 | 1.12 | 38.3 | 76.7 |
| | | 3.33 | 57.4 | 21.9 | 185 | 118 | 152 | 112.1 | 1.13 | 38.6 | 83.9 |
| | | 3.25 | 55.6 | 22.2 | 182 | 122 | 147 | 110.3 | 1.14 | 38.4 | 82.0 |
| | B | 2.98 | 51.1 | 17.8 | 177 | 100 | 168 | 109.8 | 1.07 | 33.1 | 78.3 |
| | | 2.96 | 50.8 | 21.0 | 183 | 115 | 140 | 101.4 | 1.09 | 36.1 | 74.5 |

TABLE 7-II
TEST (I)—RETEST (II) VARIABILITY OF MAXIMAL CIRCULATORY
VALUES

| | $\dot{V}O_2$ (liter/min) | | $\dot{Q}c$ (liter/min) | | Heart Rate | | Stroke Vol (ml) | | $\Delta a\text{-}VO_2$ (ml/liter) | |
|---|---|---|---|---|---|---|---|---|---|---|
| | I | II | I | II | I | II | I | II | I | II |
| $\bar{x}$ | 3.71 | 3.74 | 22.6 | 23.0 | 184 | 185 | 122 | 124 | 165 | 164 |
| sd | 0.60 | 0.49 | 3.2 | 3.6 | 7 | 5 | 17 | 20 | 17 | 18 |
| $n^a$ | 10 | | 10 | | 10 | | 10 | | 10 | |
| $\bar{d}^b$ | −0.04 | | −0.44 | | −0.7 | | −2.1 | | 0.8 | |
| Percent Error$^c$ | 4.3 | | 6.6 | | 1.7 | | 6.4 | | 9.6 | |

[a] Treadmill and bicycle data combined giving ten comparisons.
[b] None of the $\bar{d}$ was significant.
[c] Percent error $= \dfrac{SEM}{\bar{x}} \times 100$.

Minute ventilation and respiratory exchange ratio were similar during maximal work on the treadmill and bicycle (Table 7-IV). However, both $PaCO_2$ and $P\bar{v}CO_2$ were significantly higher during running.

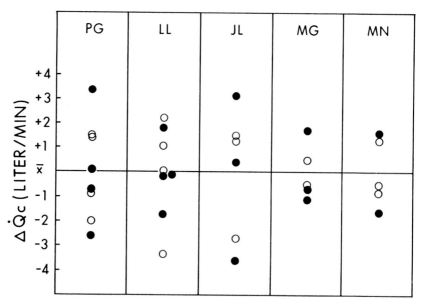

Figure 7–1. Intraindividual variability of $\dot{Q}c$ max determinations expressed as differences from individual mean values for the treadmill (filled circles) and bicycle (open circles).

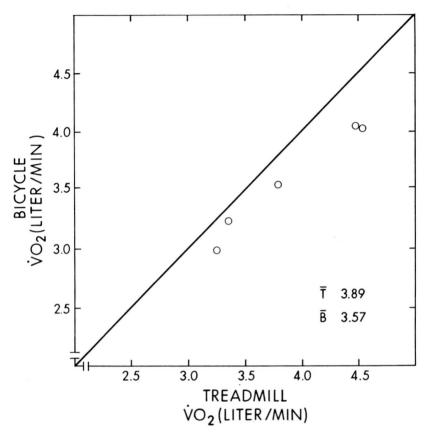

Figure 7–2. Comparison of $\dot{V}O_2$ max between bicycle and treadmill work.

TABLE 7-III
CIRCULATORY COMPARISON OF MAXIMAL TREADMILL (T) AND
BICYCLE (B) EXERCISE

| | $\dot{V}O_2$ (liter/min) | | $\dot{Q}c$ (liter/min) | | Stroke Vol (ml) | | Heart Rate | | $\Delta a\text{-}VO_5$ (ml/liter) | |
|---|---|---|---|---|---|---|---|---|---|---|
| | T | B | T | B | T | B | T | B | T | B |
| x̄ | 3.89 | 3.57 | 23.8 | 21.7 | 127 | 120 | 188 | 181 | 164 | 165 |
| sd | 0.60 | 0.47 | 3.5 | 2.9 | 19 | 17 | 5 | 4 | 18 | 8 |
| d̄ | 0.32** | | 2.1* | | 7 | | 7** | | 1 | |
| Δ% | 8.2 | | 8.8 | | 5.5 | | 3.7 | | 0.6 | |

* P < 0.05.
** P < 0.01.

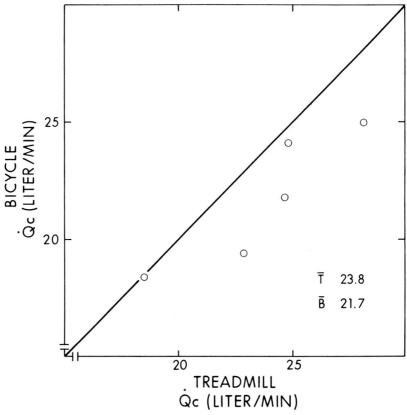

Figure 7–3. Comparison of $\dot{Q}c$ max between bicycle and treadmill work.

TABLE 7-IV

RESPIRATORY COMPARISON OF MAXIMAL TREADMILL (T)
AND BICYCLE (B) EXERCISE

|  | $\dot{V}e\ BTPS$ (liter/min) | | $PaCO_5$ (mmHg) | | $P\bar{v}CO_5$ (mmHg) | | RER | |
|---|---|---|---|---|---|---|---|---|
|  | T | B | T | T | T | B | T | B |
| $\bar{x}$ | 136.9 | 137.9 | 33.8 | 30.3 | 79.2 | 73.4 | 1.09 | 1.08 |
| sd | 22.5 | 18.8 | 2.9 | 3.4 | 3.2 | 4.4 | 0.03 | 0.03 |
| $\bar{d}$ | −1.0 | | 3.5* | | 5.8* | | 0.01 | |
| $\Delta\%$ | 0.7 | | 10.4 | | 7.3 | | 0.9 | |

* P 0.05.

## Discussion

The SEM (6.6 percent) of $\dot{Q}c$ max by "$CO_2$ rebreathing" is only slightly higher than that reported by Hanson and Tabakin[7] for the dye-dilution method. This indicates good reproducibility considering that, in the present study, $\dot{Q}c$ max was determined on different days and includes not only technical error of the measurement but true $\dot{Q}c$ variability from day to day and from $\dot{V}O_2$ max variations (SEM 4.3%).

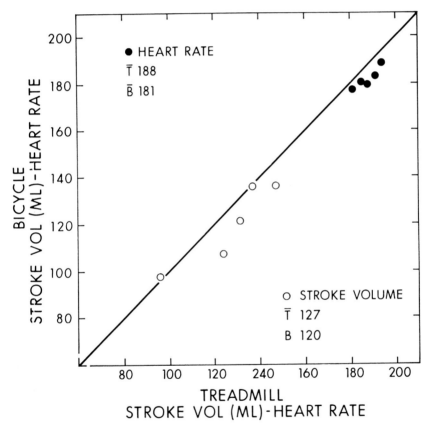

Figure 7–4. Comparison for maximal heart rate and stroke volume between bicycle and treadmill work.

Differences of $\dot{V}O_2$ max between treadmill and bicycle work ranging from 5 to 15 percent have been reported.[2,3,6,8,9] Hermansen, Ekblom and Saltin[9] found that a 6 percent higher $\dot{V}O_2$ max running was accompanied by an equivalent increase in Qc max with little variation in the a-v$O_2$ difference. Also, no differences were noted in maximum minute ventilation or lactic acid. Rephrasing their explanation, one could suggest that cycling may involve a higher relative tension in the working muscles evoking a rise in arterial pressure which could be secondary to an even greater rise in peripheral resistance. The combination of these two factors would result in a lower cardiac output during cycling.

As stated by Hermansen, Ekblom and Saltin,[9] and supported by the present data, the difference in $\dot{Q}c$ max between maximal cycling and running is relatively small and is within the error of measurement of $\dot{Q}c$, whether this be determined by the dye-dilution or "$CO_2$ rebreathing" techniques. Thus for most purposes either the treadmill or the bicycle is sufficient for the evaluation of maximal work. However, it would seem prudent not to employ maximal bicycle exercise to test hypotheses concerning $\dot{Q}c$ as a limiting factor to attaining $\dot{V}O_2$ max

## References

1. Asmussen, E., and Nielsen, M.: *Acta Physiol. Scand.* 38: 1, 1956.
2. Astrand, P.-O., and Saltin, B.: *J. Appl. Physiol.* 16: 977, 1961.
3. Chase, G.A., Grave, C., and Rowell, L.B.: *Aerospace Med.* 37: 1232, 1966.
4. Defares, J.G.: *A Study of the Carbon Dioxide Time Course During Rebreathing* (thesis). Utrecht Kemink en Zoon NU, 1956.
5. Ferguson, R.J., Faulkner, J.A., Julius, S. and Conway, J.: *J. Appl. Physiol.* 25: 450, 1968.
6. Glassford, R.G., Baycroft, G.H.Y., Sedgwich, A.W., and Macnab, R.B.J. *J. Appl. Physiol.* 20: 509, 1965.
7. Hanson, J.S., and Tabakin, B.S.: *J. Appl. Physiol.* 19: 275, 1964.
8. Hermansen, L. and Saltin, B.: *J. Appl. Physiol.* 26: 31, 1969.
9. Hermansen, L., Ekb!om, B. and Saltin, B.: *J. Appl. Physiol.* 29: 82, 1970.
10. Karlsson, J., Astrand, P.-O., and Ekblom, B.: *J. Appl. Physiol.* 22: 1061, 1967.
11. Klausen, K.: *J. Appl. Physiol.* 20: 763, 1965.

# Chapter 8

# The Intensity of Training

NORMAN GLEDHILL
ROBERT B. EYNON

R esearchers have shown conclusively that cardiorespiratory fitness may be elevated by training, and thus a topic of major practical concern is the determination of optional training procedures. Previous investigations support the theory that there is a training effect only beyond a threshold stimulus. However, they propose a continuum of minimal training stimulus intensities extending from a low of 120 beats/min, to the highest reported minimum threshold of 150 beats/min.

This study assessed the effect on selected parameters of cardiorespiratory fitness, of training at intentities eliciting heart rates of 120, 135 and 150 beats/min. The relative cardiorespiratory fitness of the subjects was also investigated to determine whether this variable affected the intensity question.

## Methods and Materials

Thirty-two clinically healthy male university students were classified prior to the pretest as being above or below the group median (which was almost identical to the mean) in cardiorespiratory fitness, based solely upon their maximal oxygen intake in ml/kg/min. The resultant two groups were then both randomly subdivided into one control and three experimental subgroups, with four subjects in each of the eight subgroups.

The training sessions, which consisted of twenty minute bicycle ergometer rides at 120, 135 or 150 beats/minute were repeated five days a week for five weeks. The subjects were connected by electrocardiograph leads to a cardiotachometer

97

which monitored a plainly visible dial reading of their heart rate. The training sessions began with a warm-up period of approximately three minutes duration, which was designed to elicit the prescribed intensity as near as possible to the end of the third minute. The timing of the actual twenty minute ride did not commence until the assigned heart rate was achieved. On occasions when the subject was premature or overdue in reaching the required heart rate, the timer was adjusted so that the training time at desired intensity was identical for all subjects. During the twenty minute training rides, the subjects pedalled at a cadence and load which was sufficient to maintain their heart rates continuously at the prescribed intensity.

## Results

Table 8-I contains a description of the division of the subjects into two cardiorespiratory fitness classifications, based on their maximal oxygen intake in ml/kg/min.

TABLE 8-I
CLASSIFICATION OF THE SUBJECTS ON THE BASIS OF THEIR
MAXIMAL OXYGEN INTAKE IN ML/KG/MIN

| Classification | Range | Median | Mean |
|---|---|---|---|
| All Subjects | 27.8–63.2 | 40.2 | 40.4 |
| Below Median | 27.8–39.9 | 33.7 | 34.0 |
| Above Median | 40.7–63.2 | 45.4 | 46.8 |

A summary of the data is presented in Table 8-11. The significance of the difference between and within groups was determined by a 2 x 2 x 4 analysis of variance. When a significant F was attained for the interaction effects in the analysis of variance, post hoc comparisons were made using Duncan's New Multiple Range Test.

The analysis of the maximal oxygen intake data indicated that there was a significant ($p < .01$) difference in the training effect produced by the various intensities. There was no significant change in either the control subjects or the subjects who trained at 120 beats/minute, but those subjects who trained at 135 beats/minute and 150 beats/minute made sig-

## TABLE 8-II
## SUMMARY OF THE DATA

| Classification | N. | $\dot{V}O_2$ ml/kg/min Pre | Post | Diff. | End. Performance (min) Pre | Post | Diff. | Resting HR Pre | Post | Diff. | HR at 1500 kpm Pre | Post | Diff. |
|---|---|---|---|---|---|---|---|---|---|---|---|---|---|
| **Below Median** | | | | | | | | | | | | | |
| Control | 4 | 33.9 | 34.4 | 0.5 | 16.5 | 16.5 | 0.0 | 58 | 58 | 0 | 173 | 172 | −1 |
| 120 | 4 | 35.2 | 38.2 | 3.0 | 14.9 | 16.2 | 1.3 | 65 | 62 | −3 | 167 | 161 | −6 |
| 135 | 4 | 34.4 | 39.1 | 4.7 | 16.3 | 16.8 | 0.5 | 61 | 60 | −1 | 172 | 167 | −5 |
| 150 | 4 | 32.5 | 38.8 | 6.3 | 15.8 | 16.7 | 0.9 | 59 | 58 | −1 | 183 | 176 | −6 |
| **Above Median** | | | | | | | | | | | | | |
| Control | 4 | 49.6 | 50.6 | 1.0 | 16.6 | 16.6 | 0.0 | 54 | 55 | +1 | 171 | 170 | −1 |
| 120 | 4 | 47.7 | 47.9 | 0.2 | 17.2 | 17.2 | 0.0 | 52 | 52 | 0 | 174 | 169 | −5 |
| 135 | 4 | 43.5 | 49.2 | 5.7 | 17.0 | 17.4 | 0.4 | 55 | 54 | −1 | 185 | 178 | −7 |
| 150 | 4 | 46.3 | 51.2 | 4.9 | 16.5 | 17.7 | 1.2 | 56 | 54 | −2 | 177 | 168 | −9 |
| **Combined** | | | | | | | | | | | | | |
| Control | 8 | 41.7 | 42.4 | 0.7 | 16.6 | 16.6 | 0.0 | 56 | 56 | 0 | 172 | 171 | −1 |
| 120 | 8 | 41.5 | 43.0 | 1.5 | 16.0 | 16.7 | 0.7 | 58 | 57 | −1 | 171 | 165 | −6 |
| 135 | 8 | 38.9 | 44.1 | 5.2 | 16.6 | 17.1 | 0.5 | 58 | 57 | −1 | 178 | 172 | −6 |
| 150 | 8 | 39.4 | 45.1 | 5.7 | 16.1 | 17.2 | 1.1 | 58 | 56 | −2 | 180 | 172 | −8 |

nificant (p<.01) improvements in maximal oxygen intake. However, the improvements of the 135 beats/minute group and the 150 beats/minute group did not differ significantly from one another, and the initial cardiorespiratory fitness of the subjects had no significant effect on their response to training.

The analysis of the endurance performance data also indicated a significant (p<.01) difference in the training effect produced by the various intensities. Those subjects who trained at 150 beats/minute made significant (p<.01) improvements in endurance performance time, while there was no significant change in the control subjects or the subjects who trained at 120 and 135 beats/minute. The initial cardiorespiratory fitness of the subjects again had no significant effect on their response to training.

Although the analysis indicated that over the training period there was a significant (p<.01) improvement in both the resting heart rate and the heart rate response to a fixed submaximal load, there was no statistically significant difference between the various subgroups.

## Discussion

In order to produce a significant improvement in maximal oxygen intake, the intensity of training had to be strenuous enough to elicit heart rates of at least 135 beats/minute. This observation supports the findings of Hollmann and Venrath[2], and Horvath,[3] but the lack of a significant increase by the subjects who trained at 120 beats/minute opposes the contentions of Shephard[9] and Astrand.[1] It should be noted, however, that the 120 group did show a slight improvement in maximal oxygen intake (4%), and if the training had continued longer, or the subjects had been more sedentary prior to the training program, this increase might have become statistically significant. Although the statistical analysis of the maximal oxygen intake data does not support Astrand's[1] position that the effect of training is more pronounced as the work load increases, there is a definite trend toward greater improvements with increasing intensity. Astrand stated that the optimal aerobic training program is one in which the oxygen transport system is just taxed maximally, and in a subsequent study with Karlsson,[4] he established this point at approximately 80 percent of the maximal work load.

The lack of a statistically significant difference between the improvements of the two fitness classifications does not support the hypothesis that the discrepancy between previously reported training thresholds was the result of a dissmilarity in the initial cardiorespiratory fitness of their subjects. It is interesting to note however, that although the improvements in the mean maximal oxygen intake of the 150 and 135 groups were comparable for the two fitness classifications, the below median 120 group increased substantially more than did the above median 120 group (3.0 ml/kg/min, as compared to 0.2 ml/kg/min), and if the period of training had been extended, a statistically significant difference might have been observed. The implication here is that individuals who possess a low level of cardiorespiratory fitness may have a low threshold of training. This is in agreement with the findings of Shephard,[8] who stated, in reference to the cardiorespiratory improvements which took place during a training program, that, "the magnitude of these changes could be related to initial 'fitness.'"

The significantly different improvement in endurance performance time recorded for the group which trained at an intensity of 150 beats/minute, is in concurrence with the findings of Karvonen[5] and Sharkey,[7] who observed that the intensity of training must be greater than 150 beats/minute in order to elicit cardiorespiratory fitness improvements. Although the improvements in the endurance performance times of the 135 and 150 groups were comparable for both the above median and below median fitness classifications, the below median 120 group increased substantially more than did the above median group. Though their difference was not statistically significant, this observation supports the theory that individuals who possess a low level of cardiorespiratory fitness may have a low threshold of training.

Although the changes in resting and working heart rate

recorded for the training groups did not differ significantly from those recorded for the control groups, it is evident that the training groups did make substantial improvements in these parameters. Also there was a trend toward greater improvements with increasing intensity similar to that reported by Karvonen.[6]

## References

1. Astrand, P.O.: *Canad. Med. Assoc. J.* 96:12, 793, 1967.
2. Hollmann, W., and Venrath, H. In: Korbs, W. u.a., Carl Diem Fet-Schrift, Frankfurt a. M./Wein 1962.
3. Horvath, S.M.: *Canad. Med. Ass. J.* 96:12, 791–793, 1967.
4. Karlsson, J., Astrand, P.O., and Ekblom, B.: *J. Appl. Physiol.* 22:1061–1065, 1967.
5. Karvonen, M.J.: *Work and the Heart*, Rosenbaum, F.F., Ed. New York, Hoeber, 1959 pp. 199–210.
6. Karvonen, M.J., Kentala, E. and Mustala, O. *Ann. Med. Exp. Feen.* 35:307–315, 1957.
7. Sharkey, B.J., and Holleman, J.P.: *Res Quart.* 38:698–703, 1967.
8. Shephard, R.J.: *Ergonomics* 9:3–16, 1966.
9. Shephard, R.J.: *Canad. Med. Assoc. J.* 96:12, 899, 1967.

# Laboratory Measurements Applied to the Development and Modification of Training Programs

JAMES S. THODEN
MAURICE JETTE

This paper is oriented less toward the presentation of results from a specific experiment than it is to outlining an application of laboratory measurements in training athletes. In so doing, a description of the preliminary development and possible uses of the approach will be presented and the following paper will demonstrate its application to a specific sport.

Awareness of this as a problem requiring study has become most acute in recent years following the success of some international athletes who have been involved in laboratory programs. The opportunity for our laboratory to become involved in training programs came when we were approached at first by individual athletes and then by coaches who were looking for assistance in assessing functional capacities. This was attractive to us because we have always had difficulty in gaining the continued cooperation of athletic teams in connection with our more research-oriented programs. We therefore began to explore the possibility of organizing and augmenting our test batteries to include the type of information which could be valuable to the coach as well as to ourselves in connection with other programs.

In order that the various coaches who were involved would be able to develop the proper perspective with regard to the information that we could supply, we conceptualized physical

*Note:* Appreciation is extended to J.A. Spence and P.H. Bélanger for their invaluable assistance in collecting and calculating data.

103

performance as the product of interaction among a large number of inputs including biological, environmental, and psychological variables and their many facets (Fig. 9–1). We wanted them to understand that, because the social, barometric, and physical characteristics of the environment are largely uncontrollable, there would be little point in assessing them, at least for the present. We also wanted them to understand that while moti-

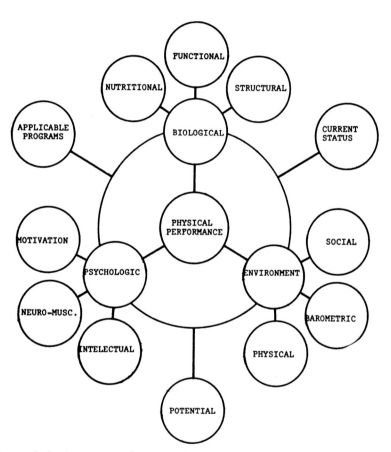

Figure 9–1. A conceptual approach to the identification of components which interact to affect physical performance. The performance of any physical activity will depend upon the current status of biological, psychological and environmental factors and their potential for improvement as promoted through applicable programs.

vational and intellectual characteristics have long been suggested as major factors in the process of separating winners from also-rans, examples of their isolation and quantification are limited to a small number of activities. We therefore explained that little use could be made of psychometric data at this time but that its collection might eventually be used in constructing profiles of developing athletes. Recognition was made of the inevitable superiority of the coach in assessing the neuromuscular skills connected with his particular activity and therefore only superficial attempts have been made to assist him through the provision of video tape equipment. Perhaps some attempts at biomechanical analysis will be made in the future if and when the program is expanded.

It may be expected by the tactic of progressive exclusion employed thus far that we felt there was a better chance of immediately categorizing our subjects primarily on the basis of biological variables. We proposed to do this by examining the functional capacities connected with energy production and strength, by quantifying structural characteristics, and by superficially assessing nutritional and biological adequacy. Thus we felt that the current status of an athlete might be established relative to his local, national, and international peer group, at least within the limits set by a paucity of normative data.

Unfortunately, the really useful information from the coaches' point of view was that which would assess the potential of an individual with regard to meeting environmental circumstances or modifying psychological and biological variables. This, of course, offered a problem which was somewhat more complex than the simple measurement of functional capacities. Many investigators have attempted to relate championship performances to one or a small number of physical characteristics and have succeeded only in proving the lack of precision through such measurements. The explanation for this can probably be related to acquired compensations for the deficiency of particular requirements through the assertion of other qualities. Unfortunate though it may be, the combination of these qualities is usually unique to an individual but it does seem logical that there will be a limit to the applicable qualities that can be described and we have expressed to the coaches the hope of eventually developing some "selection" guidelines.

Of the possible compensating factors certainly skill performance and personality structure will hold prominent positions, especially in view of the high levels of biological excellence usually displayed by most athletes of international caliber. It seems justifiable then to consider that the analysis of a longitudinally oriented testing program which covers a broad spectrum of psychological as well as biological variables will yield some insight into the major ingredients of success and thus provide some basis for categorizing the potential of an athlete.

In addition, it soon became apparent that the principles of training employed by most coaches were not necessarily a product of their own ingenuity and empirical methods, but rather had been taken from the programs of other successful performers and applied without real knowledge of the reasons underlying their use. As a result, if programs were to be altered because of our test results, we must also accept in part the responsibility for interpreting this material and training principles into workable programs. This also implies the necessity for continuing our measurements longitudinally in order to assess the effectiveness, or lack of it, following any modification.

Thus the problem had been expanded from its original concept to include not only the assessment of biological capacities but also the construction of biological and psychological profiles for successful athletes and the design of programs which would allow them to maximize their potential.

### Methods and Procedures

The tests with which we proposed to begin this program are summarized in Table 9-I. Social and attitudinal qualities are assessed by Cattel's sixteen personality factor test and some attempt at assessing neuromotor response is made through reaction-time measurements. We are currently working with psychologists to expand this program. Structural qualities are recorded by skeletal, tissue, and body build dimensions according to accepted criteria.[4,10] Functional measurements include

TABLE 9-I
TESTING FORMAT

*Psychological*
Cattel's 16 PF
Reaction Time measurements
*Biological*
Structural—skeletal and tissue dimensions
—fat and fat free body weight (skinfold method)
—somatotyping
Functional—resting: caloric cost, 12 lead ECG, pre-ejection interval, lying and
standing HR and BP, Schneider bench-step, hematology
(Na, K, Cl-, $CO_2$, Total protein, Albumin, Ca, Total Bilirubin, BUN, SGOT, Hb, Hct, Cholesterol)
—maximum: strength: grip strength, arm strength, back and leg
strength plus measures specific to each sport
flexibility: CAHPER hip flexibility plus range of movements specific to the sport
aerobic performance: intermittent 8.6% grade runs with
progressively increasing speed; to be supple-
mented where applicable by field measurements

cardio-pulmonary and hematological determinations during rest and exercise as well as standard strength and flexibility items. The treadmill test has been adopted from one applied to athletes[6] to make it compatible with a wide range of subject types including children and females as well as athletes. In order to avoid any great changes in performance efficiencies by using only speed or treadmill grade as the work variable,[3] the treadmill is set at an 8.6% grade (based on its length) and the speed is varied at 0.5 mph or 1.0 mph increments from an initial speed of 6.0 or 7.0 mph. The subject performs for a five minute period and measurements are taken during the third and fifth minutes. After a rest period (to allow the heart rate to return to about 110 beats per min) the speed is increased and a second five minute run is conducted. The progression continues until the subject is exhausted between the third and fifth minutes. Using this test we usually demonstrate the characteristic plateauing of oxygen consumption and an r of 0.92 on repeated measurements. Specific items for strength, flexibility, and aerobic performance are also being tailored for individual sports.

Theoretically the results will have the multiple application of categorizing athletes and of providing a data bank to which multiple stepwise prediction analysis can be applied in order to isolate the most important variables. Reapplication of the test or test parts allows monitoring of the athlete's progress through a training program.

## Results and Discussion

Time and funds have restricted our major interests to skiers, swimmers, and hockey players although we have tested paddlers, football players, speed skaters and track men to date.

Table 9-II shows maximum aerobic performance data gathered from a number of groups. We have found a significant difference in results of maximum aerobic performance tests conducted on the same individuals using both bicycle ergometer and treadmill tests of the intermittent type. As European laboratories make extensive use of the ergometer but report less discrepancy in their results (5%–8%),[3] we use the treadmill almost exclusively as a source of data for comparison with other laboratories and this is supported by the comparable values for adult, active males as measured in our laboratory and in Sweden.[8]

Among the first to undergo these tests as a group were fifteen members of our school hockey team. We found that, as far as aerobic performance was concerned, they were not much higher than healthy noncompetitive males and no different from a high school cross-country interest group composed of nine sixteen-to-eighteen-year-old boys, most of whom were not competitive other than at the school level. It was also interesting to note that they were no different from a thirty-four member group made up of the 1966–68 Canadian National Hockey teams.[5] These results compare favorably with those given for varsity players in Montreal[7] and players in Europe.[9] However, there was a greater intrateam variability in the University of Ottawa players when compared with fourteen of the better national team members. As we consider hockey to be essentially a series of maximum performances linked by coasting and rest periods, we felt that the players could benefit from high aerobic capacities. The coach has accepted this suggestion and our team is now being trained with more emphasis on the development of aerobic performance. We hope that proof of its benefit may be shown in the spring play-offs.

TABLE 9-II

MAXIMUM AEROBIC PERFORMANCE—MEAN VALUES FOR SELECTED SPORTS

| Group | N | HR $\bar{x}$ | HR $\sigma$ | $\dot{V}_E$ $\bar{x}$ | $\dot{V}_E$ $\sigma$ | $\dot{V}O_2$ $\bar{x}$ | $\dot{V}O_2$ $\sigma$ | $\dot{V}O_2/kg$ $\bar{x}$ | $\dot{V}O_2/kg$ $\sigma$ | R $\bar{x}$ | R $\sigma$ | $\dot{V}O_2/kg^{1-2}$ |
|---|---|---|---|---|---|---|---|---|---|---|---|---|
| Male Adults | | | | | | | | | | | | |
| Treadmill | 6 | 182.5 | 6.1 | 159.5 | 21.0 | 4.82 | 0.48 | 67.8 | 4.5 | 1.04 | 0.06 | |
| Bike | 6 | 179.3 | 10.7 | 155.2 | 21.3 | 3.86 | 0.24 | 53.1 | 7.1 | 1.18 | 0.17 | |
| Male Adults | | | | | | | | | | | | |
| 20–30 years | | | | | | | | | | | | |
| Hockey Players | 13 | 176.7 | 7.6 | 117.0 | 23.4 | 3.22 | 0.46 | 45.8 | 5.7 | 1.13 | 0.12 | 44[1] |
| National Hockey | 15 | 177.4 | 13.3 | 141.0 | 23.0 | 4.19 | 0.56 | 54.5 | 7.8 | 1.07 | 0.16 | 55[2] |
| Team 1968 | 34 | | | | | | | 53.4 | 5.9 | | | 55[2] |
| High School | | | | | | | | | | | | |
| Track—Male | 9 | 186.4 | 9.0 | 110.5 | 8.0 | 4.02 | 0.47 | 56.4 | 5.7 | 0.94 | 0.12 | |
| Speed Skating | | | | | | | | | | | | |
| Male | 1 | 190.0 | | 135.4 | | 4.13 | | 58.0 | | 0.98 | | 78.0[1] |
| Female | 1 | 190.0 | | 123.0 | | 3.90 | | 58.7 | | 1.00 | | 54.0[1] |
| Football Players | | | | | | | | | | | | |
| Pretrain | 5 | 178.8 | 9.7 | 156.3 | 8.5 | 4.46 | 0.55 | 51.9 | 8.5 | 1.13 | 0.09 | |
| Posttrain | 5 | 188.4 | 7.0 | 188.7 | 11.7 | 4.99 | 0.58 | 59.1 | 5.9 | 0.97 | 0.07 | |
| Paddlers | 3 | 180.6 | 4.1 | 149.5 | 15.3 | 4.53 | 0.33 | 59.6 | 4.6 | 1.13 | 0.09 | 70.5[1] |
| Skiers | | | | | | | | | | | | |
| Preseason | 3 | 177.3 | 1.9 | 159.8 | 27.6 | 4.50 | 0.44 | 65.6 | 5.3 | 1.05 | 0.02 | 83[1] |
| Midseason | 3 | 181.7 | 5.3 | 163.8 | 11.8 | 4.56 | 0.40 | 66.0 | 2.3 | 1.04 | 0.07 | |

[1] From Saltin, B. (1967)
[2] From Ferguson, R.J. (1969)
* Range

In addition, by observing the ventilation, heart rate, and respiratory quotient measured during the performance of maximum aerobic tests and by noting the plateau established in oxygen consumption, it was possible to speculate as to the amount of effort the subject had expended, that is, the amount of stress that he was willing to incur. We found ourselves to be about 80 percent accurate as compared to the coaches' subjective judgment in assessing this characteristic. Such a speculation might be useful in assessing "desire" in an athlete but, because of difficulty in validation, it is stressed that this, and all of our tests for that matter, should be used only as more data input rather than as the major basis for evaluation of players. Little else has been done with the hockey players primarily because of the lack of material on which to base the quantification of their attributes. We are currently attempting to develop such criteria together with practical field tests for rapid categorization by the coach but we expect this to be a long and involved process.

Training programs for each sport generally follow traditional patterns that include an introductory "camp" followed by skill sessions and then "peaking" programs. The value of these patterns interested us and we proposed to examine them in part. This last spring a group of our varsity football players who might have been described as "just adequate" physically were gathered and trained three times weekly by one of our laboratory personnel. The intent was to evaluate their response to the training program and compare it with their response to the fall training camp as well as to the response of team members who did not train over the summer. This approach was taken because measurements on Canadian cross-country ski team members the previous fall had demonstrated little benefit from a particularly gruelling three-month period of endurance training. This suggested that either these adult skiers had already come near to their physiological limits for improvement, or that the value of high pitch training camps was open to some question, at least as a beneficial program for sports requiring high levels of aerobic ability. Unfortunately, once the training camp was completed, we found it difficult to get the players back for testing. Thus, the data is incomplete except in showing improvements by five players and in eliciting positive comments by the coach. We are currently hoping for better results by following the same rationale with our basketball and hockey players but we cannot report on them at this time.

The question of the value of high intensity training camps was more variable with respect to four national qualifying swimmers whom we have had in our laboratory during the past year. Tables 9-III and 9-IV show individual anthropometric, $\dot{V}O_2$, $\dot{V}_E$, and HR data from basal and maximum aerobic performance tests conducted seven weeks prior to, two weeks prior to and 2½ months following the national championships. Three subjects show varying improvements in aerobic performance during a five to six day per week, 1½ hour per session, maximum demand schedule. Three subjects had a low Hct and Hb and three showed a decrease in both of these variables during "peaking." Subject four who, according to the coach had been complaining of being tired, showed a decrease of 2 gm % Hb, 2% Hct, and 5 ml/kg/min in $\dot{V}O_2$. This type of change should, according to Allik,[1] have been reflected by increased levels of resting $\dot{V}O_2$ but these remained unchanged. Hematological analysis showed all other serum levels to be well within normal ranges. Our recommendation at this time was to give everyone a rest from heavy training beginning about one week before the events. Unfortunately the apprehension by these unseasoned swimmers forced them to continue the heavy program and we do not feel it to be coincidental that during the national events all swam times above their previously demonstrated capability.

Both the male and female swimmers were well below $\dot{V}O_2$ levels that have been recorded on international swimmers and this was understandable as the age range was fourteen to sixteen years. However, it was surprising that they were released by their coach for a two-month period before the recommencement of training. The result was a major drop in aerobic performance for one subject while the other two remained relatively stable where an improvement might have been expected if only by growth alone. We have therefore suggested the value of continuous training to their coach and they are currently undergoing

## TABLE 9-III
### INTRAINDIVIDUAL COMPARISON OF SELECTED ANTHROPOMETRIC STRENGTH AND RESTING DATA MALE AND FEMALE SWIMMERS

| | Test | Ht | Wt | % Fat | Strength Index | Lying Hr | Stdg Hr | $\dot{V}O_2$ | Hb | Hct |
|---|---|---|---|---|---|---|---|---|---|---|
| Subject 1 (Male) | 1 | 70.50 | 72.0 | 12.1 | 11 | 68 | 88 | 0.241 | 13.8 | 40.0 |
| | 2 | 70.50 | 72.5 | 13.0 | | 88 | 100 | 0.230 | 13.9 | 41.0 |
| | 3 | 71.00 | 76.9 | 13.0 | 13 | 64 | 96 | 0.226 | 13.7 | 40.0 |
| Subject 2 (Male) | 1 | 68.00 | 59.2 | 13.5 | 18 | 36 | 56 | 0.192 | 15.5 | 44.0 |
| | 2 | 68.00 | 57.7 | 13.7 | 18 | 40 | 48 | 0.180 | 14.6 | 52.8 |
| | 3 | 68.00 | 59.9 | 15.4 | 20 | 40 | 48 | 0.189 | 14.7 | 43.5 |
| Subject 3 (Female) | 1 | 62.75 | 53.6 | 20.6 | 10 | 101 | 92 | 0.160 | 14.0 | 40.0 |
| | 2 | 62.75 | 52.8 | 19.0 | 14 | 102 | 80 | 0.121 | 13.1 | 39.0 |
| | 3 | 62.75 | 54.3 | 20.5 | 11 | 108 | 100 | 0.150 | 13.3 | 38.0 |
| Subject 4 (Female) | 1 | 64.5 | 59.5 | 20.2 | 13 | 108 | 80 | 0.189 | 14.8 | 40.0 |
| | 2 | 64.5 | 59.1 | 19.1 | 14 | 104 | 80 | 0.170 | 12.9 | 38.0 |

TABLE 9-IV
INTRAINDIVIDUAL COMPARISON OF MAXIMAL AEROBIC
PERFORMANCE DURING TRAINING
MALE AND FEMALE SWIMMERS

| | Test | HR | $\dot{V}_E$ | $\dot{V}O_2$ | $\dot{V}O_2/kg$ | R |
|---|---|---|---|---|---|---|
| Subject 1 | 1 | 164 | 157.0 | 4.68 | 65.0 | 1.06 |
| (Male) | 2 | 162 | 156.5 | 4.92 | 68.6 | 0.97 |
| | 3 | 148 | 149.4 | 4.34 | 56.2 | 1.08 |
| Subject 2 | 1 | 190 | 178.0 | 3.42 | 57.8 | 1.23 |
| (Male) | 2 | 174 | 156.8 | 3.94 | 68.3 | 1.03 |
| | 3 | 182 | 146.2 | 4.17 | 69.7 | 0.94 |
| Subject 3 | 1 | 180 | 87.9 | 2.18 | 40.6 | 1.04 |
| (Female) | 2 | 178 | 72.5 | 2.50 | 47.3 | 0.96 |
| | 3 | 194 | 88.6 | 2.46 | 45.6 | 1.05 |
| Subject 4 | 1 | 180 | 95.8 | 3.29 | 55.3 | 0.97 |
| (Female) | 2 | 182 | 101.2 | 2.97 | 50.2 | 1.14 |

a program of an aerobic or endurance nature accompanied by weight training.

These represent only a few of the simplest practical applications which have been made of data collected in connection with various other laboratory and research programs. It is suggested that the effort required is minimal once the program has been organized and that our experience shows it to be of real value in providing us with subject material for our research activities. We also have been told by the coaches that the material is valuable to them, so much so that we feel it can be justified on its own merits even without the added benefit of providing us with subjects. More extensive use will depend upon the development of a confidence by coaches so that more extensive and repetitive measurements can be made. We feel also that the next logical step is to develop, in addition to normative data, field testing programs of a practical nature which are specific to each sport and which can be used by the coach on a weekly basis in order to establish the effects of his program.

## References

1. Allik, T.A. *et al.*: *Medical Research on Swimming*, S. Firnov and E. Jokl, Eds. Moscow, Fédération Internationale Natation Amateur, 1968.
2. Astrand, P.O.: *Physiol. Rev.* 36: 307, 1956.

3. Astrand, P.O., and K. Rodall: *Textbook of Work Physiology*, New York, McGraw-Hill, 1970.
4. Brozek, J. (Ed.): *Body Composition*, Vol. I and II. *Ann. N.Y. Acad. Sci.*, 110: 1, 1963.
5. Coyne, L.: Some physiological characteristics of the Canadian National Hockey Team. Personal communication.
6. Cureton, T.K.: *Physical Fitness of Champion Athletes*, Urbana, University of Illinois Press, 1951.
7. Ferguson, R.J., G.G. Marcotte, and R.R. Montpetit: *Med. Sci. Sports* 1(4): 207, 1969.
8. Saltin, B., P.O. Astrand: *J. Appl. Physiol.* 23: 353, 1967.
9. Seliger, V.: *Int. Z. Physiol. Eischl. Arbeitsphysiol.* 25: 104, 1968.
10. Sills, F.D.: *Science and Medicine of Exercise and Sport*, W.R. Johnson (Ed.) New York, Harper and Bros., 1962.

# Chapter 10

# A Profile of the Canadian National Cross-country Ski Team*

Maurice Jetté
James S. Thoden

Our ultimate aim in the approach we have adopted to the study of selected sports, as previously outlined by my colleague, is in essence twofold: (a) to evaluate the present status and potential of either a seasoned athlete or a budding young aspirant; (b) to assist the coach and athlete in designing a sound training program and in modifying the program, if warranted.

The task is not an easy one, for although we find a great deal of descriptive scientific information pertaining to various sports, there is a dearth of remedial information related to their specific physical, physiological, and psychological variables.

During our relatively brief endeavor of one year, we have directed our attention to the study of three sports, namely, swimming, hockey, and cross-country skiing. In respect to the latter, we have been particularly fortunate in having a good portion of the Canadian national cross-country ski team visit our laboratory. This team included the young group of boys and girls from Inuvik, N.W.T.

The information collected on these skiers has permitted us to draw a characteristic profile of their attributes and it was used in counseling individuals, and in outlining to those concerned particular deficiencies or assets.

The skiers we examined were serious, hard-working, and dedicated to the development of their sport. The training pat-

* The authors wish to express their appreciation to Mrs. Paule Bélanger and Mr. John Spence who assisted them in the data collection.

tern of these athletes is most arduous, and lasts throughout the year. A typical program starts during the summer months, termed the "off-months," and is comprised of easy work, such as hiking, or participation in a variety of sports. At the beginning of July, training becomes "serious," and lasts one to two hours per day, four times a week. It consists of running and "ski striding," an imitation of the actual technique of cross-country skiing. In August, the training is further intensified, with the program designed to enhance endurance, usually by long hiking and jogging sessions. Long-distance running of up to three hours per day dominates the program during September and October. There is much emphasis on "ski striding" using interval patterns. In late November, most of the skiers head West to get an early start at skiing on snow. Training at this stage is most strenuous, with an average time on the trail of six to seven hours per day. The aim is to ski as many kilometers per day as possible.

Interval training dominates their training program during December. The skiers start by sprinting for short distances, and progressively increase the distances. Workouts usually last between three to four hours per day.

Competitions start in early January, with a race every three or four days. At the end of January, the top skiers fly to Europe where they train and compete in preparation for the World Championships which are normally held during the second or third week of February. Three more weeks of competition in the Scandinavian countries usually precede their return to Canada, where a final race is held in Inuvik during early March. As you can see, their program is such that only a determined and dedicated person is able to endure its tempo.

### Methods and Procedures

I would now like to outline a few basic variables which we measured on these skiers last autumn. Table 70-I describes selected anthropometric measurements. The mean ag at the time of testing of the seniors and juniors was twenty-six and seventeen years respectively. The striking feature of their an-

TABLE 10-I
SELECTED ANTHROPOMETRIC MEASUREMENTS
CANADIAN CROSS-COUNTRY SKI TEAM

| Variable | Units | | Seniors x̄ Age 26.2 | Juniors x̄ Age 17 |
|---|---|---|---|---|
| 1. Height | in. | x̄ | 70.2 | 67.6 |
| | | σ | 3.2 | 4.1 |
| 2. Weight | lb. | x̄ | 155 | 127.8 |
| | | σ | 10 | 21 |
| 3. Percent Fat | % | x̄ | 13.2 | 12.8 |
| | | σ | 1.4 | .3 |
| 4. FFBW | lb. | x̄ | 135 | 111.5 |
| | | σ | 8 | 18.9 |
| 5. Hip Width | in. | x̄ | 11.2 | 10.7 |
| | | σ | .5 | 1.0 |
| 6. Chest–Normal | in. | x̄ | 37.5 | 34.7 |
| | | σ | 1.6 | 1.9 |
| 7. Abdominal Girth | in. | x̄ | 30.7 | 27.1 |
| | | σ | 1.2 | 2.2 |
| 8. Thigh Girth | in. | x̄ | 20.9 | 18.9 |
| | | σ | .9 | 2.3 |
| 9. Arm Span | in. | x̄ | 71.8 | 70.7 |
| | | σ | 2.5 | 7.1 |

thropometric measurements is their leanness as reflected by
their height, low percentage of fat, and narrow hips. Notice
also the particularly long arm span of the juniors: a good three
inches longer than their height.

## Results and Discussion

In Table 10-II, we have a few basic measurements related
to circulation. Note the low resting heart rates, both resting
supine and standing, and the rather low postexercise heart
rates (Modified Schneider test–Cureton). The hemoglobin and
hematocrit was quite low in the seniors, which was accompanied in some instances by high levels of total bilirubin. The
blood pressure in the Eskimo and Indian boys was also somewhat low. An interesting incident, in this respect, occurred
when we measured the blood pressures from lying to standing
in the Firth sisters who at fourteen years of age are the fastest
female cross-country skiers in North America. Both nearly
fainted when they stood up from the lying position for their
blood pressure measurement. (Indian children from the Inuvik
area have been reported to suffer from hypotension as a result
of poor nutrition during infancy.)

TABLE 10-II
SELECTED CIRCULATION MEASUREMENTS
CANADIAN CROSS-COUNTRY SKI TEAM

| Variable | Units | | Seniors | Juniors |
|---|---|---|---|---|
| 1. Resting HR | beat/min | x̄ | 50 | 51 |
| | | σ | 15 | 7 |
| 2. Resting SBP | mmHg | x̄ | 117 | 104 |
| | | σ | 10 | 7 |
| 3. Resting DBP₅ | mmHg | x̄ | 77 | 55 |
| | | σ | 9 | 3 |
| 4. Standing HR | beat/min | x̄ | 65 | 85 |
| | | σ | 13 | 5 |
| 5. Standing SBP | mmHg | x̄ | 119 | 104 |
| | | σ | 10 | 10 |
| 6. Standing DBP₅ | mmHg | x̄ | 90 | 83 |
| | | σ | 8 | 3.5 |
| 7. Post-Ex HR | beat/min | x̄ | 91 | 87 |
| | | σ | 39 | 11 |
| 8. Hemoglobin | g/100 ml | x̄ | 14.5 | 15.5 |
| | | σ | 1.1 | 1.0 |
| 9. Hematocrit | ml/100 ml | x̄ | 41.6 | 44.2 |
| | | σ | 3.0 | 3.1 |

The basal metabolic rates are shown in Table 10-III. The BMR of the seniors is somewhat low in relation to the Mayo Foundation Standards.[9] Those of the juniors, however, are even lower when compared to these same standards. This is most interesting since it is hypothesized that a low BMR is associated with superior performance due to a lower P/O ratio in the phospholyration process.[1,5]

TABLE 10-III
BASAL METABOLIC RATE MEASUREMENT
CANADIAN CROSS-COUNTRY SKI TEAM

| Variable | Units | | Seniors | Juniors |
|---|---|---|---|---|
| 1. BMR | cal/hr | x̄ | 77.2 | 57 |
| | | σ | 11.7 | 19 |
| 2. BMR | cal/hr/kg | x̄ | 1.090 | .968 |
| | | σ | .155 | .19 |
| 3. BMR | cal/hr/M² | x̄ | 35.7 | 36.5 |
| | | σ | 15.0 | 7.9 |

Table 10-IV outlines some work capacity measures. Note the higher heart rate and lower ventilation of the juniors as opposed to the seniors. The V̇CO₂ and V̇O₂ are quite high in both groups and are the highest as a group that we have encountered in our laboratory. However, these values are much below the maximum O₂ intakes of the Swedish national cross-country ski team reported by Saltin and Astrand in 1967.[3] Their male

TABLE 10-IV
WORK CAPACITY
CANADIAN CROSS-COUNTRY SKI TEAM

| Variable | Units | | Seniors | Juniors |
|---|---|---|---|---|
| 1. Max HR | beat/min | x̄ | 171 | 190 |
| | | σ | 11 | 8 |
| 2. V̇$_E$ BTPS | liter/min | x̄ | 160 | 139 |
| | | σ | 31 | 20 |
| 3. V̇O$_2$ STPD | liter | x̄ | 4.60 | 3.90 |
| | | σ | .36 | .62 |
| 4. V̇CO$_2$ STPD | liter | x̄ | 4.80 | 4.18 |
| | | σ | 1.0 | .8 |
| 5. V̇O$_2$ | ml/kg | x̄ | 65.5 | 67.2 |
| | | σ | 4.8 | 2.4 |

members had maximum $O_2$ intakes of 83 ml/kg/min while the female members achieved values of 64 ml/kg/min. The young Eskimo and Indian girls that we tested (average age: fifteen yrs) had maximal intakes of 57.3 ml/kg/min. Since the maximal $O_2$ intake is normally not attained until the age of eighteen, we feel that our juniors possess good potential for future international competition.

The personality test employed in our laboratory is the IPAT 16PF. We have chosen this test for a number of reasons: (a) it has been extensively applied to athletes, (b) it is oriented and standardized on normal populations, (c) it has a variety of norms, and (d) it is easy to understand and administer. Table 10-V describes the sixteen personality factors along with a graph depicting where our skiers stand (broken line) in relation to forty-one athletes (solid line) measured by Heusner at the 1952 Olympic Games.[3] It must be stated that we do not expect our skiers to have different personality traits than those of nonathletes. However, specific sports may require particular traits necessary for optimal performance. In this respect, Rushall has described what he terms the professional personality type for an athlete.[7] He feels this type of personality is most desirable for athletic success although it may not be conducive to social interaction. He singled out five factors which appear important for this type: emotionally stable (*factor C*), independent, aggressive and dominant (*factor E*), socially adventurous (*factor H*), realistic (*factor I−*), and confident (*factor O−*). Athletes of this type are said to produce reliable

## TABLE 10-V
## SIXTEEN PERSONALITY FACTOR TEST PROFILE

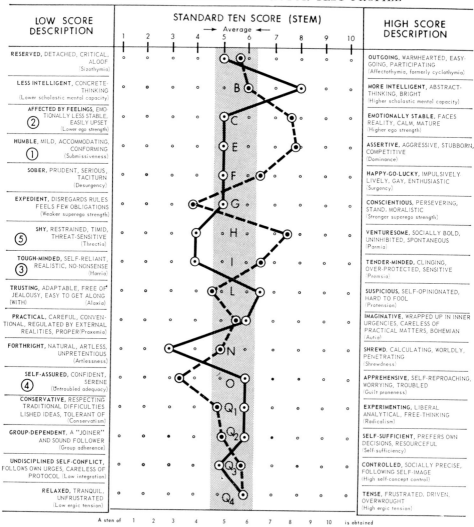

| LOW SCORE DESCRIPTION | STANDARD TEN SCORE (STEM) | HIGH SCORE DESCRIPTION |
|---|---|---|

RESERVED, DETACHED, CRITICAL, ALOOF (Sizothymia) — OUTGOING, WARMHEARTED, EASYGOING, PARTICIPATING (Affectothymia, formerly cyclothymia)

LESS INTELLIGENT, CONCRETE-THINKING (Lower scholastic mental capacity) — B — MORE INTELLIGENT, ABSTRACT-THINKING, BRIGHT (Higher scholastic mental capacity)

② AFFECTED BY FEELINGS, EMOTIONALLY LESS STABLE, EASILY UPSET (Lower ego strength) — C — EMOTIONALLY STABLE, FACES REALITY, CALM, MATURE (Higher ego strength)

① HUMBLE, MILD, ACCOMMODATING, CONFORMING (Submissiveness) — E — ASSERTIVE, AGGRESSIVE, STUBBORN, COMPETITIVE (Dominance)

SOBER, PRUDENT, SERIOUS, TACITURN (Desurgency) — F — HAPPY-GO-LUCKY, IMPULSIVELY LIVELY, GAY, ENTHUSIASTIC (Surgency)

EXPEDIENT, DISREGARDS RULES FEELS FEW OBLIGATIONS (Weaker superego strength) — G — CONSCIENTIOUS, PERSEVERING, STAND, MORALISTIC (Stronger superego strength)

⑤ SHY, RESTRAINED, TIMID, THREAT-SENSITIVE (Threctia) — H — VENTURESOME, SOCIALLY BOLD, UNINHIBITED, SPONTANEOUS (Parmia)

③ TOUGH-MINDED, SELF-RELIANT, REALISTIC, NO-NONSENSE (Harria) — I — TENDER-MINDED, CLINGING, OVER-PROTECTED, SENSITIVE (Premsia)

TRUSTING, ADAPTABLE, FREE OF JEALOUSY, EASY TO GET ALONG (WITH) (Alaxia) — L — SUSPICIOUS, SELF-OPINIONATED, HARD TO FOOL (Protension)

PRACTICAL, CAREFUL, CONVENTIONAL, REGULATED BY EXTERNAL REALITIES, PROPER (Praxemia) — M — IMAGINATIVE, WRAPPED UP IN INNER URGENCIES, CARELESS OF PRACTICAL MATTERS, BOHEMIAN (Autia)

FORTHRIGHT, NATURAL, ARTLESS, UNPRETENTIOUS (Artlessness) — N — SHREWD, CALCULATING, WORLDLY, PENETRATING (Shrewdness)

④ SELF-ASSURED, CONFIDENT, SERENE (Untroubled adequacy) — O — APPREHENSIVE, SELF-REPROACHING, WORRYING, TROUBLED (Guilt proneness)

CONSERVATIVE, RESPECTING TRADITIONAL DIFFICULTIES LISHED IDEAS, TOLERANT OF (Conservatism) — Q₁ — EXPERIMENTING, LIBERAL ANALYTICAL, FREE-THINKING (Radicalism)

GROUP-DEPENDENT, A "JOINER" AND SOUND FOLLOWER (Group adherence) — Q₂ — SELF-SUFFICIENT, PREFERS OWN DECISIONS, RESOURCEFUL (Self-sufficiency)

UNDISCIPLINED SELF-CONFLICT, FOLLOWS OWN URGES, CARELESS OF PROTOCOL (Low integration) — Q₃ — CONTROLLED, SOCIALLY PRECISE, FOLLOWING SELF-IMAGE (High self-concept control)

RELAXED, TRANQUIL, UNFRUSTRATED (Low ergic tension) — Q₄ — TENSE, FRUSTRATED, DRIVEN, OVERWROUGHT (High ergic tension)

A sten of 1 2 3 4 5 6 7 8 9 10 is obtained

by about 2.3% 4.4% 9.2% 15.0% 19.1% 19.1% 15.0% 9.2% 4.4% 2.3% of adults consistent performances, irrespective of competitive conditions. Our limited number of subjects precludes any statements related to the specific personality traits of our cross-country skiers.

A question we always ask ourselves when compiling an extensive battery of tests is which of all the tests administered reflects best the performance of the athletes in that particular sport.

Although our data and number of subjects is limited, we did compute a multiple step-wise prediction analysis to determine those variables that best predict performance. To our surprise, we found that (Table 10-VI) with two variables, 16PF Factor I+ and $\dot{V}CO_2$, we accounted for 92 percent of the total variance.

TABLE 10-VI
PERCENT RELATIVE CONTRIBUTION OF
BEST TWO PREDICTOR VARIABLES
CANADIAN CROSS-COUNTRY SKI TEAM

| Variable | B | B² | Percent Contribution | Correlation with Predictor |
|----------|-----|-----|-----|-----|
| 1. 16 PF-Factor I | −0.777 | .604 | 79 | −0.88 |
| 2. $\dot{V}CO_2$ STPD | 0.400 | .160 | 21 | 0.60 |
| Sum | | .764 | 100 | |
| $R^2$ = 92% | | | | |

This was really not as unusual as we had originally believed when we realized that the variance in the predictor (time for the 15 km race) was, except for one case, but a few seconds. Factor I+, in the analysis, accounted for 79 percent of the total variance measured, while the $\dot{V}CO_2$ accounted for the remaining 21 percent. As I mentioned earlier, the available data is too meager to prove very meaningful at this stage. However, it does emphasize our attention to these two variables.

We have confined ourselves, during this short presentation, to a limited amount of information. Other variables measured in our battery of tests include strength, flexibility, reaction time, spirometry measures, energy cost and preejection intervals of the left ventricle, a variable which we have recently initiated. We must now further evaluate this information in relation to the level of the competitor and his performance. We must gather further information to determine if a pattern can be revealed in relation to performance and laboratory data for a specific sport. More important, however, we are striving to apply this data to the benefit of the athlete by determining his potential and deficiencies, in order to assist him in designing, modifying, and evaluating his training program.

## References

1. Allik, T.A. *et al.*: *Medical Research on Swimming*, S. Firnov and E. Jokl, Eds. Moscow, Federation International Natation Amateur, 1968.

2. Cattel, R.B., and Eber, H.W.: *Sixteen Personality Factor Questionnaire*, Champaign, Illinois, IPAT, 1957.

3. Heusner, W.V.: Personality Traits of Champion and Former Champion Athletes. Unpublished M.S. Thesis, Physical Education, University of Illinois, Urbana, 1952.

4. Kane, J.E.: *International Research in Sport and Physical Education*, E. Jokl and E. Simon, eds. Springfield, C.C Thomas, 1964.

5. Jetté, M.: *Mouvement*. 5: 89, 1970.

6. Ogilvie, B.: *J.A.M.A.* 205: 780, 1968.

7. Rushall, B.S. An Interim Report on the Personality of Athletes as Revealed by the 16 PF Tests. Unpublished research, Indiana University, May, 1967.

8. Saltin, B., and Astrand, P.O.: *J Appl Physiol.* 23: 353, 1967.

9. Selkurt, E.E. (Ed.): *Physiology*, 2nd ed. Boston, Little, Brown and Company, 1966.

# Chapter 11

# Exercise and the Myocardial Fiber Capillary Ratio

R.D. Bell

R.L. Rasmussen

## Abstract

Ninety male albino (Wistar) rats, sixty of which were pre-pubescent animals four weeks of age and thirty of which were postpubescent animals fourteen weeks of age, were randomly divided into exercise and control groups as follows:

1. *Prepubescent Exercise Group*—This group of animals was exercised for six weeks before the onset of puberty.
2. *Prepubescent Control Group*
3. *Prepost Pubescent Exercise Group*—This group of animals was exercised for eleven weeks before, during, and after puberty.
4. *Prepost Pubescent Control Group*
5. *Postpubescent Exercise Group*—This group of animals was exercised for six weeks after puberty.
6. *Postpubescent Control Group*

All control groups remained in a sedentary state for the duration of the experiment.

The experimental treatment consisted of swimming the animals with 4 percent body weight attached to the tip of the tail. All experimental groups were exercised for thirty minutes daily, five days per week. Following the six or eleven week training program the animals were individually sacrificed by an overdose of ether. The abdominal and thoracic cavities were opened via a midline incision and the beating heart isolated. The inferior vena cava was clamped to reduce venous return and the aorta was cannulated. Following aortic cannulation the heart was injected with a mix-ture of Locke's Solution, carbochrome ink, and heparin. Next the heart was removed and fixed in a 10 percent formalin solution for forty-eight hours. A small midventricular section was obtained by transverse ablations of the ventricles. Paraffin tissue sections approximately 15 u thick were cut on a microtome and stained with a standard hematoxylin-eosin stain. The myocardial fiber-capillary ratio was calculated for each animal and mean F-C ratios were computed for each group.

A program of moderate intensity exercise significantly increased the myocardial capillary concentration in both the prepubescent exercise and the prepostpubescent exercise group, but not in the postpubescent exercise group. Thus it appears that exercise can significantly increase the capillarization of the heart but only during specific stages of development.

During the past decade much attention has been focused on coronary heart disease and its role as North America's leading cause of death. The premature loss of productive citizens has great personal and economic significance and has stirred research interests into investigating feasible methods of modifying the course of coronary heart disease. It is now well recognized that coronary heart disease is a multifactorial disease and that lack of regular, vigorous physical activity is one of the factors contributing to the increasing incidence of coronary heart disease. Several epidemiological studies[3,7,8,9,13] have indicated that physically active individuals have a lower incidence of coronary heart disease and a lower mortality rate following myocardial infarction than do sedentary individuals. The current increase of interest in jogging and physical fitness in general, has seemed to promote a renewed scientific interest in the effects of exercise on various cardiovascular parameters. However, studies concerned with the effects of exercise on the myocardial fiber-capillary ratio (F-C ratio) have been relatively few and diverse. The present study was designed to determine the effects of a moderate exercise program on the F-C ratio in prepubescent, postpubescent, and prepostpubescent male albino rats. It was hoped that this study would provide further evidence about the potential protective function of physical exercise in the etiology of coronary heart disease.

Wearn[17] was probably the first researcher to successfully inject and count the number of capillaries in both human and animal hearts. Petren *et al.*[10] also studied the effects of physical training on the capillarization of cardiac muscle. They concluded that intensive physical training led to the formation of new capillaries causing an increased myocardial capillary density. Petren's experiment was repeated by Hakkila[4] but he was not able to verify Petren's results. Roberts and Wearn[13] studied the quantitative changes in the F-C ratio in human myocardial tissue during various stages of growth and hypertrophy. They calculated the F-C ratio at birth to be approximately 6:1. This ratio changed during the growth process until at maturity it was approximately 1:1 where it remained throughout adult life. This was in agreement with values reported by Ankelakos *et al.*[1]

In 1966, Poupa and Rakusan[11] studied the myocardial capillary bed in both "athletic" (wild Norwegian Rats) and "non-athletic" (white domesticated) animals. They concluded that the myocardial capillary density in the athletic animals was greater than the myocardial capillary density in the nonathletic animals. They attributed the difference to the fact that the wild infant animals of athletic parents were exposed to a greater activity load when accompanying their parents. In the prepubescent stage of life a load was placed on the heart when it could still react by numerical growth. In an earlier study Rakusan and Poupa[12] found a decreased muscle fiber atrophy. Leon and Bloor[6] also concluded that daily exercise significantly increased the myocardial F-C ratio in the experimental animals. Following the cessation of exercise the myocardial F-C ratio remained significantly greater in all exercised animals for at least forty-two days postexercise. In agreement with Tepperman and Pearlman[16] Stevenson *et al.*[14] found that in the rat forced physical exercise caused an increase in apparent coronary tree size provided the exercise was not too strenuous or frequent.

## Methods and Materials

Ninety male albino rats (Wistar), sixty of which were prepubescent animals four weeks of age and thirty of which were postpubescent animals fourteen weeks of age, were randomly divided into exercise and control groups as follows:

1. Prepubescent Exercise Group. This group of animals was exercised for six weeks before the onset of puberty.

2. Prepubescent Control Group. This group remained in a relatively sedentary state for six weeks.
3. Prepost Pubescent Exercise Group. This group of animals was exercised for a total of eleven weeks before, during, and after puberty.
4. Prepost Pubescent Control Group. This group of animals remained in a relatively sedentary state for the eleven weeks.
5. Postpubescent Exercise Group. This group of animals was exercised for six weeks after puberty had been completed.
6. Postpubescent Control Group. This group of animals remained in a relatively sedentary state for six weeks.

All exercise groups were subjected to a moderate physical exercise program which consisted of a thirty minute swim daily, five days a week for either six or eleven weeks duration. Water temperature was maintained at approximately 30° C. A weight equal to 4 percent body weight was attached to the tip of the tail of each animal during each exercise period. All animals received a standard laboratory chow and water ad libitum throughout the duration of the experiment.

Following the respective training programs all animals were individually anaesthetized with an overdose of ether. After anaesthesia the animal was fastened to a dissection board and the abdominal and chest cavities were opened via a midline incision.

The inferior vena cava was clamped with a hemostat to reduce venous return to the heart. The abdominal aorta was then exposed, isolated, and cannulated with an 18 gauge needle against the normal flow of blood. The needle was attached to a 3 mm diameter polyethylene tubing which was connected to the perfusing apparatus. When the aorta was successfully cannulated the heart was perfused at a pressure of approximately 65 mm Hg for several moments until it was uniformly dark on the surface or judged to be as completely perfused as possible. The perfusate was a solution of 2.0 percent carbochrome ink, 0.2 percent heparin, and 97.8 percent Locke's Solution. The perfusate was maintained at a temperature of 30° C. When the perfusion process was complete a few drops of carbachol (Merck and Co. Inc. Rahway, New Jersey) were topically administered to stop the heart in full diastole. The heart was then tied off around the base, removed from the animal, and fixed in a 10% formalin solution for twenty-four hours. Next a midventricular section approximately 1 cm thick was obtained by a transverse ablation of the ventricles and embedded in paraffin. A minimum of two tissue sections, each approximately 15 u thick, were cut on a Leitz microtome. All tissue sections were stained simultaneously with a standard hematoxylin and eosin stain (Fig. 11–1).

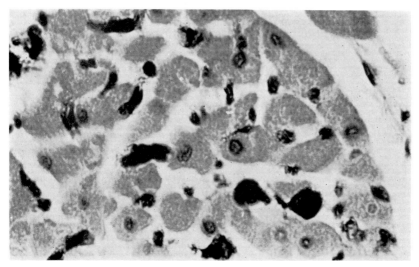

Figure 11–1. Cross section of the rat endocardium showing myocardial muscle fibers and capillaries.

## Results

Myocardial F-C ratios were determined for ten animals of each exercise and control group in accordance with the procedures described by Wearn.[17] A mean F-C ratio was then calculated for each of the six experimental groups (Table 11-I).

The mean F-C ratio for the prepubescent exercise group was 0.894 while the mean F-C ratio for the prepubescent control group was 0.620. Calculations for the postpubescent exercise and control groups yielded mean F-C ratios of 1.044 and .960 respectively. Similarly, F-C ratios for the prepost pubescent group were 1.296 and 1.089 for the exercise and control groups respectively.

TABLE 11-I

MEAN MYOCARDIAL F-C RATIOS FOR EXERCISED AND
NONEXERCISED MALE ALBINO RATS OF VARYING AGES

| | Prepubescent | Pre-postpubescent | Postpubescent |
|---|---|---|---|
| Exercise | .894 | 1.296 | 1.044 |
| Control | .620 | 1.089 | .960 |

A three by two Analysis of Variance (Table 11-II) revealed significant differences in the F-C ratio for the various ages of the animals as well as for exercised groups versus the sedentary control groups. A new Multiple Range Test was then employed in order to determine specifically what these significant differences were.

The capillary concentration of the prepubescent control group (0.620) was significantly lower than the other five experimental groups. However the prepubescent exercise group had

TABLE 11-II

THREE BY TWO ANALYSIS OF VARIANCE OF THE MEAN MYOCARDIAL
F-C RATIO FOR EXERCISED AND NONEXERCISED MALE ALBINO RATS
OF VARYING AGES

| Source | DF | SS | MSS | F |
|---|---|---|---|---|
| Age | 2 | 1.903 | .952 | $F_2, 54 = 56.00^*$ |
| Exercise | 1 | .532 | .532 | $F_1, 54 = 31.29^*$ |
| Interaction | 2 | .078 | .039 | $F_2, 54 = 2.294$ |
| Error | 54 | .927 | .017 | |
| Total | 59 | 3.440 | | |

\* Significant at .05 level of significance.

a slightly higher capillary concentration (0.894) which was significantly different from only both the exercise and control groups of the prepost pubescent treatment. The postpubescent exercise and control groups were significantly different only from the prepost exercise group. Lastly, the prepost pubescent control group had a significantly lower concentration (1.089) when compared to the prepost pubescent exercise group (1.296) (Table 11-II).

## Discussion

The increased capillary concentration of all five treatment groups, when compared to the prepubescent control group may, in part, be attributed to the aging process. During the developing years of life the internal structure of the heart is in a state of constant change.[13] The myocardial fiber-capillary ratio reflects this changing status as it develops from an approximate 6:1 ratio if the stress of exercise is not an added factor. Our values for the prepost pubescent control group and the postpubescent control groups are in agreement with this 1:1 ratio. However, the stress of exercise can have a marked effect on this F-C ratio, especially if the increased activity load is placed on the heart during the formative years. This, of course, would be during the prepubescent and pubescent stages of development.

Under the conditions of this particular exercise program the fiber capillary ratio of the heart was significantly altered. Both the prepubescent exercise group and the prepost pubescent exercise group developed a significantly higher myocardial capillary concentration than did their respective control groups. This was not the case when the postpubescent exercise group was compared to the postpubescent control group. This finding was in agreement with the work of Poupa and Rakusan.[11] However, no attempt was made to vary either the intensity or the frequency of exercise. Stevenson *et al.*[14] suggested that moderate exercise with adequate rest resulted in more of an increase in coronary tree size than did heavy frequent exercise. Observation of the animals during the exercise periods suggested that the exercise program was, in fact, a moderate one as most of the animals completed the one-half hour swim with ease. Research in this area has been generally in agreement with the role of exercise in increasing the myocardial capillary concentration, but the specific frequencies and intensities of exercise which best accomplishes this task remains unknown.

Furthermore, the exact stimulus for an increased capillary concentration as a result of exercise remains unknown, and further research is necessary to establish this factor as an actual scientific phenomenon.

It would appear that exercise of a moderate intensity is

capable of increasing the myocardial capillary concentration, especially if the exercise program is administered before and/or during puberty. It also appears that moderate exercise has a limited value during the postpubescent period of life as far as increasing the coronary capillary concentration is concerned. Exercise, then, should be considered as a significant preventative in the etiology of coronary heart disease. Properly administered at the appropriate time of life, regular exercise should significantly lower the incidence and severity of coronary heart disease.

## References

1. Ankelakos, E.T., Bernandini, P., Barrett Jr., W.C.: *Anat Rec.* 149:671, 1964.
2. Edwards, A.L.: *Experimental Design in Psychological Research*, 7th ed. New York, Rhinehart, 1950.
3. Frank, C.W., Weinblatt, E., Shapiro, S., and Sager, R.V.: *Circulation.* 34:1022, 1966.
4. Hakkila, J.: *Ann. Med. Exp. Biol. Fenn. Helsinki.* 33, Suppl. 10. 1955.
5. Johnson, T.: *Fed. Proc.* 18:77, 1959.
6. Leon, A.S., and Bloor, C.M.: *J Appl Physiol.* 24:485, 1968.
7. Morris, J.N., Heady, J., and Raffle, P.A.B.: *Lancet.* 2:569, 1956.
8. Morris, J.N., Heady, J., Raffle, P.A.B., Roberts, C.G., and Parks, J.W.: *Lancet.* 2:1053, 1953.
9. Morris, J.N., and Crawford, M.D.: *Brit. Med. J.* 2:1485, 1958.
10. Petren, T., Sjostrand, T. and Sylven, B.: *Arbeitsphysiologie.* 9:376, 1936.
11. Poupa, O., Rakusan, K.: *In Physical Activity in Health and Disease.* Baltimore, Williams and Wilkins, 1966, pg. 18.
12. Rakusan, K., and Poupa, O.: *Gerontologia.* 9:107, 1964.
13. Roberts, J.T., and Wearn, J.T.: *Amer. Heart J.* 21:617, 1941.
14. Stevenson, J.A.F., Feleki, V., Rechnitzer, P., Beaton, J.R.: *Circ. Res.* 15:265, 1964.
15. Taylor, H.L.: *J. Sports Med.* 2:73, 1962.
16. Tepperman, J., and Pearlman, D.: *Circ. Res.* 9:576, 1961.
17. Wearn, J.T.: *J. Exp. Med.* 47:273, 1928.
18. Winick, Myron: *Nutrition in Preschool and School Age*, edited for the Swedish Nutrition Foundation by Gunnary Blix, 1969.

# Chapter 12

# The Influence of Training Upon the Distribution of Cardiac Output

R. SIMMONS
ROY J. SHEPHARD

## Abstract

Ten sedentary men performed arm ergometer exercise at 80 percent of aerobic power for thirty minutes biweekly. At the end of one month, the directly measured maximum oxygen intake had increased by 8 percent, and there was also some decrease of postural work, with an improved mechanical efficiency. The maximum cardiac output, as measured by an acetylene rebreathing method, increased from 17.8 to 19.3 1/min. This increase was due entirely to an augmentation of stroke volume, and in submaximum exercise there was a decrease of both heart rate and arteriovenous oxygen difference. Peripheral blood flow was measured by twin mercury in rubber strain gauges. With training, the total flow to the forearm increased. There was a large increase in the flow to muscle, and a smaller decrease of skin flow. The latter probably reflects development of alternative methods of heat dissipation. Practical application of these findings to sports medicine and athletic training is briefly discussed.

When the athlete makes the final spurt of maximum effort, the skin blood flow is dramatically reduced. The flushed face becomes ashen grey in color, and there is obviously intense cutaneous vasoconstriction. But in the preceding minutes of an endurance effort, the skin is hot and receives a substantial fraction of the total cardiac output. We may estimate the distribution of blood flow from the respective weights of muscle, skin, and viscera, the total arteriovenous difference, and the expected arteriovenous difference of the three tissue types.[1] The results of such a calculation are shown in Fig. 12–1. In this example,

| MUSCLE | 28 | 4550 | 87 | 24.5 | 186 |
| SKIN | 10 | 12 | 60 | 6.0 | 2 |
| OTHER | 32 | 138 | 4.7 | 1.5 | 92 |
| | | | | | |
| OVERALL | 70 | 4700 | 45.7 | 32 | 147 |

Figure 12–1. The estimated volume (l.), oxygen consumption (ml/min STPD) unit blood flow (ml/100 ml/min), total blood flow (l./min) and arteriovenous oxygen difference (ml/l.) in three tissue compartments during maximum exercise.

the skin receives about 25 percent of the total cardiac output. The purpose of the large skin flow is to dissipate body heat through radiation and convection. If alternative methods of heat dissipation are developed with training, then the athlete should be able to reduce his skin blood flow, and thus to improve his performance by directing a larger blood flow to the active muscles.

## Methods and Materials

We have recently tested this hypothesis in a group of ten sedentary young men who undertook a one month conditioning program involving thirty minutes of arm ergometer exercise at 80 percent of aerobic power, twice per week. Cardiac outputs were measured by an acetylene method that involved seven seconds rebreathing of a 1 percent acetylene mixture.[2,3] Skin and muscle flows were measured at the immediate end of the exercise periods, using twin strain gauges around the upper and lower parts of the forearm.[4]

## Results

The directly measured maximum oxygen intake[5] increased by an average of 8% over the course of the training program (Fig. 12–2). This is as good if not better than would be expected with a month of leg exercise of comparable intensity,[6] suggesting that arm exercise of this type may have a useful

$\dot{V}O_2$(max) l/min. STPD

| INITIAL | FINAL | |
| 2.76 | 2.99 | +0.223 |
| | | ±0.100 |

t8 = 7.07
P < 0.001

Figure 12–2. The change in aerobic power produced by repeated exercise on an arm ergometer.

place in the maintenance and restoration of cardiorespiratory fitness in patients with injuries to the lower half of the body. The oxygen consumption during rest and submaximum exercise decreased with training (Fig. 12–3). The change in the "resting" readings probably reflects a reduction of postural tension while sitting on the bicycle ergometer. There was also a small but statistically significant increase in mechanical efficiency, as can

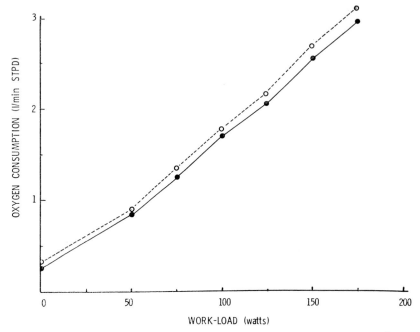

Figure 12–3. The influence of repeated exercise on the efficiency of arm ergometer work. Broken line: before training, Solid line: after training.

be seen from the progressive divergence of the pre- and post-training lines.

The slope of the cardiac output/oxygen consumption line was similar before and after training (Fig. 12–4), but the relationship was displaced significantly to the left by conditioning. The resting cardiac output showed a small decrease of 4.7 percent

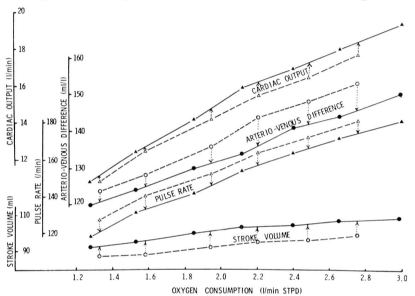

Figure 12–4. The influence of training upon responses to arm ergometer work—data for cardiac output, arterio-venous difference, stroke volume and pulse rate. Broken lines: before training, Solid lines: after training.

over the course of the program, but the maximum cardiac output increased, from 17.8 to 19.3 l/min. This increase was due entirely to an increase of stroke volume, there being no change in the maximum heart rate. On the other hand, because of the greater stroke volume, the pulse rate/oxygen consumption line for submaximum exercise was displaced to the right (Fig. 12–4). There was also a significant decrease of arteriovenous oxygen difference at rest and during submaximum exercise (Fig. 12–4).

Training was associated with a small, but statistically significant increase of forearm volume, from 1147 to 1157 ml. This presumably reflects the small degree of muscle hypertrophy over the course of this program.

The initial forearm flow was 5.6 ml/min per 100 ml of tissue at rest, and increased to 32.6 ml/min per 100 ml immediately following maximum exercise (Fig. 12–5). After training, all except the resting readings were greater. Partition of the blood

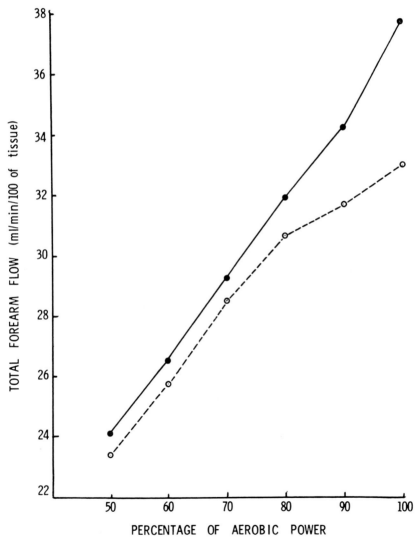

Figure 12–5. Total forearm flow immediately following exercise at specified percentages of aerobic power. Broken lines: before training, Solid lines: after training.

flow into muscle and skin component (Fig. 12–6) showed that muscle flow increased by 25 percent at 50 percent to 80 percent of aerobic power, and by as much as 56 percent at 90 percent to 100 percent of aerobic power. On the other hand, the skin flows decreased, by 35 percent at 50 percent to 80 percent of aerobic power, and by 25 percent at 90 percent to 100 percent of aerobic power.

## Discussion

We may thus conclude that training improves the blood flow to the forearm muscle, and that this improvement is achieved partly through an increase in maximum cardiac output and partly through a reduction of skin blood flow. Since our data are based not on exercise, but on the immediate recovery period, they probably represent a minimum estimate of the redistribution of blood flow away from the skin. Presumably, the body acquires an ability to dissipate heat through earlier and more vigorous sweating, and this may explain the partial interaction between heat acclimatization and cardio-respiratory training. It also emphasizes the danger of "doping" an athlete with amphetamines; drugs of this class cause a similar diversion of blood flow away from the skin, but the body lacks development of sweat secretion, and the athlete is subjected to a potentially dangerous heat load.

It is somewhat surprising that training was associated with an increase of cardiac output during submaximum exercise. We feel the explanation lies in a peripheral limitation of effort during arm work. The maximum cardiac output is no more than 70 percent of what the same subject could achieve during leg exercise.[5] A substantial volume of blood was pooled in the leg veins during this experiment, and it may be that training decreased such orthostatic pooling, thereby allowing our subjects to develop a larger stroke volume. A second possible factor is that there was difficulty in perfusing muscles that were contracting at a large percentage of their maximum voluntary force.[7] Training leads to an increase of maximum voluntary force through both hypertrophy of the muscles and distribution of a given task among a larger number of motor units. It could

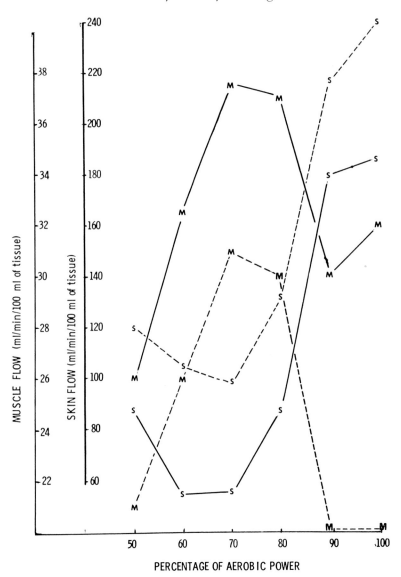

Figure 12–6. Skin and muscle blood flow to forearm immediately following exercise at specified percentages of aerobic power. Broken lines: before training, Solid lines: after training.

thus ease the perfusion of actively contracting fibers, permitting the development of a greater cardiac output at a given work load.

From the practical point of view, those who have a responsibility to improve the fitness of physically lazy and yet overbusy Canadians may draw some comfort from the fact that a useful gain of cardiorespiratory fitness can be achieved by as little as two exercise sessions per week, providing that the individuals concerned are initially in poor condition and they are exercised at high percentage of their aerobic power.

## References

1. Shephard, R.J. *J. A. M. A.* 205: 150, 1968.
2. Simmons, R. *Some Effects of Training Upon Cardiac Output and Its Distribution.* M.Sc. Thesis, University of Toronto, Toronto, Ont., 1970.
3. Simmons, R., and Shephard, R.J. *Int. Z. Angew. Physiol.* In Press, 1971.
4. Whitney, R.J. *J. Physiol.* 121: 1, 1953.
5. Shephard, R.J., Allen, C., Benade, A.J.S., Davies, C.T.M., diPrampero, P.E., Hedman, R., Merriman, J.E., Myhre, K., and Simmons, R. *Bull. W.H.O.* 38: 757, 1968.
6. Shephard, R.J. *Endurance Fitness.* University of Toronto Press, 1969.
7. Kay, C., and Shephard, R.J. *Int. Z. Angew. Physiol.* 27: 311, 1969.

# Chapter 13

# The Effect of Swimming Training on Selected Aspects of the Pulmonary Function of Young Girls—A Preliminary Report

J. A. Gibbins
D.A. Cunningham
D.B. Shaw
R.B. Eynon

Experimental evidence concerning the effect of physical training on pulmonary diffusing capacity for carbon monoxide (DLCO) is inconclusive. Several studies[3,4,6,7,8,10] have shown that athletes possess higher values for DLCO than non-athletes. Mostyn et al.[9] discovered that olympic swimmers had higher DLCO's than other athletic and nonathletic groups. However, Anderson and Shephard[1] and Reuschlein et al.[11] showed that physical training did not affect DLCO. On the other hand, Rosenberg[12] and Newman et al.[10] (who trained only one subject) found that training substantially increased DLCO. It appears therefore, that some disagreement exists as to whether the superior values of DLCO in athletes, particularly in swimmers, are due to training or were inherited. The purpose of the present investigation was to study the effect of six months of swimming training on the DLCO's of six girl swimmers (9–10 years) compared with six age-matched controls (non-swimmers). In addition, total lung capacity (TLC), vital capacity (VC), functional residual capacity (FRC), forced expiratory volume in the first second ($FEV_{1.0}$) and the physical work capacity at a heart rate of 150 beats per minute were measured before and after training.

*Note:* This study was supported in part by a grant from the Fitness and Amateur Sport Directorate, Ottawa and in part by a grant from the Faculty of Social Science, The University of Western Ontario.

## Methods and Materials

### *Pulmonary Diffusing Capacity*

DLCO was calculated, before and after training, at three submaximal work loads on the bicycle ergometer (100, 200, and 300 Kpm/min) using a steady-state technique similar to the method of Donevan *et al.*[5] A value for the dead space (VD) was predicted from knowledge of the subject's height (Ht) and tidal volume (VT) according to the following regression line determined by Andrew[2]: $VD = -21.8 + .77$ $(ht - cm) + .110 (VT - ml)$, SE $= \pm 71.0$. The pulmonary midcapillary partial pressure of carbon monoxide ($\overline{PC}_{CO}$) was determined by a CO — rebreathing technique. Pulse rate and $FE_{O_2}$ were monitored during each test. All subjects rode for six minutes at each of the three work loads. After three minutes of riding the subject was considered to be in a steady-state and, at this point, the subject began inhaling .1310% CO in air. During the fourth minute of exercise the inspired minute ventilation and mixed expired $O_2$ and CO were measured. The respiratory rate was counted automatically. Each subject was allowed to rest ten minutes between rides.

### *Lung Volumes and Capacities*

VC and $FEV_{1.0}$ were measured with a 9-litre Collins spirometer. FRC was determined by a closed circuit helium dilution technique.

### *Physical Work Capacity*

$PWC_{150}$ was calculated by extrapolation or interpolation, of the line joining the heart rates for the second and third work loads, to a heart rate of 150 beats/min.

## Results

### *Cardio-respiratory Fitness*

The heart rate response to exercise for the subjects is graphically illustrated in Figure 13–1. Both before and after the

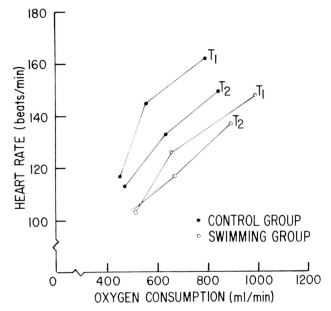

Figure 13–1. Heart rate vs. oxygen consumption: training effects.

training period, the mean heart rates of the swimmers and the controls increased with increasing work load at approximately the same rate. However, the mean heart rates of the swimmers were at a much lower level than the controls for all of the work loads. Although the percent increase in $PWC_{150}$ during the six month training period was the same for both groups, the swimmers began in better condition and maintained their superiority after training.

### Pulmonary Diffusing Capacity

The means and standard deviations for the DLCOs of the control group and the swimming group at the three work loads before and after training are presented in Table 13-I. The values of "t" for the group comparisons of DLCO before and after training are presented in Table 13-II. None of the values of "t" were found to be significant. In addition to this, none of the "F" ratios derived from the variance analysis were found to be significant.

TABLE 13-I

GROUP MEANS ($\overline{X}$) AND STANDARD DEVIATIONS (S) FOR DIFFUSING
CAPACITY (ml/min per mmHg) BEFORE (T1) AND AFTER (T2) TRAINING

| Work Load | Swimmers ($n = 6$) | | | | Controls ($n = 6$) | | | |
| | T1 | | T2 | | T1 | | T2 | |
| (Kpm/min) | $\overline{X}$ | S | $\overline{X}$ | S | $\overline{X}$ | S | $\overline{X}$ | S |
|---|---|---|---|---|---|---|---|---|
| 100 | 18.7 | 4.4 | 20.3 | 5.1 | 19.6 | 2.4 | 21.3 | 7.9 |
| 200 | 19.7 | 6.1 | 25.5 | 7.6 | 19.9 | 4.5 | 21.8 | 4.7 |
| 300 | 23.3 | 4.8 | 24.5 | 7.4 | 21.3 | 4.5 | 22.2 | 4.5 |

TABLE 13-II

VALUES OF "t" FOR GROUP COMPARISONS OF DIFFUSING CAPACITY
AT EACH OF THE THREE WORK LOADS BEFORE (T1) AND AFTER
(T2) TRAINING

| | Work Load (Kpm/min) | | |
| | *100* | *200* | *300* |
|---|---|---|---|
| T1 | .44 | .06 | .75 |
| T2 | .26 | 1.01 | .65 |

*Note:* A t value of 2.571 is necessary for significance

## Lung Volumes and Capacities

None of the measured lung volumes or capacities were affected by training.

## Discussion

The results of this study tended to agree with those of Anderson and Shephard[1] and Reuschlein *et al.*[11] who found that DLCO was not affected by physical training. According to the statistical analysis, a significant difference between the control group and the swimmers, with respect to DLCO, was not shown before or after training. In addition to this, the analysis of variance did not not demonstrate any significance between group changes as a result of training. The large difference between the means at the second work load may be due to an increased scatter of the DLCO values found for the swimmers.

Before training, the mean DLCO's of both groups, for the second work load, are very nearly the same. However, after training there is a divergence of the swimmers' mean DLCO away from the mean DLCO of the control group and toward a value which would be significantly higher than that of the controls. This trend is also reflected in the "t" scores at the second work load before and after training (Table 13-II). The fact that there was no difference between the swimming group and the control group before training with respect to DLCO, coupled with an apparent trend of divergence demonstrated at the second and third work loads after training may indicate that with further training large and significant differences as observed by other investigators[8,9] would be found.

## References

1. Anderson, T.W., and Shephard, R.J.: *Int. Z Angew. Physiol.* 25: 198, 1968.
2. Andrew, G.M.: Unpublished material.
3. Bannister, R.G., Cotes, J.E., Jones, R.S., and Meade, F.: *J. Physiol.* 152: 66P, 1960.
4. Bates, D.V., Boucot, N.G., and Dormer, A.E.: *J. Physiol.* 129: 237, 1955.
5. Donevan, R.E., Palmer, W.H., Varvis, C.J., and Bates, D.V.: *J. Appl. Physiol.* 14: 483, 1959.
6. Heinonen, A.O., Karvonen, M.J., and Ruosteenota, R.: *J. Physiol.* 142: 54P, 1958.
7. Holmgren, A.: *Acta Physiol. Scand.* 65: 207, 1965.
8. Magel, J.R., and Andersen, K.L.: *Med. Sci. Sports* 1 (3): 131, 1969.
9. Mostyn, E.M., Helle, S., Gee, J.B.L., Bentivoglio, L.G., and Bates, D.V.: *J. Physiol.* 18: 687, 1963.
10. Newman, F., Smalley, B.F., and Thomson, M.L.: *J. Appl. Physiol.* 17: 649, 1962.
11. Reuschlein, P.S., Reddan, W.G., Burpee, J., Gee, J.B.L., and Rankin, J.: *J. Appl. Physiol.* 24: 152, 1968.
12. Rosenberg, E.: *Int. Z. Angew. Physiol.* 24: 246, 1967.

# Chapter 14

# The Effect of Frequency of Exercise Upon Physical Work Performance and Selected Variables Representative of Cardiorespiratory Fitness

K.H. Sidney
R.B. Eynon
D.A. Cunningham

A weakness common to nearly all frequency studies[1,2,3,4,5,6] is their failure to eliminate differences in the total quantity of work performed by the various exercise groups during training. For example, persons assigned to a group which trained four times weekly would perform approximately twice as much work per week as those persons who trained only twice weekly.

The purpose of the present study was to determine the effects of training four times, two times and once per week upon measures of physical work and cardiorespiratory fitness, both after four weeks of training, and after a period of training during which all exercise groups completed equal amounts of work on the bicycle ergometer.

## Methods and Procedures

Twenty-four male university students volunteered for this investigation. Three exercise groups and one control group, each consisting of six subjects, were equated on max. $\dot{V}_{O_2}$ Group 1X exercised one day per week, Group 2X exercised two

*Note:* This study was supported in part by a grant from Faculty of Social Science, University of Western Ontario and in part by a grant from Fitness and Amateur Sport Directorate, Ottawa.

days per week, and Group 4X exercised four days per week. The members of Group 4X trained for a total period of four weeks, but the members of Groups 2X and 1X continued to train until they completed the same total amount of work in kpm as did the members of Group 4X.

All subjects were tested before and after four weeks of training. The members of Groups 2X and 1X (and the control group) were further tested at the completion of their respective training programs. Heart rates, $\dot{V}_{O_2}$ and performance time were determined from a step-increment type of maximal work capacity test administered on a Monark bicycle ergometer.

Training sessions consisted of fifteen minutes of bicycle ergometer pedaling preceded by a standard five minute warm-up. The initial ergometer load setting was that work level which had elicited a heart rate of 150 beats/min on the pretest work capacity test. Subjects were instructed to complete as many revolutions as possible during the session at the specified work load. Whenever a subject completed nine hundred revolutions during a training session, the load was increased by 1 kp for the following session. Work performed during the fifteen minutes of training was calculated in Kpm.

## Results After Four Weeks of Training

*Total Work Performed.* After four weeks of training the accumulative total amount of work performed by each of the three exercise groups was nearly directly proportional to frequency.

*Work Performed in Fifteen Minutes.* The percentage increases in work performed in fifteen minutes of training were 54 percent, 27 percent and 13 percent for Groups 4X, 2X and 1X respectively. These increases were nearly directly proportional to exercise frequency.

*Performance Time to Exhaustion.* The changes in the length of the bicycle ergometer ride to exhaustion were 44 percent, 26 percent and 12 percent for Groups 4X, 2X and 1X respectively. These increases were also nearly directly proportional to exercise frequency.

*Cardiorespiratory Variables.* When $O_2$ uptake values were expressed in ml/kg x min, the 10 percent increases in max. $\dot{V}_{O_2}$ were significant for the three exercise groups. All experimental groups showed parallel 9 percent decreases in exercise heart rate which were nonsignificant. On $PWC_{170}$ Groups 4X and 2X showed significant increases of 25 percent and 20 percent respectively. In addition, the control group's increase was just significant. There were no significant differences between groups on any of these cardiorespiratory variables after four weeks of training.

The comparisons between groups after the completion of equal amounts of work in training were based upon only five subjects per group.

*Total Work Performed.* The accumulate total work performed by each of the three exercise groups while training on the bicycle ergometer was 1.65 x $10^6$ kpm. Group 2X required only fifteen training sessions to complete this quantity of work and Group 1X required 15.8 sessions.

*Work Performed in Fifteen Minutes.* The increases in mean amount of work performed in fifteen minutes appeared directly related to exercise frequency. The percentage improvements were 56 percent, 35 percent and 29 percent for groups 4X, 2X and 1X respectively.

*Performance Time to Exhaustion.* Groups 4X and 2X both increased performance time to exhaustion by 50 percent as compared to only 20 percent for Group 1X.

*Cardiorespiratory Variables.* Groups 4X and 2X differed significantly from Group 1X on max. $\dot{V}_{O_2}$. This significant post-training difference between groups was a result of Groups 4X and 2X increasing on max. $\dot{V}_{O_2}$ values and Group 1X decreasing. Although the difference between Group 4X and 2X was not significant, the percentage changes on max. $\dot{V}_{O_2}$ were directly related to exercise frequency.

There was no significant difference between groups after training on either heart rate at 900 kpm/min or $PWC_{170}$. None of the exercise groups demonstrated a significant decrease in working heart rate and only Group 2X demonstrated a significant increase on $PWC_{170}$.

## Discussion

The relationship of total work performed to the effects of exercise frequency has not been examined in studies on frequency. Observed posttraining differences in dependent variables were automatically attributed to frequency differences.

The results of this study clearly indicate an interaction between exercise frequency and total work performed. Increases in the capacity to perform work were directly and nearly proportionately related to both frequency and total work performed.

When the confounding effect of exercise work differences is removed, the evidence suggests that exercise frequency is the important factor for the improvement of work performance, and not the actual performance of work per se. Even though all groups completed an equal quantity of work, Groups 4X and 2X demonstrated a higher performance level and greater increases than Group 1X on work capacity measures. It thus appears that it is the frequency at which work is performed that determines the response to training and not the quantity.

After four weeks of training, the changes in the physiological variables were apparently not directly related to frequency or total work performed. After the completion of equal amounts of work, only changes in max. $\dot{V}_{O_2}$ were related to exercise frequency.

The interpretation of max. $\dot{V}_{O_2}$ results is difficult since Groups 2X and 1X both showed a level of max. $\dot{V}_{O_2}$ lower at the study's completion than at the end of four weeks of training. A significant decrease in max. $\dot{V}_{O_2}$ with training, such as that witnessed in Group 1X, is rarely if ever reported in the literature.

After four months of training Group 1X improved significantly only in the amount of work completed in fifteen minutes and decreased significantly on max. $\dot{V}_{O_2}$. It seems that once a week training, even in an all-out manner, is little better than not training.

The results of this experiment did not indicate whether Group 4X was superior to Group 2X, but rather there appears to be an optimal frequency for training greater than once a week. Further experimentation is needed to determine at which frequency the gains in physical work performance and cardio-respiratory fitness are greatest.

## References

1. Churdar, J.B.: A study of the effect of four different frequencies of a specific exercise program on physical fitness. Unpublished Ed.D dissertation. Tallahassee, Florida State University, 1967.
2. Jackson, J.H., Sharkey, B.J. and Johnston, L.P.: *Res. Quart.* 39(2): 295, 1968.
3. Johnson, R.C.: *Res. Quart.* 40(1): 93, 1969.
4. Joseph, J.J.: *J. Phys. Educ.* 61(4): 28, 1963.
5. O'Brien, R.F.: The effects of frequency of training on cardio-respiratory conditioning. Unpublished Ph.D. dissertation. Ohio State University, 1967.
6. Pollock, M.L., Cureton, T.K., and Greninger, L.: *Med. Sci. Sports.* 1(2): 70, 1969.

# Chapter 15

# Characterization of Physiological Modifications Occurring During Interval Training

Jacques Damoiseau
Ginette Hunnebelle
Paul Houssière

## Introduction

Interval training is a method of physical training generally used in certain sports and especially in track and field. Although this method is known to be intense[6,7] few studies have been undertaken in order to objectify the athlete's reactions during his usual training. On the field, heart rate measured with the hand at the radial artery is used as the only criterion.

Studies in which the athlete is asked to produce efforts which do not correspond to the type of work he performs during his training are subject to criticism since it is well known that for a same work level cardiorespiratory adjustments can vary according to the exercise execution modalities.[2,5,8,9]

The purpose of this study was to follow the evolution of certain cardiorespiratory parameters known to give valid information on the athlete's behavior during interval training sessions. One of our main concerns was to respect the type and rhythm of work done by the runners and to reproduce as much as possible these conditions in the laboratory.

*Note:* Information on training programs and personal records of the examined athletes were given by Mr. J. Boudart, coach at the R.F.C. of Liège, whose collaboration and interest were consistent throughout the study. The authors take this opportunity to thank him.

## Methods and Procedures

Thirteen[13] subjects regularly engaged in competitive track and field participated in the experimentation. Their physical characteristics and their best performance are shown in Table 15-I. A previous medical examination excluded anyone with lung or heart abnormalities liable to make the competition harmful for the subject.

TABLE 15-I

BIOMETRIC DATA AND PERFORMANCES

Individual data and mean age, height and weight are noted according, on the one hand, to the usual scoring system (time required to cover a distance), and, on the other hand, to the appreciation method proposed by the International Athletic Federation.[20]

| Subjects | Age Year, Month | Height (cm) | Weight (kg) | Best Performances Distance (m) | Time Min | Sec | Appreciation by F.I.A.A. |
|---|---|---|---|---|---|---|---|
| P.H. | 30,00 | 173.5 | 62.0 | 5000 | 14. | 55. 0 | 851 |
| A.G. | 21,06 | 176,0 | 66.5 | 800 | 2. | 01. 1 | 729 |
| T.R. | 24,11 | 170.0 | 56.5 | 3000 | 8. | 57. 8 | 767 |
| J.D. | 21,01 | 174.5 | 63.0 | 1500 | 4. | 10. 7 | 730 |
| J.M. | 19,08 | 176.5 | 69.0 | 800 | 2. | 05. 1 | 663 |
| C.O. | 19,08 | 175.0 | 57.5 | 800 | 1. | 58. 9 | 767 |
| H.R. | 18,11 | 181.0 | 65.0 | 1500 | 4. | 18. 8 | 669 |
| C.V. | 18,06 | 174.5 | 64.0 | 800 | 2. | 04. 0 | 681 |
| Y.B. | 23,08 | 173.5 | 66.0 | 800 | 2. | 09. 8 | 592 |
| J.S. | 23,08 | 173.0 | 66.0 | 800 | 2. | 06. 0 | 650 |
| G.W. | 20,08 | 184.0 | 73.5 | 400 | . | 52. 0 | 720 |
| D.U. | 23,08 | 167.5 | 59.5 | 1500 | 3. | 44. 9 | 953 |
| W.V. | 20,05 | 182.0 | 74.5 | 800 | 1. | 53. 1 | 874 |
| X̄ | 22,05 | 176.2 | 64.4 | | | | 742 |

The treadmill ergometer was used horizontally at various speeds which could be hydraulically increased from 2 to 36 km/hr within four seconds.

Ventilation was continuously measured with two 200-liter Tissot bells. The subject wore a nose-clip and was connected by a mouthpiece to a set of low resistance valves. The subject alternately expired into each of the bells. The reading was taken at 0.25 liters.

Mean $pO_2$ of expired air was measured with a paramagnetic oxymeter (SERVOMEX) of which the accuracy has been shown.[3] An expired air sample was continuously collected through an even flow pump. The air sample was passed over sodium asbestos to remove its $CO_2$ and water vapor contents. With $pO_2$ variations of 100 to 160 mm Hg at the mouthpiece level, nineteen seconds were required to obtain a 90 percent response. A fifteen-second systematic correction was made to compensate for this time lag.

The $O_2$ consumption was measured every thirty seconds, according to the method proposed by Margaria *et al.*[13]

The heart rate was registered with an electrocardiograph (Hellige) at a paper speed of 25 mm/sec. A bipolar derivation of the type V6–V6R or V5–V5R gave satisfactory readings. Mean heart rate was measured from ten successive peaks.

The values were expressed according to international standards: the $O_2$ consumption in $ml_{STPD}$ ($O°$ C, 760 mm Hg, dry); the ventilation in $liters_{BTPS}$ ($37°C$, water saturated and ambiant pressure). The heart rate was expressed in beat/minute whereas ventilation and $VO_2$ values were calculated over periods of thirty seconds. The oxygen utilization coefficient represents the number of ml of $O_2$ consumed for each liter of inspired air (ml/1) whereas $O_2$ pulse is the number of ml of $O_2$ carried by the blood at each heart beat (ml/beat).

Each subject ran and walked several times on the treadmill at various speeds in order to get used to the ergometer. When the subject showed sufficient coordination, especially during accelerations and decelerations, he was given a thirty-minute rest in a sitting position in order to reduce at maximum all disturbances pertaining to familiarization exercise.[17] Individual working intensities were determined on the basis of each training program. The treadmill speed was calculated on the basis of the time required for a 200-meter run; the treadmill run lasted thirty seconds for all subjects, which introduced an approximative error of 7.5 percent (Table 15-II).

Figure 15–1 presents the conduct of the experiments. Each subject carried out without interruption:

a six-minute walk at a speed of 4 km/hr;
a thirty-second run at a speed of 22, 24 or 26 km/hr, according to the training program of the subject;
a five-minute walk at a speed of 4 km/hr;
a thirty-second run;
a five-minute walk at a speed of 4 km/hr;

TABLE 15-II

QUANTITY OF WORK DONE

The thirteen subjects are divided into four groups according to their type of training. The number of periods represents the number of runs and walks at 4 km/hr. Three of the thirteen subjects did fifteen repetitions. Although the training consists of 200-meter runs, we are introducing an error of approximately fifteen meters by imposing a thirty-second run on the treadmill. The training time is comparable for all athletes but the intensity differs as it can be noticed from the various distances run.

| *Number of Subjects* | *Number of Periods* | *Running Speed Km/hr* | *Distance in 30 sec Meters* | *Total Distance of the Run Km* | *Total Distance Run Km* | *Total Time of Exper Min–Sec* |
|---|---|---|---|---|---|---|
| 1 | 20 | 22 | 184 | 4 | 6,6 | 51 |
| 7 | 20 | 24 | 200 | 4,4 | 7,1 | 51 |
| 3 | 15 | 24 | 200 | 3,4 | 5,7 | 43,30 |
| 2 | 20 | 26 | 215 | 4,7 | 7,3 | 51 |

a series of fifteen or twenty (according to the subjects) thirty-second runs punctuated by one-minute walk periods; a five-minute walk at a speed of 4 km/hr (recovery).

The experiment is so designed as to determine the following:

1. The moment when the cardiorespiratory equilibrium is reached during the warm-up phases. This happens when the parameter variations become significantly less than the individual random error; this is determined by successively comparing means and variances obtained with ($N-n_i$) measures, where N is the maximum number of measures taken during each warm-up phase (that is 12, 10, 10 and 8) and where $n_i$ varies from O to (N–2) with an interpolation of 1.

Means were compared by calculating a Student's "t" factor, variances by calculating a Snedecor's "F" factor ($f = V_1/V_2$.[19]

The individual variance of the different parameters for the first two running periods was estimated on the basis of the values obtained for the runs punctuated with long walking periods.

2. The possible changes in parameters during the twenty (or 15) runs and intercalated walks.

These variations were determined by comparing the four (or 3) means obtained after grouping the results by five. The calculation of a Snedecor's F factor made the com-

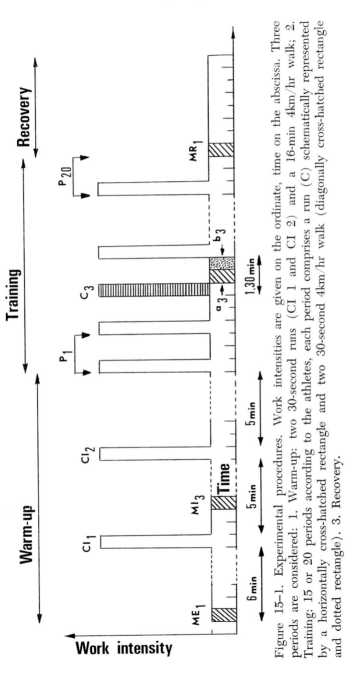

Figure 15–1. Experimental procedures. Work intensities are given on the ordinate, time on the abscissa. Three periods are considered: 1. Warm-up: two 30-second runs (CI 1 and CI 2) and a 16-min 4km/hr walk; 2. Training: 15 or 20 periods according to the athletes, each period comprises a run (C) schematically represented by a horizontally cross-hatched rectangle and two 30-second 4km/hr walk (diagonally cross-hatched rectangle and dotted rectangle). 3. Recovery.

parison possible. One can equally easily determine the exact moment when this equilibrium (as defined in 1) is lost.

3. The moment when the cardio-respiratory equilibrium was reestablished during the recovery period; this was done through successive checks as in 1.

## Results

Biometrical data, individual performances and mean values are shown in Table 15-I. Except for P.H., all athletes examined were under twenty-five years of age. Seven of the thirteen runners examined preferred the 800 meters. The last two subjects (D.V. and V.W.) had the highest performances (953 and 874 points); incidentally, the two athletes underwent a harder training program (Table 15-II). According to the F.I.A.A. cotation, the mean value of the group was 742 points.

During the 4 km/hr walk the mean energy expenditure of the group was 1.3 1/min (630 ml per 30 second), whereas the mean heart rate was 90. The two intercalated runs transitorily modified the constant values (Fig. 15–2) obtained during the walking period. The heart rate reached its maximal value during the run, then decreased as ventilation and VO2 kept on increasing. This phenomenon disappeared during the repetition of efforts (Fig 15–3).

During the training period, the obtained values were low, as shown in Table 15-III. Most of the subjects did not reach a heart rate of 160 beats/minute. The energy expenditure expressed in 1 of $O_2$/30 seconds was around 1.5 and the mean ventilation was approximately 56 1/min. (28 1/30 sec.) The high respiratory equivalents (extreme values of 61.9 and 45.3 during the runs) indicate a high respiratory exchange efficiency.

During the last thirty seconds of walking immediately prior to the next running effort, most of the values were different from those obtained during walking at steady state. While the mean heart rate during the walking exercise was 90 beats/min, it increased to 105 and 102 during the walking periods. Changes observed at the level of respiratory parameters were distinctly

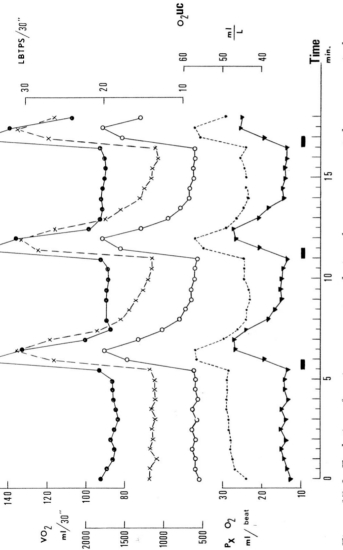

Figure 15–2. Evolution of various parameters during the warm-up period are successively considered: heart rate (dark circles, continuous lines), ventilation (crosses, interrupted lines), oxygen consumption (clear circles, continuous lines), oxygen utilization coefficient (black dots, pointed lines), oxygen pulse (triangles, continuous lines). Black rectangles indicate runs.

While maximal heart rates are reached in the end of runs, ventilations, oxygen consumptions, oxygen utilization coefficients oxygen pulse values are higher during the first thirty seconds of walk. On the other hand cardiac deceleration is quicker than that of ventilatory parameters. A clear-cut divergence can be seen between circulatory and ventilatory parameter behaviors.

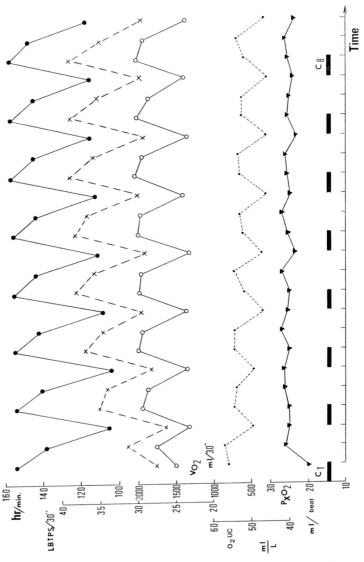

Figure 15–3a,b,c. Evolution of various parameters during interval training and recovery. Symbols are identical to those of Figure 15–1. Hyperventilation is a function of the number of repetitions; it is observed during the eight first trials after what it stabilizes. The delayed hyperventilation of the first thirty seconds of run disappears with repeated efforts. In these conditions a parallelism sets in between circulatory and ventilatory parameters. During the last thirty seconds of walk heart rate progressively increases with the number of repetitions.

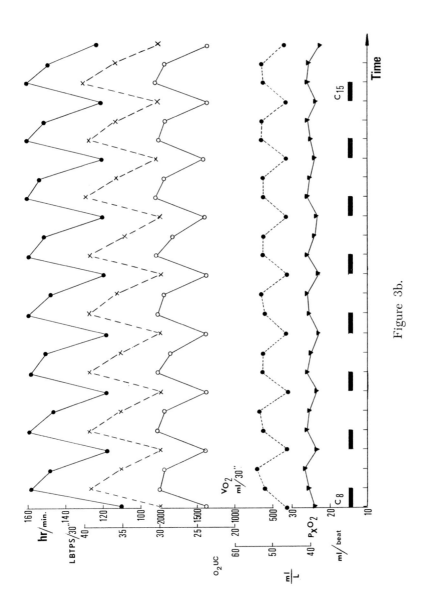

Figure 3b.

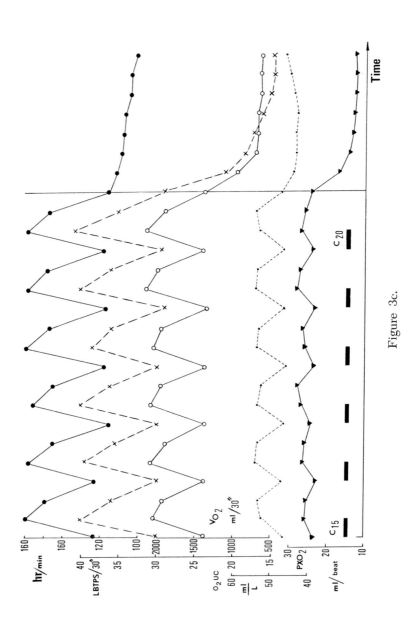

Figure 3c.

## TABLE 15-III

### INDIVIDUAL VALUES AND MEANS REGISTERED DURING THE WALK AND THE REPEATED EFFORTS

Heart rate, ventilation, oxygen consumption, oxygen utilization coefficient and oxygen pulse are taken during the steady state attained while walking at 4km/hr (m), during the thirty seconds of running (C) and during both thirty-second periods following the run (a and b respectively). The results registered during and after the runs are averaged for each speed ($\bar{x}$) while the general mean ($\bar{X}$) is calculated for the values obtained during the 4 km/hr walk. In a and b heart rate progressively decreases in relation to the run (C) which is not the case for ventilation nor oxygen consumption. This behavior divergence between the circulatory and ventilatory parameters is reflected by a net increase in the oxygen pulse in a and b relatively to C.

| Subjects | Heart Rate Beat/min | | | | Ventilation 1/30 sec | | | | O₂ Consumption ml/30 sec | | | | O₂ utilization coefficient ml/l | | | | O₂ Pulse ml/beat | | | |
|---|---|---|---|---|---|---|---|---|---|---|---|---|---|---|---|---|---|---|---|---|
| | m | c | a | b | m | c | a | b | m | c | a | b | m | c | a | b | m | c | a | b |
| **22 km/hr** | | | | | | | | | | | | | | | | | | | | |
| P.H. | 72 | 125 | 111 | 64 | 16.7 | 18.9 | 27.5 | 23.7 | 680 | 1126 | 1568 | 1178 | 42.3 | 59.9 | 57.3 | 49.7 | 20.5 | 18.0 | 28.1 | 37.0 |
| **24 km/hr** | | | | | | | | | | | | | | | | | | | | |
| A.G. | 78 | 152 | 130 | 88 | 14.2 | 28.0 | 32.1 | 26.3 | 710 | 1731 | 1915 | 1303 | 48.5 | 61.0 | 59.8 | 49.7 | 20.5 | 22.8 | 29.4 | 30.0 |
| T.R. | 76 | 162 | 116 | 85 | 14.0 | 30.7 | 33.5 | 25.0 | 560 | 1626 | 1736 | 1095 | 44.6 | 52.9 | 51.9 | 44.0 | 18.5 | 20.1 | 30.1 | 25.6 |
| J.D. | 93 | 163 | 140 | 102 | 16.5 | 39.7 | 31.3 | 29.3 | 680 | 1998 | 1681 | 1299 | 42.0 | 50.5 | 53.7 | 44.4 | 18.5 | 24.5 | 24.1 | 25.4 |
| J.M. | 102 | 153 | 139 | 112 | 13.5 | 27.3 | 30.1 | 23.0 | 640 | 1598 | 1869 | 1222 | 47.5 | 58.7 | 62.0 | 53.1 | 16.0 | 20.9 | 27.0 | 21.9 |
| C.O. | 96 | 157 | 139 | 120 | 15.5 | 26.0 | 34.0 | 30.7 | 690 | 1500 | 1925 | 1584 | 44.8 | 57.9 | 56.6 | 51.6 | 14.5 | 19.1 | 27.7 | 26.3 |
| H.R. | 92 | 157 | 143 | 92 | 16.0 | 26.7 | 32.9 | 28.2 | 730 | 1654 | 1917 | 1392 | 45.5 | 61.9 | 58.3 | 49.4 | 16.0 | 21.1 | 26.8 | 30.3 |
| C.V. | 88 | 142 | 128 | 97 | 17.2 | 26.6 | 35.0 | 29.1 | 690 | 1496 | 1960 | 1395 | 41.0 | 56.2 | 56.0 | 48.0 | 15.8 | 21.0 | 30.6 | 28.7 |
| Y.B. | 108 | 151 | 147 | 120 | 16.5 | 22.7 | 27.5 | 25.4 | 760 | 1182 | 1547 | 1358 | 45.7 | 52.1 | 56.3 | 54.4 | 14.0 | 15.7 | 21.0 | 21.6 |
| J.S. | 98 | 152 | 133 | 99 | 16.3 | 24.2 | 27.9 | 23.4 | 540 | 1243 | 1583 | 1117 | 43.7 | 51.4 | 56.8 | 50.4 | 12.7 | 16.4 | 23.8 | 23.9 |
| G.W. | 107 | 158 | 163 | 130 | 15.8 | 30.6 | 31.8 | 29.2 | 670 | 1587 | 1825 | 1407 | 48.3 | 51.9 | 57.3 | 48.4 | 12.5 | 20.1 | 22.1 | 21.7 |
| $\bar{x}$ | — | 155 | 138 | 105 | — | 28.3 | 31.6 | 27.0 | — | 1562 | 1796 | 1323 | — | 55.5 | 56.9 | 49.3 | — | 20.2 | 26.3 | 25.5 |
| **26 km/hr** | | | | | | | | | | | | | | | | | | | | |
| W.V. | 85 | 156 | 140 | 105 | 16 | 33.0 | 34.8 | 29.1 | 630 | 1493 | 1891 | 1432 | 48.0 | 45.3 | 54.3 | 49.3 | 18.0 | 19.2 | 27.0 | 27.3 |
| D.U. | 91 | 162 | 144 | 98 | 12 | 24.1 | 28.7 | 23.6 | 490 | 1308 | 1543 | 1064 | 40.6 | 54.6 | 53.9 | 45.2 | 10.7 | 16.2 | 21.5 | 21.7 |
| $\bar{x}$ | — | 159 | 142 | 102 | — | 28.5 | 31.7 | 26.4 | — | 1400 | 1717 | 1248 | — | 50.0 | 54.1 | 47.8 | — | 17.7 | 24.3 | 24.5 |
| $\bar{X}$ | 90 | | | | 15.4 | | | | 630 | | | | 44.0 | | | | 14.9 | | | |

greater. The ventilation increased from 15.4 1/30 sec. to 26.4–27.0 1/30 sec. Table 15-III $V_{02}$ approximately doubled as did $O_2$ pulse; these values were respectively 630 ml/30 sec and 14.9 ml/beat during walking at steady state. During the last thirty seconds of intercalated walks, the values were 1400–1500 ml/30 sec and 25 ml/beat. This phenomenon is also shown in Figure 15–3.

In this figure, a disparity between the average behavior of the parameters appears. During the first eight repetitions (Fig. 15–3a), an important hyperventilation sets in as a function of the number of repetitions, while the heart rate mean values were relatively constant from one effort to the other. The statistical analysis (Table 15-IV) also shows an almost systematic hyperventilation which accompanied the repeated runs as compared to the ventilation obtained during the isolated running exercises. The delayed systolic hyperventilation observed immediately after the warm-up running exercises disappeared during the repeated runs (Fig. 3a, b and c).

The characterization of the individual behavior during interval training is shown in Table 15-V where the number and the percentage of statistically different values are given for each parameter and subject.

The different parameters of subject P.H. were remarkably constant due to the low work intensity to which he was submitted.

Behavioral divergencies appeared depending on the subjects and on the parameter considered. During the repeated runs, ventilation and VO2 were systematically affected by the number of repetitions while the heart rate during the last thirty seconds of walking showed considerable variance. The difference between the behavior of energy expenditure as represented by VO2 and of the heart rate was also illustrated by the high percentage of statistically different $O_2$ pulses recorded during the first thirty seconds of walking following each running session (Table 15-V).

### Discussion

Peculiarities of interval training were reproduced on the treadmill. However, two systematic errors related to method-

## TABLE 15-IV
### SIGNIFICANT VENTILATORY VARIATIONS DURING THE RUNS

Table 15-IV gives an example of statistical analysis. The ventilation mean is calculated with data obtained from two intercalated runs and from the first training session run. These values are not influenced by repetition. Confidence intervals are calculated (s. pr. 0.05) and noted under each subject's initials. A cross in a column indicates that it is a value statistically different from the values not influenced by repetition. The number and the percentage of ventilation values significantly different are calculated for each subject.

| | P.H. | A.G. | T.R. | J.D. | J.M. | C.O. | H.R. | C.V. | Y.B. | J.S. | G.W. | W.V. | D.U. |
|---|---|---|---|---|---|---|---|---|---|---|---|---|---|
| | 19 | 28,3 | 30,7 | 39,7 | 27,3 | 26 | 26,7 | 26,6 | 22,7 | 24,2 | 30,6 | 33 | 24 |
| Repetitions | >30 | >33,2 | >32,8 | >55 | >31 | >33 | >28 | >30,1 | >28 | >27,4 | >34,5 | >33,7 | >32,2 |
| 2 | | | | | × | × | × | × | × | × | × | × | × |
| 3 | | × | | | × | × | × | × | × | × | × | × | × |
| 4 | | × | × | | × | × | × | × | × | × | × | × | × |
| 5 | × | × | × | | × | × | × | × | × | × | × | × | × |
| 6 | × | × | × | | × | × | × | × | × | × | × | × | × |
| 7 | × | × | × | | × | × | × | × | × | × | × | × | × |
| 8 | | × | | | × | × | × | × | × | × | × | × | × |
| 9 | × | × | × | | × | × | × | × | × | × | × | × | × |
| 10 | | × | | | × | × | × | × | × | × | × | × | × |
| 11 | | × | × | | × | × | × | × | × | × | × | × | × |
| 12 | | × | | | × | × | × | × | × | × | × | × | × |
| 13 | | × | × | | × | × | × | × | × | × | × | × | × |
| 14 | | × | | | × | × | × | × | × | × | × | × | × |
| 15 | × | × | × | | × | × | × | × | × | × | × | × | × |
| 16 | × | × | × | | × | × | × | × | | | × | × | × |
| 17 | × | × | × | | × | × | × | × | | | | × | × |
| 18 | | × | | | × | × | × | × | | | | × | × |
| 19 | | × | × | | × | × | × | × | | | | × | × |
| 20 | | × | | | × | × | × | × | | | | × | × |
| N | 7 | 18 | 11 | 0 | 19 | 19 | 19 | 19 | 14 | 14 | 14 | 19 | 19 |
| % | 37 | 95 | 57 | 0 | 100 | 100 | 100 | 100 | 100 | 100 | 100 | 100 | 100 |

## TABLE 15-V
### BEHAVIOR OF INDIVIDUAL PARAMETERS DURING INTERVAL TRAINING

Heart rate, ventilation, oxygen consumption, oxygen utilization coefficient and oxygen pulse are successively considered. For each subject and parameter, the number (N) and the percentage of the statistically different values are taken for the run (C), for the first thirty seconds (a) and the last thirty seconds (b) of the 4 km/hr walk. The three subjects Y.B. J.S. and G.W. (marked with an *) did but fifteen repetitions of which fourteen influenced each other.

| Subjects | | | P.H. | A.G. | T.R. | J.D. | J.M. | C.O. | H.R. | C.V. | Y.B.* | J.S.* | G.W.* | W.V. | D.U. |
|---|---|---|---|---|---|---|---|---|---|---|---|---|---|---|---|
| HR | C. | N. | 0 | 2 | 16 | 9 | 12 | 0 | 17 | 19 | 14 | 14 | 0 | 11 | 4 |
| | | %. | 0 | 11 | 84 | 47 | 63 | 0 | 89 | 100 | 100 | 100 | 0 | 57 | 21 |
| | a. | N. | 0 | 12 | 19 | 13 | 16 | 16 | 8 | 12 | 11 | 14 | 11 | 15 | 19 |
| | | %. | 0 | 63 | 100 | 68 | 84 | 84 | 42 | 63 | 79 | 100 | 79 | 79 | 100 |
| | b. | N. | 0 | 3 | 12 | 12 | 12 | 12 | 15 | 19 | 8 | 14 | 14 | 10 | 15 |
| | | %. | 0 | 16 | 63 | 63 | 63 | 63 | 79 | 100 | 57 | 100 | 14 | 52 | 79 |
| Vent. | C. | N. | 7 | 18 | 11 | 0 | 19 | 19 | 19 | 9 | 14 | 14 | 14 | 19 | 19 |
| | | %. | 37 | 95 | 57 | 0 | 100 | 100 | 100 | 47 | 100 | 100 | 100 | 100 | 100 |
| | a. | N. | 0 | 0 | 0 | 19 | 16 | 0 | 14 | 10 | 0 | 14 | 14 | 9 | 3 |
| | | %. | 0 | 0 | 0 | 100 | 84 | 0 | 74 | 52 | 0 | 100 | 100 | 47 | 16 |
| | b. | N. | 5 | 0 | 7 | 0 | 19 | 19 | 8 | 19 | 14 | 14 | 3 | 10 | 2 |
| | | %. | 26 | 0 | 37 | 0 | 100 | 100 | 42 | 100 | 100 | 100 | 21 | 52 | 11 |
| VO₂ | C. | N. | 0 | 8 | 19 | 0 | 11 | 5 | 19 | 2 | 11 | 14 | 14 | 19 | 19 |
| | | %. | 0 | 42 | 100 | 0 | 57 | 26 | 100 | 16 | 79 | 100 | 100 | 100 | 100 |
| | a. | N. | 0 | 0 | 0 | 11 | 12 | 2 | 0 | 0 | 3 | 11 | 0 | 17 | 3 |
| | | %. | 0 | 0 | 0 | 57 | 63 | 11 | 0 | 0 | 21 | 79 | 0 | 89 | 16 |
| | b. | N. | 0 | 6 | 0 | 0 | 0 | 6 | 2 | 17 | 0 | 12 | 0 | 0 | 5 |
| | | %. | 0 | 32 | 0 | 0 | 0 | 32 | 11 | 89 | 0 | 86 | 0 | 0 | 26 |
| O₂UC | C. | N. | 0 | 10 | 0 | 0 | 19 | 0 | 9 | 3 | 0 | 14 | 12 | 0 | 19 |
| | | %. | 0 | 52 | 0 | 0 | 100 | 0 | 47 | 21 | 0 | 100 | 86 | 0 | 100 |
| | a. | N. | 5 | 0 | 0 | 19 | 19 | 0 | 0 | 19 | 0 | 14 | 4 | 0 | 0 |
| | | %. | 26 | 0 | 0 | 100 | 100 | 0 | 0 | 100 | 0 | 100 | 29 | 0 | 0 |
| | b. | N. | 15 | 0 | 0 | 0 | 15 | 0 | 0 | 0 | 0 | 0 | 0 | 0 | 0 |
| | | %. | 79 | 0 | 0 | 0 | 79 | 0 | 0 | 0 | 0 | 0 | 0 | 0 | 0 |
| Px O₂ | a. | N. | 16 | 11 | 13 | 0 | 19 | 19 | 19 | 19 | 14 | 14 | 14 | 19 | 15 |
| | | %. | 84 | 57 | 68 | 0 | 100 | 100 | 100 | 100 | 100 | 100 | 100 | 100 | 79 |
| | b. | N. | 0 | 9 | 14 | 3 | 0 | 13 | 15 | 7 | 0 | 1 | 8 | 11 | 12 |
| | | %. | 0 | 47 | 74 | 16 | 0 | 68 | 79 | 37 | 0 | 7 | 57 | 57 | 63 |

ological difficulties were made: an approximative error of 7.5 percent on the distance covered by the athletes (Table 15-II) and an underestimation of the work normally produced on the track due to the air resistance absence.

Although precise informations on individual peculiarities of training have been obtained it was impossible to evaluate the intensity of the warm-up normally done by the athletes which consisted of jogging and short runs. The time varied however from one individual to the other. By standardizing the warm-up to a sixteen-minute walk and two thirty-second runs we were able to register values which could be compared with the values obtained during the interval training as such.

The two systematic errors mentioned above cannot explain by themselves the low ventilation, VO2 and heart rate values registered during the runs. The shortness (30 sec) of the runs did not allow to reach a steady state and can therefore explain the low values obtained. The ergometer would eventually be responsible for these low values; however[16] obtained a higher $O_2$ consumption during treadmill running than track running. If we admit with Kreuzer[11] that an international class long distance runner must attain maximal VO2 values of 5.0 liters; working ventilation values of 150 liters and minute heart rate values of two hundred beats, the physiological stimulation of the cardiorespiratory system seems moderate during reproduction of efforts comparable to those regularly produced on the field. One must however note that the simulated training was a precompetition season training where the work intensity is progressively decreased. If the values proposed by Kreuzer[11] are too high for the type of examined athletes,[4] the values registered during the interval training remain nevertheless definitely inferior to their maximal attainable values. During an interval training, Yokobri[21] and Miyashimata[15] have respectively registered heart rates superior to 180 with hockey players and swimmers whose level of physical preparation was not mentioned.

The two runners with the best performances (Table 15-I) trained themselves harder (26 km/hr runs). However the behavior of their parameters is not significantly different from that of the whole group examined (13 runners). The quality of their performances can partially be explained by a higher efficiency.

During the warm-up period, ventilation and VO2 values were higher during the thirty seconds immediately following the runs than during the runs themselves. This confirms observations made by Reindell,[18] Leclerq,[12] Menier[14] and Assailly[1]. The last author has also observed immediately after pedalling on a bicycle ergometer a compensatory hyperventilation related to a tidal volume increase of 400 to 600 ml. This compensatory hyperventilation is interpreted as a result of a thoracic blocking during exercise. It is worth noting that this particular ventilatory behavior disappears after repeated runs (Fig. 3a-b-c), which indicates a faster and more adequate respiratory adjustment to the effort.

Statistical analysis shows numerous modifications during the repetition of running exercises. The athlete undertakes new efforts in progressively less favorable conditions. Heart rate seems mostly affected during the second thirty-second period following the runs while the ventilatory function is mostly affected during the runs and the first thirty-second period immediately following the runs (Table 15-V). Although it seems justifiable to consider the heart rate prior to a new effort in order to estimate the recovery state of an athlete doing interval training, it appears that this parameter can provide but partial information on the athlete's state of fatigue. The divergence among the parameters studied would be accentuated if the working intensity was increased.

It seems that the optimal training intensity could be determined by confronting the trainer's observations with absolute values and mainly with the athlete's behavior while performing efforts comparable to those he achieves on the track.

## References

1. Assaily, P.: *Amer. Entr. Franc. Athl. 22:* 5, 1970.
2. Bobbert, A.C.: *J. Appl. Physiol. 15:* 1007, 1960.
3. Cotes, J.E., and Wooimer, R.F.: *J. Physiol, 163:* 36, 1962.

4. Damoiseau, J.: *Kinanthropologie. 2:* 1970, sous presse.
5. Damoiseau, J., Deroanne, R. and Petit, J.M.: *J. Physiol. 55:* 235, 1963.
6. Fox, E.L., Robinson, S. and Wiegman, D.L.: *J. Appl. Physiol. 27:* 174, 1969.
7. Harper, D.D., Billings, C.E. and Mathews, D.K.: *Res. Quart. 40:* 239, 1969.
8. Hermansen, L., Exblom B. and Saltin B.: *J. Appl. Physiol. 29:* 82, 1970.
9. Hermansen, L. and Saltin B.: *J. Appl. Physiol. 26:* 31, 1969.
10. Krautchenko, J. and Gordon S.: *La Médecine Sportive,* ed. en langues étrangères, Moscou, 1960, p. 289.
11. Kreuzer, F.: *Rev. Suisse Méd. Sportive, 14:* 7, 1966.
12. Leclercq, J.: *Méd. Educ. Phys. Sport, 2:* 57, 1961.
13. Margaria, R., Meischia, G. and Marro, F.: *J. Appl. Physiol. 6:* 776, 1954.
14. Menier, P.: *Méd. du Sport. 2:* 90, 1969.
15. Miyashita, M.: *Proceed. of Int. Congress of Sport Science 1964,* ed., Kitsuo Kato, Tokyo, 1966, p. 493–494.
16. Nakanishi, M., Tsukagoshi, K., Yorikane, Y. and Aoki, J.: *Proceed. of Int. Congress of Sport Science, 1964* ed., Kitsuo Kato, Tokyo, 1966, p. 446–448.
17. O.M.S.: Epreuves d'effort et fonction cardio-vasculaire Rap. technique n° 388, 1968, 3Ip.
18. Reindell, H.: *Sport. 5:* 23–31 1959.
19. Schwartz, D.: *Flammarion Paris,* 1963.
20. *SCORING TABLE FOR MEN'S TRACK AND FIELD EVENTS I.A.A.F.,* 1962, 54 p.
21. Yokobori, S.: *Proceed. of the Int. Congress of Sport Science,* 1964 ed. Kitsuo Kato, Tokyo, 1966, p. 294–495.

# Chapter 16

# The Urinary Elimination of Vanilmandelic Acid Before and After a Standard Exercise in Trained and Untrained Men

Serge Dulac

Catecholamines are secreted by the adrenal medulla and the nerve endings of the sympathetic nervous system.[5,6] Many studies were done on the secretion of catecholamines into the blood[4,14] and their elimination in urine[7,11,15] after exercise. Few studies have been done in order to differentiate trained and untrained men for urinary elimination of catecholamines before and after exercise. In the study of Kärki[7] there is no measure of the work load, while in the study of Von Euler and Hellner[15] there is no statistical comparison between the work loads and the catecholamine excretion. Klepping, Didier and Escousse[8] found that the urinary elimination of vanilmandelic acid at rest and after exercise was less in trained men than in the untrained ones. However, in their study the evaluation of the degree of fitness of the subject was poor, and also the exercise varied in intensity and duration.

The basic purpose of this study was to study the urinary elimination of vanilmandelic acid (VMA) before and after a standard exercise in trained and untrained young men.

## Methods and Procedures

The subjects (N=21) were young men (18 to 30 years old) having less than 20 percent of their body weight as fat.

Note: Work done at the biokinetic laboratory of the school of physical education and recreation of the Ottawa University for the degree, master of sciences in kinanthropology.

*First Testing Session.* At subject arrival, some anthropometric measurements were taken (weight, height, age), and the thickness of skinfolds were measured according to the procedures of Pascale *et al.*[9] for predicting the fat-free body weight.

The subject was then tested for maximal oxygen intake on a Monarch bicycle ergometer. The test consisted of a step increase of the work load at every two minutes until the subject was unable to continue for a further work load.

The maximal oxygen intake was used mainly to classify the subjects into three groups: trained (N=5), untrained (N=5), intermediary (N=11).

*Second Testing Session.* Taking into consideration the data of Elmadjian, Larson and Neri,[2] of Kärki,[7] of Reton and Weil-Malherbe,[10] of Sunderman *et al.*[12] and of Von Euler, Hellner-Björkman and Orwen[16] on diurnal variations in the urinary elimination of catecholamines, it was decided that the test involving urine samples would be done in the morning between 8:30 and 11:30.

The subjects were allowed to take a light breakfast before the testing session, but were submitted to the following alimentary restrictions: for two days before the urine collection they had to abstain from medication, coffee, tea, chocolate and bananas.

At subject arrival, he was asked to empty his bladder as completely as possible. The time was noted and the subject had to drink 250 ml of water in order to favor the diuresis.

Thirty minutes later, a first urine sample (before exercise) was collected in a bottle and refrigerated. The time was noted and again the subject was asked to drink 250 ml of water.

The subject then performed a standard exercise (900 kpm/min for 30 minutes) on the bicycle ergometer.

About two hours after the beginning of exercise, the subject urinated into a second bottle which was then refrigerated and the time was noted.

*Determination of Urinary Vanilmandelic Acid.* The urine specimens were thawed and the volume was measured. Then, the VMA concentration was determined according to the method of Sunderman *et al.*[12] The total urinary VMA content was divided by the time of collection in order to obtain the urinary

VMA elimination in $\mu$g/min. For the postexercise urine sample, the urinary VMA output corresponding to the work period was computed as had Klepping, Didier and Escousse.[8]

The following statistical tests were used in the appropriate circumstance: "t" test, variance or covariance analysis. Furthermore, maximal oxygen intake was predicted from the heart rate at the thirtieth minute of exercise, or from resting VMA urinary values.

## Results

The trained group does not differ from the untrained one in regard to age and height (Table 16-I). However, the trained group is significantly heavier than the untrained group, even if we take off the influence of body fat.

At maximal work load, the pulmonary ventilation, oxygen intake, oxygen intake per kg of body weight, and $O_2$ pulse are higher in trained than in untrained men.

During the standard exercise, the trained group is characterized by a lower heart rate and respiratory equivalent, and by a higher oxygen pulse than the untrained group.

TABLE 16-I

PHYSICAL AND PHYSIOLOGICAL CHARACTERISTICS OF THE
TRAINED AND UNTRAINED GROUPS

| | Trained Group (N = 5) | Untrained Group (N = 5) | Signifi- cance Level |
|---|---|---|---|
| Physical Characteristics | | | |
| Age (years) | 24.2 ± 3.19 | 23.2 ± 3.19 | p > .05 |
| Height (inches) | 69.65 ± 2.21 | 68.3 ± 2.4 | p > .05 |
| Weight (kg) | 71.75 ± 4.94 | 63.82 ± 3.2 | p < .05 |
| Fat free body Weight (kg) | 63.03 ± 3.02 | 55.97 ± 2.11 | p < .01 |
| Physiological Characteristics | | | |
| a) Maximal Work load | | | |
| $\dot{V}$ E max (liter/min) | 158.86 ± 24.37 | 98.44 ± 15.18 | p < .01 |
| $\dot{V}$ $O_2$ max (liter/min) | 4.00 ± 0.06 | 2.70 ± 0.14 | p < .001 |
| $\dot{V}O_2$ max/body weight (ml/kg) | 56.04 ± 4.17 | 42.51 ± 3.43 | p < .01 |
| Max. $O_2$ pulse (ml $O_2$/beat) | 22.46 ± 1.53 | 15.11 ± 0.83 | p < .001 |
| b) Standard Exercise | | | |
| Heart rate (beat/min) | 128.2 ± 8.5 | 160.2 ± 13.8 | p < .01 |
| $O_2$ pulse (ml $O_2$/beat) | 16.65 ± 1.95 | 13.12 ± 1.68 | p < .05 |
| Respiratory equivalent | 22.15 ± 3.53 | 28.25 ± 3.53 | p < .05 |
| urinary output before exercise | 0.85 ± 0.35 | 1.22 ± 0.52 | p > .05 |
| (ml/min) after exercise | 0.94 ± 0.31 | 1.09 ± 0.79 | p > .05 |

Before exercise, there is no significant difference between the two groups in regard to the urine output/minute (Table 16-I). Also, the variance analysis demonstrates that exercise has no effect on this variable.

Before exercise, the trained men eliminated significantly less VMA (p<.001) than the untrained one (Fig. 16–1). The covari-

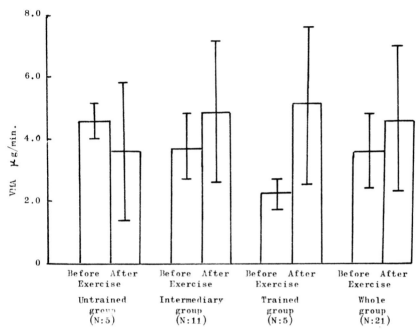

Figure 16–1. Urinary elimination of vanilmandelic acid (VMA) before and corresponding to the work period (after) for the untrained, trained, intermediary, and whole group.

ance analysis shows that the standard exercise did not affect significantly the urinary elimination of VMA in either groups. However, this analysis demonstrates that the effect of exercise is different in the two groups (p<.001). In the trained group, there was an elevation of that variable (121.4%) while in the untrained group, there was a decrease (19.9%).

The mean values for urinary elimination of VMA at rest and corresponding to the exercise period for the untrained, the trained, the intermediary, and the whole group are illustrated in Figure 16–1. We can see that the values for the intermediary group fall between the values of the trained and the untrained groups, and also, they are almost identical to those of the whole group.

## Discussion

The trained man has heavier active mass than the untrained (63.03 vs 55.97kg).

The trained group has higher values for physical working capacity, maximal pulmonary ventilation, maximal oxygen intake, maximal oxygen pulse, and for oxygen pulse during the standard exercise, and lower values for heart rate and respiratory equivalent during the standard exercise. According to Astrand and Rodahl[1] and Van Den Bossche and Marneffe,[13] such results are characteristic of the training state, and this confirms the value of our classification into trained and untrained.

Before exercise, the resting urine output was approximately the same in the trained and in the untrained groups (Table 16-I). The standard exercise had no significant effect on this variable. All these results agree with the data of Schoeman.[11]

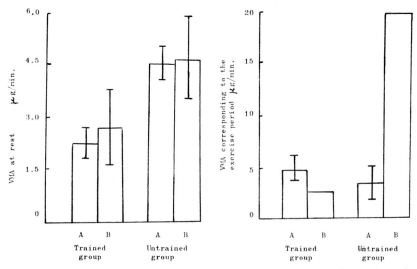

Figure 16–2. Comparison of the results of the present study (A) with those of Klepping, Didier et Escousse (1966) (B) in regard to the influence of exercise and physical fitness level on the VMA urinary elimination.

At rest, before exercise, the trained group eliminated significantly less VMA than the untrained one, and if we look at Figure 16–2, we see that the results of this study are in agreement with those of Klepping, Didier and Escousse.[8] These authors explain their results by the fact that for the untrained group, the exercise in the near future is a greater psychological stress than for the trained group.

Our results do not confirm the study of Schoeman[11] who did not find any difference in the resting urinary elimination of epinephrine and norepinephrine between an active and a sedentary group. However we can doubt the value of their classification, because their active group has a predicted maximal oxygen intake per kg of 45.8ml/kg in comparison to our predicted values of 64.2ml/kg.

In summary, the trained subject eliminated less vanilmandelic acid in urine at rest, before exercise, and this could be explained by one or many of the following suggestions:

1. Lower basal secretion.
2. Smaller psychological stress resulting from the exercise in a near future.
3. Changes in metabolic pathways.

If we look at Figure 16–1, we can see that the urinary elimination of VMA at rest seems to be discriminative only when there is a marked difference in the fitness level.

If we consider exercise as a stressing situation, an increase in urinary catecholamines can be expected.[3] However, the results of this study do not confirm this hypothesis: exercise did not cause a significant increase in the urinary elimination of vanilmandelic acid. However, if we look closely at Figure 16–1, we can see that the standard exercise caused a 121.4 percent increase in urinary VMA in the trained group and a 19.9 percent decrease in the untrained one. This difference of response between the two groups is statistically significant ($p < .001$). These results seem to be more meaningful than those of Klepping, Didier and Escousse,[8] because, according to the law of initial value,[17] the resting levels of VMA of the untrained being two times those of the trained, the same amount of physical stress will have less effect on that parameter in the untrained group than in the trained one.

The correlations obtained between the resting VMA values and the numerous criterions of the training state (Astrand and Rodahl[1]) being significant in many cases, we have made comparisons between the predictions of maximal oxygen intake from exercise heart rate and from resting urinary VMA values. As illustrated in Figures 16–3 and 16–4, the VMA values obtained at rest before exercise are as precise as heart rate measured at the thirtieth minute of exercise to predict the maximal oxygen intake.

## Conclusions

The following conclusions seem to be justified:

1. At rest, before exercise, the urinary elimination of VMA was less in the trained group than in the untrained one.
2. The standard exercise did not modify significantly the elimination of VMA in either group.

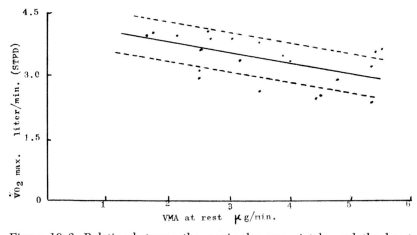

Figure 16–3. Relation between the maximal oxygen intake and the heart rate at the thirtieth minute of the standard exercise and representation of the regression line and the standard error of estimation of maximal oxygen intake from heart rate

r : −0.67

regression equation: Y : −.02X + 6.33

standard error of estimation: 0.3704 liter of oxygen

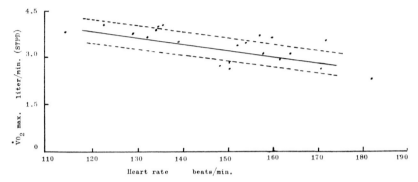

Figure 16–4. Relation between maximal oxygen intake and the urinary elimination of VMA at rest (before exercise) and representation of the regression line and the standard error of estimation of maximal oxygen intake from the values of urinary VMA elimination at rest

r : —0.52

regression equation: Y : —.21X + 4.1872

standard error of estimation: 0.4261 liter of oxygen

3. Urinary elimination of VMA was affected differently by exercise in the trained and in the untrained groups.

4. The prediction of maximal oxygen intake from the resting values of VMA urinary elimination seems as precise as prediction from the heart rate during the standard exercise, this within the limits of this study.

## References

1. Astrand, P.-O., and Rodahl, K.: *Textbook of Work Physiology.* New York, McGraw-Hill, 1970.
2. Elmadjian, F., Lamson, E.T., and Neri, R.: *J. Clin. Endocr.* 16:222, 1956.
3. Frankenhaeuser, M.: *Försvarsmedicin.* 6:17, 1970.
4. Gray, I., and Beetham, W.P., Jr.: *Exp. Biol. Med.* 96:636, 1957.
5. Guyton, A.C.: *Textbook of Medical Physiology.* Philadelphia, Saunders, 1956.
6. Iverson, L.L.: *The Uptake and Storage of Noradrenaline.* Cambridge, University Press, 1967.
7. Kärki, N.T.: *Acta Physiol. Scand.* 99: Suppl. 132, 1956.
8. Klepping, J., Didier, J.-P., and Escousse, A.: *Revue Suisse de Médecine Sportive.* 14:266, 1966.

9. Pascale, L.R. *et. al.: Hum. Biol.* 28:165, 1950.
10. Renton, G.H., and Weil-Malherbe, H.: *J. Physiol.* 131:170, 1956.
11. Schoeman, J.H.: *The Catecholamine Excretion during Rest, Maximal and Submaximal Exercise in Active, Semi-active and Sedentary Subjects.* M.A. Thesis, Physical Education, 1968, University of Alberta, 58 pp.
12. Sunderman, F.W., Jr. *et al.: Amer. J. Clin. Pathol.* 34:293, 1960.
13. Van Den Bossche, F., and Marneffe, O.: *Sport.* 11:176, 1968.
14. Vendsalu, A.: *Kgl. Fysiograf. Sällskap. Lund. Fors.* 29:45, 1959. *Chem. Abstracts.* 54:9048d, 1960.
15. Von Euler, U.S., and Hellner, S.: *Acta Physiol. Scand.* 22:161, 1951.
16. Von Euler, U.S., Hellner-Björkman, S., and Orwen, J.: *Acta Physiol, Scand.* 33: Suppl. 118, p. 10, 1955.
17. Wilder, J.: *Ann. N.Y. Acad. Sci.* 98:1211, 1962.

# Chapter 17

# Effect of an Anabolic Steroid at the Molecular Level

M.E. Houston

G.T. Tomlinson

## Abstract

Studies were undertaken to determine the site of action of the anabolic steroid Danabol (Methandrostenolone) at the molecular level. Initial studies were carried out using male Wistar rats. Blood analyses indicated that Danabol-treated rats had increased serum glutamic oxalacetic transaminase (SGOT) activities. Furthermore, incubation of serum from untreated rats with Danabol did not alter SGOT activities, nor did Danabol alter the activity of isolated glutamic oxalacetic transaminase.

Subsequent experiments were undertaken to determine whether Danabol influenced adenyl cyclase in rat liver and muscle in a manner analogous to natural hormones. Results of these studies indicated that Danabol had no effect on rat liver and muscle adenyl cyclase.

The use of anabolic steroids by athletes has become a topic of widespread concern to many people associated with sport. Recently, the physicians who comprise the National Collegiate Athletic Association Committee on Competitive Safeguards and Medical Aspects of Sports have condemned their use by athletes.[9]

Danabol (Methandrostenolone) has found extensive application as a therapeutic agent in the management of a wide variety of disorders characterized by protein depletion. Clinical use of Danabol resulted in a decrease in urinary nitrogen, induced bromsulphalein retention,[7] excretion of 17-ketosteroids and 17-hydroxycorticosteroids[5] and increased serum transaminase activity, notably serum glutamic oxalacetic transaminase (SGOT).[5,6,11,13]

In the past few years, countless studies employing catecholamines and other hormones have provided evidence for a hypothesis concerning a two messenger system for the action of hormones.[12] Varied stimuli acting on the endocrine glands elicit specific hormones. The hormone, or first messenger, acts on the cells of the target organ, specifically on an enzyme in the cell membranes of the target tissue. The enzyme, called adenyl cyclase, acts on ATP and produces a compound known as cyclic AMP. The cyclic AMP is the second messenger and elicits the required response in the particular tissue. So rapid has data accumulated implicating cyclic AMP as an intermediate in the action of hormones that it is now conceivable that the biological effects of a wide variety of pharmacological agents may be soon understood in terms of cyclic AMP action.[3]

The purpose of this investigation was to examine the effects of Danabol at a molecular level. Initial studies concerned the effects of Danabol on rat SGOT activity. Subsequent experiments were designed to determine whether Danabol acts via a cyclic AMP mechanism.

## Method and Materials

Male Wistar rats (200 to 250g) were divided into a control and a Danabol-treated group. Both groups were fed Purina Rat Chow *ad libitum,* while the Danabol-treated rats received daily 250 micrograms of Danabol, fed orally.[4] Blood samples were taken by cardiac puncture, and analyzed for their SGOT activity by a spectrophotometric procedure proposed by Amador and Wacker.[1] Purified pig heart glutamic oxalacetic transaminase, a product of Mann Research Laboratories, New York, was employed to determine the effect of Danabol on the isolated enzyme.

Rat liver and gastrocnemius muscle cell membranes were isolated and purified according to the procedure of Neville.[10] Adenyl cyclase was assayed by the method of Bär and Hechter.[12] Adenyl cyclase activity is expressed as percent conversion of

ATP-$\alpha$-[32]P to [32]P-cyclic AMP per milligram of cell membrane protein per milliliter of cell membrane suspension per twenty minutes of assay time. Protein was determined by the Lowry procedure[8] with crystalline bovine albumin as standard.

## Results and Discussion

The initial experiments were designed to indicate whether the Danabol-produced changes in SGOT levels were due to a steroid-induced increase in the SGOT activity, or rather were due to either increased synthesis of the enzyme or decreased breakdown of existing enzyme. As shown in Table 17-I, Danabol-treated rats had significantly higher SGOT values than the untreated rats. However, addition of Danabol to the assay mixture did not increase the enzyme activity. Furthermore, when purified pig heart glutamic oxalacetic transaminase was assayed alone, and in the presence of Danabol, there was no increase in the activity of the enzyme.

TABLE 17-I
EFFECT OF DANABOL ON RAT SGOT

| | Sgot Concentration $\Delta$ $O.D_{340}$ per minute $\times$ 100 | |
| Diet | No Danabol | Danabol Incubation |
|---|---|---|
| Normal | $5.9 \pm 1.1$ | $5.7 \pm 1.3$ |
| Normal Plus Danabol | $7.8 \pm 1.5$ | $7.5 \pm 1.7$ |

Concentration of SGOT measured as the rate of disappearance of absorption at 340 nm
Values expressed are Means $\pm$ 1 S.D. for six assays

Thus Danabol does not appear to influence enzyme activity *per se*, but must somehow increase the synthesis of new SGOT, or retard the degradation of preexisting glutamic oxalacetic transaminase.

In view of the well-documented evidence for an adenyl cyclase mechanism for the action of many hormones,[3] further studies were performed on the rats to determine whether Danabol acts by a similar mechanism. Adenyl cyclase assays were performed on homogenates obtained from the liver and gastrocnemius muscle of both the control and Danabol-treated rats.

$10^{-2}$M sodium fluoride, known to produce immediate and drastic changes in adenyl cyclase activity, was added to one of the four assay mixtures.[2] In addition, Danabol and sodium fluoride were added together to determine if the effects produced by one could be influenced by the presence of the other.

As shown in Table 17-II, the Danabol (20 micrograms) alone had no significant effect on the activity of the adenyl cyclase obtained from either rat liver or muscle. Furthermore, NaF produced the typical response with both tissues. When both Danabol and NaF were incubated in the assay mixture anomalous results were obtained. While there was no change in the effect of the NaF on the adenyl cyclase of rat liver, an appreciable decrease in the response of the muscle adenyl cyclase

TABLE 17-II
EFFECT OF DANABOL ON RAT LIVER
AND MUSCLE ADENYL CYCLASE

| Tissue | Diet | Control | Danabol Incubation | NaF Incubation | NaF + Danabol Incubation |
|---|---|---|---|---|---|
| | | | *Adenyl Cyclase Activity Percent Conversion per mg Protein per ml per 20 Minutes* $\times$ *100* | | |
| Muscle | Normal | $0.3 \pm 0.08$ | $0.4 \pm 0.02$ | $2.5 \pm 0.4$ | $1.8 \pm 0.6$ |
| | Normal Plus Danabol | $0.3 \pm 0.05$ | $0.3 \pm 0.04$ | $2.6 \pm 0.6$ | $1.9 \pm 0.5$ |
| | Normal | $2.0 \pm 0.8$ | $2.2 \pm 1.1$ | $12.5 \pm 3.3$ | $12.6 \pm 3.5$ |
| Liver | Normal Plus Danabol | $1.9 \pm 0.9$ | $1.8 \pm 1.2$ | $14.0 \pm 3.4$ | $13.1 \pm 3.9$ |

Values reported are means $\pm$ 1 S.D. for five determinations

to sodium fluoride occurred. This decrease may be due to weak competitive inhibition by the Danabol for the NaF binding site on the enzyme.

The results of this study indicate that Danabol alters the concentration of SGOT in rats. However, the mode of action of Danabol does not appear to involve cyclic AMP.

# References

1. Amador, E., and Wacker, W.E.C.: *Clin. Chem.* 8:343, 1962.
2. Bär, H.P., and Hechter, O.: *Anal. Biochem.* 29:476, 1969.
3. Breckenridge, B.M.: *Ann. Rev. Pharm.* 10:19, 1970.
4. Danabol, from CIBA Pharmaceuticals, Dorval, Quebec.

5. Friis, T.H., and Sparevohn, S.: *Acta Med. Scand.* 180:77, 1966.
6. Johnson, L.C., and O'Shea, J.P.: *Science.* 164:957, 1969.
7. Liddle, G.W., and Burke, H.A.: *Helv. Med. Acta.* 27:504, 1960.
8. Lowry, O.H., Rosenbrough, N.J., Far, A.L., and Randall, R.J.: *J. Biol. Chem.* 193:265, 1951.
9. N.C.A.A. News. 6:11, 1969.
10. Neville, D.M., Jr.: *Biochem. Biophys. Acta.* 154:540, 1968.
11. O'Shea, J.P.: *Nutr. Rep. Int.* 1:337, 1970.
12. Sutherland, E.W., Øye, I., and Butcher, R.W.: *Recent Progr. Hormone Res.* 21:623, 1965.
13. Wynn, V., Landon, J., and Kawerau, E.: *Lancet.* January 14, 1969, p. 69.

Chapter 18

# Comparisons Between Athletes, Normal and Eskimo Subjects from the Point of View of Selected Biochemical Parameters

Robert Carrier
Fernand Landry
Robert Potvin
Claude Bouchard

A scientific approach to training implies the consideration of a matrix of interrelated and complementary factors. The athlete who trains systematically over a number of years mobilizes adaptation mechanisms in rather specific patterns. However it is difficult to differentiate between the relative influence of inherited characteristics and those which might have been brought about by certain habits of life or might result from regular physical training.

The present report deals with only a portion of a broad research project aiming at identifying the physical, physiological and psychological characteristics of athletes of various specialties and of different categories of physically active and physically inactive normal population. More specifically, it purports to analyze observed differences between normal sedentary people, well-trained cyclists and Eskimos from northern Quebec from

*Note:* The authors wish to express their gratitude to the following persons who have contributed to this study: Doctors Paul Bédard, Jean-Marcel Boucher and Pierre Langelier, to MM. Marcel Boulay, Pierre Houde, Marcel Larue, Jean-Claude Mondor, Pierre Savary and to Miss Marie-Christine Thibault.

the point of view of the parameters of total serum cholesterol and immunoelectrophoresis of the serum proteins.

## Methods and Procedures

The data which can be judged useful in the description of physical, physiological or psychological characteristics of normal persons and athletes are obviously many and varied.

General information pertaining to age, sex, family history, description of past and current habits relative to physical activity or training are essential.

A full-scale medical examination including the description of current health and life habits such as diet, sleep, use of tobacco, tranquilizants, stimulants or dietary supplements is also judged essential.

Anthropometric and body measurements (height, weight, surface area, subcutaneous fat, etc.) always with body density are normally included as well as cardiocirculatory and respiratory parameters at rest (hemoglobin, heart rate, blood pressures, heart volume and respiratory profile).

The measurement of the physical working capacity and of its associated variables ($\dot{V}_E$, $\dot{V}_{O_2}$, $\dot{F}_C$, $\dot{V}_{O_2}/\dot{F}_C$), both in relative steady state and in maximal performance, retains our particular attention. Lastly, we normally complete the data with significant serum electrolytes, lipids and enzymes.

In this study we have chosen to illustrate certain biochemical aspects dealing more specifically with serum cholesterol and immunoelectrophoresis of serum proteins.

Five cyclists and four adult Eskimo subjects were used in this study.

The serum cholesterol was determined by the Liebermann-Burchardt reaction[1] consisting in colorimetric reaction resulting from a condensation of the cholesterol molecule at 3′ position in the presence of sulfuric acid, acetic acid and acetic anhydride.

The immunoelectrophoresis was done according to the method of Grabar and Williams[2] modified by Scheidegger.[3] It consists in a starch gel electrophoresis followed by diffusion against antihuman protein serum of rabbit.

## Results

Well-trained individuals, according to their specialty, present many characteristics which distinguish them from normal untrained individuals.

In the case of our cyclists, the serum lipids including the electrophoresis of lipoproteins, and the enzyme profile including the isoenzymes of lactic dehydrogenase, were for the practical purposes comparable to the values normally found in healthy but untrained subjects.

Table 18-I points out the part that it is the aerobic capacity capacity which reveals the well-known organic efficiency of cyclists.

TABLE 18-I

SELECTED PHYSICAL AND PHYSIOLOGICAL VARIABLES
OF THE CYCLIST

| Subjects | Age (Years) | Height (cm) | Weight (kg) | Subcutaneous Fat (%) | $\dot{V}_{O_2}$ Max. | $\dot{V}_{O_2}$ ml/kg | Hb% | Blood Glucose (mg%) |
|---|---|---|---|---|---|---|---|---|
| 0009 | 16 | 186,0 | 85,7 | 6,10 | | | 15,9 | 92 |
| 0006 | 22 | 169,0 | 64,6 | 3,50 | 4,44 | 68,7 | 15,7 | 92 |
| 0012 | 25 | 172,0 | 66,1 | 2,70 | 3,15 | 47,6 | 15,6 | 86 |
| 0011 | 16 | 176,5 | 75,0 | 4,50 | 3,97 | 52,9 | 14,9 | 90 |
| 0010 | 19 | 172,0 | 64,1 | 4,00 | 3,97 | 61,9 | 15,1 | 78 |
| X* | 20 | 175,1 | 71,1 | 4,16 | 3,88 | 57,7 | 15,4 | 88 |

*Mean

The serum cholesterol levels measured in this study indicated that both the athletes and cyclists stayed within the normal expected range, i.e. between 140 and 200 mg%. However Table 18-II reveals a tendency for the athletes to have values slightly lower than those of the two other groups.

TABLE 18-II

RANGE OF THE SERUM CHOLESTEROL LEVELS

| Groups | Age Range (Years) | Serum Cholesterol (mg%) |
|---|---|---|
| Normal People | 15 to 60 | 140 to 260 |
| Athletes | 16 to 25 | 153 to 184 |
| Eskimos | 23 to 38 | 182 to 254 |

Table 18-III illustrates the fractions of the classical immuno-electrophoresis which showed the most noticeable variations. Figure 18–1 illustrates one immunoelectrophoresis from the

TABLE 18-III
SEMIQUANTITATIVE VARIATIONS OF SERUM PROTEINS
AS REVEALED BY IMMUNOELECTROPHORESIS

| | Groups Studied* | | |
|---|---|---|---|
| Protein fractions | Normal | Athletes | Eskimos |
| IgG | → | ↑ | ↑ |
| IgA | → | ↑ | ↑ |
| IgM | → | ↑ | ↑ |
| Haptoglobin | → | ↑ | → |
| Other Fractions | → | → | → |

* Legend: → Normal
      ↑ Higher values

serum of an Eskimo subject. The normal standard appears at
the lower part of the figure. It can be clearly noted that the
three main immunoglobulins IgG, IgA and IgM are definitely
augmented in the Eskimo subject. The high occurrence of both
acute and chronic infections of the respiratory tract in the
Eskimo population of northern Quebec may account for this
fact.

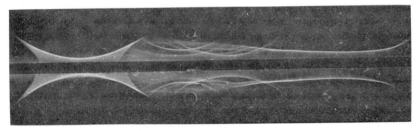

Figure 18–1. Immunoelectrophoresis of an Eskimo's serum ( #232–6).

Figure 18–2 illustrates an immunoelectrophoresis obtained
from the serum of one athlete. An evident hyperglobulinemia
implying fractions IgG, IgA and IgM as well as haptoglobin

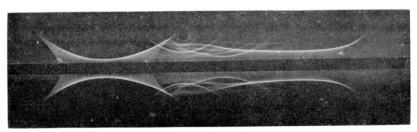

Figure 18–2. Immunoelectrophoresis of a cyclist's serum ( #242-B).

can be seen. The case history of the athletes failed to show evidence of infectious diseases, liver pathology or dysproteinemia which could account for the noted augmentations of the globulin fractions. As concerns the fraction haptoglobin, we could not find evidence of an inflammatory state or condition which could account, as would traditionally be expected, for the augmentation.

## Discussion

### 1. Serum Cholesterol

The serum cholesterol levels observed in our athletes and Eskimo subjects were situated within the normal limits generally accepted. The values of the five cyclists were however lower than those of the Eskimos. The application of the Mann-Witney U test[4] for nonparametric statistics showed that the observed difference was statistically significant ($p = 0,008$).

### 2. Immunoelectrophoresis

One would be tempted to relate the hyperhaptoglobinemia of the athlete, if it were not associated to an augmentation of the immunoglobulin fractions, to a certain amount of purely physical hemolysis, not yet resorbed, and resulting from the aggression of training. Also feasible would be a relative shortening of the life of the erythrocytes which could lead to an important resorption of plasma hemoglobin.

However, we should not discard the hypothesis of a simple mechanism responsible for both the hyperhaptoglobinemia and the hyperimmunoglobulinemia, an account of the importance of the maintenance of the equilibrium of the autoantibodies. Obviously, an athlete in training improves the function of his tissues and of his organs ultimately manifested in a physiological hypertrophy of the target-organs.

Volume increments of tissues and organs must involve their glycoprotein supports as well as the globulins previously mentioned. In this manner the need for the maintenance of the equilibrium of the autoantibodies could account for the hypertrophy of the globulin support without modifying the overall aptitude to immunity.

## References

1. Cook, R.P.: *Cholesterol*. New York, Academic Press, 1958.
2. Grabar, P., and Williams, C.A., Jr.: *Biochim. Biophys. Acta.* 10:193, 1953.
3. Scheidegger, J.J.: *Int. Arch. Allerg.* 7:103, 1955.
4. Siegel, S.: *Nonparametric Statistics for the Behavioral Sciences*. New York, McGraw-Hill, 1956.

# B. PSYCHO—SOCIOLOGICAL ASPECTS

# Psychology of the Superior Athlete

BRYANT J. CRATTY

While early philosophical writings concerning broad psychological questions appear in nineteenth century literature, scientific approaches to the study of the superior athlete, using the tools of the behavioral scientists, are primarily found in twentieth century writings. At this date, only a few scientists have even begun to explore this potentially useful, but extremely complex, topic area.

At this point in time I believe it is more correct to talk about the potential of psychological methodology in exploring the parameters which contribute to performance of the superior athlete . . . which suggests that a more appropriate title of this paper might be "Psychology *and* the Superior Athlete," rather than "Psychology *of* the Superior Athlete." An even more correct approach would be to use the plural term "athletes" rather than the singular, because most of the work carried out to date indicates that superior athletes not only appear in many different somatotypes, but that their psychological makeups also vary to a marked degree.

The interest in the psychology of superior athletes is widespread. For example, at the present time the International Society for Psychology in Sport has a membership of about 1500. Several types of scholars in the countries of the world have focused their interest on the athlete, and at the same time, many types of routes have been taken to illuminate the interactions between athletic performance and various psychological variables. In some countries there has been long-term interest focused upon athletes, by psychologists, marked by fervor and dedication usually seen only in the political arena. In other

189

countries a few psychologists or psychiatrists write in a leisurely way about the psychical states of athletes, with little data to support their often philosophical meanderings.

Within some countries, the United States is one of these, there are relatively few individuals devoting themselves to the study of superior athletes. In this same country a large number are interested in studying various other aspects of motor activity, motor learning and motor development. In other countries, superior behavioral scientists, physiologists, and physicians are in close contact with the coaches of the national teams, and together their constant aim is to elicit better performances from the athletes representing their nation. In many of these latter nations, the study of psychology of sport is often linked with the study of various aspects of bravery and courage which are important to efficient military performance, and also to studies of relationships of exercise and fitness to factory work.

This latter emphasis points to the fact that a study of the various factors impinging upon the superior athlete, and the manner in which the athlete overcomes adversity, also may disclose important information concerning how men and women meet life's stresses in a general way, not just within the sports arena.

As a younger man, I once or twice had speculated (fortunately never in writing) that I was somehow "above" or at least different from philosophers, who seemed to me, at that time, to pour out endless and not very important drivel. More recently, however, I have perhaps matured into the realization that one's philosophical viewpoint either covertly or overtly permeates most of what one does. It is usually best to consciously refer to a set of values prior to embarking on some type of scientific venture, while one is engaged in data collection, and also at the termination of a project.

With this framework in mind I would like to pose several questions to you concerning psychology of the superior athlete.

1. With whose primary welfare in mind should the psychologist carry out his duties? What if the poor mental health of the athlete actually contributes to his performance

while at the same time detracting from his daily relationships with society, his family, and with himself? Should the psychologist attempt to rehabilitate the performer to the detriment of his performance, and perhaps the consternation of his coach? An associated question is, of course, "to whom is the psychologist responsible? . . . his athlete-client, or to the total social subsystem in which the athlete resides?"

2. Should the psychologist be mainly concerned with eliciting maximum performance from a youth, or should he be more responsive to the long-term needs of the individual after his years of competition come to an end?

In addition to such moralistic questions there are others which the behavioral scientist should attempt to deal with when taking the time of athletes and coaches in the execution of research studies. For example:

1. If time is extended for studies of the athletes within a specific setting, just how valid will the findings be in helping both the athletes and coaches within the same setting? How much does the investigator intend to give back to those to whom he has obligated himself. Will the information be extended in a diplomatic manner and in a useable form?

2. Are the frequently encountered one-time studies of athletes, usually a restricted number within a specific setting, really worth carrying out? Can one really generalize from the findings of such a study? Most important, does a study of this nature represent a facet within a total program of research, or is it simply a device through which the psychologist is trying to solve an immediate problem facing him professionally? Or is the personal interest of the scientist only transitory and superficial?

I have not the answers to these queries, for I once read that to appear wise one needs only to pose important questions! At the same time I realize that the present company will be readily able to come to grips with the points I have mentioned.

I also realize that many of you are awaiting more specific answers to questions which concern those who are only beginning to become interested in the psychology of athletes, but whose primary interests lie elsewhere . . . i.e. in the physiological or medical parameters of athletic performance. Your questions are perhaps less philosophical, and more pointed. A scientist accustomed to finding a physiological-neurological mechanism underlying most of the behavior he studies is perhaps already skeptical of anyone engaged in the study of perception or motivation in athletes. It is difficult, of course, to isolate the specific structures within the brain which mediate these rather diffuse human characteristics. Others of you are perhaps cognizant of the various neurological models which attempt to explain human learning; however, if you are deeply enough into the literature, you are also aware that these models are only somewhat poorly-defined theories. They are not viable laws, such as the rather predictable principles which govern the transmission of nutrients through cell membranes, or which predict the manner in which the hydraulics within the cardiovascular system operate in athletes and in nonathletes as they engage in vigorous exercise.

I will thus attempt to briefly summarize in the time left some of the more pertinent findings about superior athletes, to outline some of the ways in which these findings were derived, and finally to illumiate some of the strategies employed by several clinical psychologists when attempting to apply these findings when working with superior athletes.

Much of the following information is contained in a book which I had the pleasure of collaborating on with Miroslav Vanek.* He was the Psychologist for the Czechoslovakian Olympic Team in 1968, and holds a chair in Sports Psychology at Charles University in Prague.

The history of experimental studies in the psychology of sport began in the 1920's when laboratories in Russia were established. During the past fifty years, studies in Eastern Europe as well as

---

* To be truthful, I acted as Dr. Vanek's transcriber and typist, while the primary content is from his research, clinical experiences, and theoretical postulations.

in other parts of the globe have continued to explore various aspects of the subject. Some of the experimental strategies employed have included:

1. Investigations of the type in which various performance tests conducted in laboratories and in the field predict athletic performance.
2. Studies of the personal attributes which seem to be prevalent within a group of athletes engaged in specific sporting activity.
3. Studies of the perceptual as well as the motor attributes of athletes, and their relationship to superior performance.
4. Investigations of some of the social psychological attributes within sports groups competing internationally.
5. Investigations of the manner in which the athlete may activate or deactivate himself prior to top-flight competition. Perhaps protocol used in these studies will be clearer upon reviewing some of the following slides.

The results of these and other investigations suggest that the following major findings are reasonably valid at the present time:

1. There appears to be no singularly identifiable "athletic type" of personality. Rather, the data available indicate that within specific events or types of events there are common types of personality traits found in groups of superior athletes. For example, there seems to be a common group of personality traits associated with events involving hard physical contact with others (wrestling or linemen in American football) just as another complex of personality traits seems common to individuals engaging in the aesthetic events of free-exercise gymnastics and figure skating.
2. Based upon some emerging data, one is able to develop a general topology of sport activities based upon the type of stress inherent in the performance of each activity. Vanek has developed a five-category classification, with subcategories including sports in which injury or death are possible, those requiring total body coordination, those in which a single burst of power is important, those involving only

hand-eye coordinations, and sports in which one must antici-
pate the movements of another individual(s). It is obvious
that several sports combine one or more of the classifications
of attributes.

3. Athletes can be aided in improving performance by expos-
ing them to techniques intended to either activate them or
calm them down to the levels of arousal needed to perform
their event in an optimal manner.

4. The motives for just why superior athletes strive with the
vigor they do, are varied. To work well with a superior
athlete, a clinician must attempt to employ a variety of
tools with which to assess his value system. Complicating
the matter is the fact that a single value or group of values
may at a given moment impinge upon the athlete's performance. A different value or group of values may, at
another time prompt him to perform well.

5. Acquainting athletes with the intellectual components of
the events in which they are to participate should prove
helpful. These cognitive elements may include knowledge
of their unique psychological and physiological makeups,
knowledge of the unique strategies and/or mechanics of
the skills they are to master, as well as the potential social-
cultural forces which are likely to impinge upon them prior
to competition.

6. Potentially useful for coaches training athletic teams, is
an attempt to duplicate the psychological stresses as far as
possible in practice, which the same teams are likely to
encounter in competition. These stresses may be introduced
in the form of crowd noise, unusual or expected competitive situations as well as various "catch-up" or "hand-on"
problems encountered by "front-runners" (or swimmers)
or those holding back within individual racing competitions.

7. Assessing the potential of athletes through relatively
simple and standard laboratory tests of various kinds is
not very helpful in predicting their performance under
complex competitive conditions. Studies have shown that

complex field tests similar to the sport abilities they must later evidence are more helpful in this regard.

There are, of course, further problems in attempting to relate research findings of this type to the realities of sports competition. For example, the criterion a psychologist uses to label his subjects "athletes" within his investigation, may not be the criterion used to select the individuals for a team competing for national honors. At the same time the language used by the psychologist in explaining his findings may prove difficult for some members of the coaching fraternity to interpret.

It is difficult to decipher why professional team members, upon whom millions of dollars are spent, and amateur teams competing within international competitions, do not have the benefit of consultation with a psychologist or psychiatrist when the unusual pressures to which they are subjected become too great to bear. Within the professional organization it would seem to be good business, while within the amateur Olympic ranks it would appear to be not only humane, but should also contribute to the superior performances usually desired by the country's inhabitants who sponsor the teams with their tax dollars or out of their personal pocketbooks. Yet in 1968 in Mexico City, only two psychologists were officially assigned to national teams, and one of these appeared only a few days before the competition, to test athletes the evening before each competed.*

Most important is the general consensus of opinion that the most productive team of scientists within an athletic team consists of the triad of coach, physician (physiologist), and psychologist. It is hoped that this type of potentially fruitful model for action, in the years ahead, is seen to an increased degree within superior sports groups.

### References

1. Beisser, Arnold R.: *The Madness in Sports.* New York, Appleton-Century-Crofts, 1967.

* The second was Professor Vanek who had worked continuously with the Czech team for three years prior to competition, accompanying them on two previous training expeditions to Mexico City's high climate.

2. Kenyon, Gerald (Ed.): *Proceedings of the Second International Congress for Sports Psychology*. Washington, D.C., Athletic Institute, Chicago, Illinois, October, 1968.
3. Knapp, B.: *Skill in Sport*. London, Routledge & Kegan, 1963.
4. Scott, Jack: *Athletics for Athletes*. Hayward, California, Quality Printing Service, 1969.
5. Vanek, Miroslav and Cratty, Bryant J.: *Psychology and the Superior Athlete*. London, Macmillan, 1970.

# Chapter 20

# Race and Sport in Canada

GARRY SMITH
CARL F. GRINDSTAFF

In the past, Canadians have taken pride in the assertion that minority group relations in their country were much better than the racial situation which prevailed in the United States. Prejudice and discrimination against minority groups were less common in Canada because of the more "mature and civilized" outlook of the economic, political, religious and social groups of the society. In recent years, however, this contention that minority groups in Canada are treated in a more equitable manner than in the United States has come under severe attack, especially in regards to racial minorities such as Indians and blacks. As one West Indian said in Toronto: "The fundamental difference between Canada and the United States *vis a vis* the black man is not that you are less prejudiced—you just have fewer black people."[5]

There are indeed broad structural differences in black-white relationships when comparing Canada and the United States. Absolute numbers and proportions, historical backgrounds, socio-economic positions, concentrations of population—all make meaningful comparisons very difficult. For these and other reasons, little research has been undertaken to examine the extent of prejudice and discrimination against blacks in Canada. We feel, however, that such research can and should be undertaken and valid comparisons made if the findings of investigations can be generalized to both countries. In this paper, we intend to make such an examination employing both objective and subjective criteria in one general area of Canadian life, sports, and in one specific sport, professional football. The objective is two-fold. First, we desire to determine, irrespective of comparisons with the United States, if prejudice and discrimination do exist in Canadian football, both on and off the field. We then want to find if our results can be applied to other institutions in Canadian society. Secondly, we want to compare Canada to the United States, using professional football as the bench mark.

Two recent books have documented in a thorough manner the extent of prejudice and discrimination in the United States against the black athlete, particularly football players. These two works are: Jack Olsen, *The Black Athlete*[4] and Harry Edwards, *The Revolt of the Black Athlete*.[1] We will use some of the same techniques and variables that they did in illustrating the situation—i.e. team roster, "stacking," and central vs. noncentral positions. In addition, we interviewed several players, both black and white, and we will discuss the subjective perceptions of the situation in Canadian football from the point of view of both races. As W. I. Thomas indicated, the perception of a situation and how individuals define that situation (even when the perception of the situation is not an accurate one from an objective standpoint) has very important consequences for concomitant and future attitudes and behavior.[6]

In our opinion, the importance of this paper is quite evident. In sports, it is presumably the individual's skills, or more accurately, the quality of his performance, that is the criterion for judgment as to whether or not he "makes the team." Unlike many other performances in society, the quality of a professional football athlete's performance is subject to rather precise quantification—speed, points, completions, receptions, interceptions, yardage, etc. Thus, if prejudice or discrimination on the basis of race exists in the area of sports where quality is somewhat measurable and all important, we might assume that such findings would be an indication of similar attitudes and behavior patterns in the society as a whole where quality of performance is not measured quite so easily or precisely.

This is not to say that quality in a sports performance is completely standardized, nor that quality in other fields such as teaching, sales, acting, etc. are completely unstandarized—only that in comparison to many other occupations in the society, it is easier to determine the quality of the participant in a sporting

event. In addition, a team sport such as football requires cooperation between individuals on the same team as well as competition
against another team. In some ways, the competitive-cooperative
aspects of team sports parallel the type of society we live in. If
race is found to be a discriminating criterion on the athletic field,
it is likely to be an important factor in other areas of the society.

## Methods and Materials

Erland[2] estimates that there are between 75,000 and 100,000
blacks in Canada today. This would place the percentage of
blacks in the total population somewhere near one-half of one
percent. This estimation takes into account a certain percentage
of people who racially are Negro, but who chose to report themselves to census enumerators under a different label. Although
only an approximate number of the Negroes in Canada is known,
the point to be made is that they represent currently a very small
part of the country's total population.

There are few Negroes in Canadian sports, but more than
their numbers in the population would indicate. This is because
most black athletes in Canada come from the United States.
There are a few native born Negro Canadians who have achieved
fame in the international sports world, the most prominent being
Harry Jerome (a world class sprinter from 1960–68) and
Ferguson Jenkins (an outstanding baseball pitcher for the
Chicago Cubs of the National League). As mentioned, the great
majority of Negro athletes in Canadian sport are American
citizens who are brought in by sports promoters to play some
professional sport. Of the three main professional sports in
Canada, only professional football has a large number of black
athletes. In the 1969 season, approximately one-sixth of all the
players in the Canadian Football League were Negro. Because
of this significant representation of the black athletes in the
C.F.L., this study is confined to this group.

First of all, it must be recognized that the sport of Canadian
professional football is largely controlled by Americans. Six of
the nine general managers are American as are all nine head
coaches and thirty-one of the thirty-two assistant coaches. When

the point of American control is mentioned, it is not thought of in terms of economic control (all teams are Canadian owned either by persons of wealth as in Montreal and Ottawa, or by the community as is the case for teams in the Western Conference), but more in the sense of control of the day to day operations of the teams. The management people who are in closest contact with the players are the coaches and general managers, the majority of whom are Americans.

One of the major effects of this American monopoly in the C.F.L. is that the American system is applied to a Canadian sport. The American system of training has large budgets and a reservoir of manpower from which to draw, and as a result is highly regarded for producing top caliber football players and coaches. However, built into the system are attitudes of the society, and in relation to minority group players, this is expressed in the social problems of prejudice and discrimination.[1,3] Thus, one might assume that with American coaches and general managers predominating in the C.F.L. that the situation concerning prejudice and discrimination in Canadian football would be similar to the situation in American college and professional football.

This leads to the formation of the first major hypothesis:

1. Negroes on C.F.L teams will be subject to the same occupational discrimination practices that exist on professional football teams in the United States. We refer to the specific discriminatory practices (a) the quota system, i.e. only so many members of a minority group allowed; (b) stacking, i.e. playing minority players only at certain positions and having them compete with each other; (c) concentration at "noncentral" positions and (d) no access to the league's "power structure," i.e. coaching and managing.

The question of social discrimination against black athletes in Canada will also be examined. As indicated in the introduction, Canadians have a reputation of being tolerant and liberal toward Negroes. This reputation dates back to the mid-eighteen hundreds when Canada was a haven for runaway slaves from the United States. In some circles, Canada is looked upon as a country "in contrast to the United States, that is unfettered by the chains of racial injustice."[7] The consensus seems to be that discrimination against Negroes is not a major social problem. It may exist to some degree, but the situation in Canada is better than in the United States.

In Canada, the general climate which can lead to discrimination against blacks is difficult to ascertain for it can be shown by example that it ranges from perceived equality to severe oppression. There is the case of Toronto Argonaut footballer Dave Raimey who states: "I've never been happier in any city in the United States or Canada. I haven't experienced a single case of blatant discrimination during the six months I've lived in the city. I'm comfortable here."[7] In contrast to this situation is the blemish of Africville, the black shanty town of Halifax. Although on a smaller scale, it was Canada's Newark.

In all likelihood, the degree of racial discrimination that is experienced by the average Negro in Canada lies somewhere between these two extremes. In a positive sense, it is noted that Canada has been relatively free of black militancy, although there has been recently a vocal minority contending that Canada is as racist as any other Western country.[8] Rarely, however, have there been altercations or even vociferous protests on the part of blacks in Canada. This could mean that blacks feel that they are treated with relative dignity and equanimity in Canada, or it may merely mean that there are so few blacks in Canada and they are so geographically scattered, that they have failed to unify and present grievances with a common voice. It is known that groups such as the Canadian Civil Liberties Association and the Ontario Human Rights Commission are working industriously in an effort to combat any racial discrimination that may exist. So far, their efforts have met with some success, particularly with landlords and employers.

On the other hand, blacks are limited professionally and socially. Frequently, they must take jobs that are beneath their education and training levels.[7] Many social and athletic clubs bar blacks and there are still many landlords who have rented their apartments "a few moments ago" when blacks apply. There is not a great deal of exaggeration in the statement once made by Sammy Davis, Jr.[7] in referring to the black Canadian male: "In Canada, you're born a Pullman Porter and you die a Pullman Porter."

Perhaps Canadian whites have been too smug and self-satisfied in their outlook toward blacks. Few Canadian racial problems come to the attention of the mass media. For example, the Human Rights Commission in Ontario settles most racial discrimination cases out of court and they refuse to publicize their activities in the areas of prejudice and discrimination. As a result, many Canadians are content to congratulate themselves on their humanistic outlook toward blacks. Unfortunately, self-pride is not a precise gauge for measuring the scope of this problem. Very few Canadians have been placed in a position where they have had to make a decision which has affected a black person, e.g. should I hire him? Should I rent to him? Should I let him take out my daughter? It would be interesting to see if their actual behavior was related to their vocal pronouncements.

At least two black Canadians are of the opinion that Canada's liberal label when applied to her treatment of Negroes is a myth. Campbell[7] claims "that black people in Canada are suffering from white tokenism. This society is basically racist." Koné sums up the racial situation in Canada as seen through the eyes of blacks when he states: "It's always lurking there in the background. You can't see it and it strikes you when you least expect it. It's subtle."[7]

This leads to the formulation of our second hypothesis:

2. Negroes on C.F.L. teams will be confronted with various types of social discrimination. The forms of social discrimination may not be as numerous, nor the extent as severe as those documented for black athletes in the United States[1,3] nevertheless they will exist. We refer particularly to the following discriminatory practices: (a) restricted housing, (b) bans on interracial dating, (c) lack of occupational opportunities to further themselves outside of professional football, and (d) restrictions on joining social and athletic clubs.

## Results and Discussion

An examination of the nine C.F.L. team rosters during the period 1954–69, revealed the following information.

a. The number of Negroes in the league has risen from a low of twelve in 1955 to a high of fifty in 1969. There is some conjecture as to why the number of black athletes has increased so remarkably. The most logical reasons appear to be:

(i) The total number of United States imports allowed per team has increased from eight to fourteen.

(ii) During this fifteen year period there have been many outstanding black football players in the C.F.L., to some extent their outstanding play has paved the way for the increased numbers.

(iii) There is a greater social awareness on the part of coaches, managers, and fans, as a result there is a more liberal racial climate now as compared to fifteen years ago.

b. Very few teams have more than six blacks on their mid-season roster. The usual number is four or five. The teams that have had the largest number of black players on their teams over the years have been the Eastern conference teams, Toronto, Montreal and Hamilton. The teams with the fewest number of black players have been the Western Conference teams, Regina, Winnipeg and Vancouver. Ottawa, Calgary and Edmonton lie between the two extremes.

It appears that all C.F.L. teams at one time or another have restricted the number of black players. Recent indications are that this may be changing, as black players are coming into the league in greater numbers.

The reason for the discrepancy in numbers of black football players between the east and the west is not known. There are two schools of thought on the question. One school is of the opinion that difference in numbers is strictly a function of the racial attitude of the particular coach and general manager. A city like Regina is cited, which had black baseball players in the forties and early fifties, but it wasn't until 1956 that they had a black football player. Thus it appears that a lack of black players on the team isn't related to the city, rather it is the product of a racist management.

The other school of thought contends that the larger cities in the league have more Negroes, that they are more cosmopolitan, that it is easier for Negroes to assimilate or, if you will, easier for them to hide. This being the case, the management of the big-city teams are less inhibited about bringing in black football players.

c. Negroes are concentrated at the positions of offensive halfback, offensive end and defensive halfback. In terms of the categories used by Loy and McElvogue[3] in their analysis of racial segregation the United States pro-football these positions would be classified as noncentral. On the other hand, there have been very few Negroes in the central (and therefore more important) offensive positions of quarterback, center and offensive guard.

Defensively the placement of black athletes at noncentral positions was not substantiated, as black players were not underrepresented in the central linebacker positions.

d. There was no indication that stacking was a major problem in the C.F.L. This is probably due to the constitutional limitations on the number of American players allowed per team. Teams generally bring in a large number of black and white American players to try for certain positions and yet they can retain only fourteen. If stacking is a problem it is just as much for American whites as it is for blacks, and in this regard is a form of American-Canadian discrimination rather than white vs. black.

e. Perhaps the hottest racial issue of all is the black athletes have been denied access to the power structure of the C.F.L. The meager total of two assistant coaches (only one currently active) is the extent of their representation. Exclusion on the basis of lack of qualification does not appear to be justified.

## Interview Analysis Summary

### *Black Football Players*

The black players felt that the Canadian racial situation was slightly better than the United States. They still, however, experienced prejudice and discrimination, both on and off the field. Specifically, they saw quota systems and stacking as methods to limit black participants in the C.F.L. They expressed bitterness that white players were able to obtain better jobs while playing football even though they weren't necessarily better qualified. They especially felt that black players were treated unfairly when it came to employing them in the league's power structure. To a man they felt they were short-changed.

### *White Football Players*

The white players were of the opinion that the racial scene in Canada was much quieter than in the United States. They did feel, however, that there was some obvious discrimination against black football players both off and on the field. They did not come on as strong, obviously, as did the black players in their mention of grievances, but they did feel that the black players were at a disadvantage in trying to make the team, strictly because of their color.

It would appear that the position of the black athlete in the C.F.L. has improved in the past fifteen years, at least on the field. The number of players has increased from fourteen to fifty, they are playing some leadership positions (especially on defense), and many blacks are rated both by the fans and by their teammates as being among the top players in the league. On the other hand, black players are discriminated against both socially and occupationally, and generally are not given equal treatment with the white players. In short, conditions for the black athelete have had some progress, but not to the point where they could be termed satisfactory by any means. From the point of view of the black player, there is still a long way to go.

In translating the black experience in Canadian sport to the larger Canadian society, which is at best a tenuous undertaking, we conclude that although racism is not overtly present to the extent that it is in the United States, the bases for prejudice and discrimination are there in the society, but they are more subtle and they do not often come into the open. Housing problems, employment discrimination, racial slurs, personal acrimony, all of these are documented in our study. However, it would appear that the development of any serious racial problems has been limited, primarily because the black population is so small and dispersed.

## References

1. Edwards, H.: *The Revolt of The Black Athlete.* New York, The Free Press, 1969.
2. Erland, A.: The new blacks in Canada. *Saturday Night,* Jan. 1970, p. 18.
3. Loy, J.W., and McElvogue, J.P.: Racial segregation in American sport. Paper presented at International Seminar on Sociology of Sport in Macolin, Switzerland, Sept. 1969.
4. Olsen, J.: *The Black Athlete: A Shameful Story.* New York, Time-Life Inc., 1968.
5. O'Malley, M.: Blacks in Toronto. In Mann, W.E.: *The Underside of Toronto.* Toronto, McClelland and Stewart, 1970, p. 132.
6. Thomas, W.I., and Znaniecki, F.; *The Polish Peasant in Europe and America.* Chicago, Univeristy of Chicago Press, 1920, vol. 1.
7. *Time,* Special issue on "Black America," Can. Ed., p. 6, April 6, 1970.
8. *Toronto Globe and Mail,* Magazine Section, "The Blacks of Canada— A Special Survey," February 15, 1969.

# Chapter 21

# The Relationship of Need Achievement and Test Anxiety to Performance of Physical Tasks

J.G. ALBINSON

Several studies have been done in the past to show the predictive power of the need: Achievement motive (n Ach) and text anxiety (TAQ) for mental, verbal and paper and pencil tasks.[1,2,6] Under achievement-oriented conditions those who score high on n Ach and low on TAQ will perform better than those who score low on n Ach and high on TAQ with the high high and low low group in between. The effects of n Ach are shown when achievement arousing instructions are given for the task.[2]

Use of sports oriented pictures for assessing n Ach have been reported by Rosenstien[7] and Daugert.[3] Rosenstien's three sport-oriented pictures were too achievement-oriented to gain useful differentiations from the scores. Daugert used two pictures that were event specific (swimming) when she studied the effects of n Ach and TAQ on learning to swim with high school girls. She also used a general sports activity anxiety scale and an event specific (learning to swim oriented) anxiety scale.

Daugert found event specific n Ach was predictive of amount of learning for S's with no previous swimming ability. Traditional n Ach was not predictive. Both anxiety scales showed inverse relationship with amount of learning.

The purpose of the present study was to determine the relationship of need achievement and test anxiety toward performance of selected sport related physical tasks. Need achievement and text anxiety were assessed in the traditional manner and by use of physical activity oriented pictures and test anxiety questionnaires.

*Note:* This study was partially supported by the U.S. National Institute of Health (Grant No. NIGMS-RGB GM 11266), J.A. Faulkner, Director.

## Methods and Materials

The subjects for this study were forty senior and graduate students at a large midwestern American university. None of the subjects were or had been varsity athletes while at college.

Performance on a six hundred yard run, a basketball lay up test and the end of exercise heart rate in a treadmill test were the physical variables studied.

The psychological data, the six hundred yard run and the basketball lay up test data were collected at one session. Subjects were given the impression that the psychological and the physical parts were unrelated. The end of exercise heart rate data were collected at a second session as part of another study.[4]

The stories for the need achievement test were written under neutral conditions followed by the completion of the test anxiety questionnaires. When the psychological tests were completed the subjects changed to gym clothes and proceeded to the gym in groups of seven where they were given achievement arousing introductions to the physical tasks.

In all cases the basketball lay-up test[5] (two 30-second periods, total number to count) was completed first. All scoring was done by nonsubjects. The six hundred yard run was done in groups of seven.

Each type of n Ach score was obtained from stories written about two pictures. For the assessment of achievement motivation in the traditional manner (n Ach (T)) the pictures used were (a) the "inventors" and (b) "man working at a typewriter with books" (1. p. 832). For the assessment of achievement motivation oriented toward sports (n Ach (S)), the two pictures were (a) a boy standing on a tennis court, with city buildings in the background and (b) two boys leaning backwards over the side of a sailboat traveling at a high speed, with open water and the shoreline in the distance.

The traditional test anxiety score [TAQ (T)] was obtained from the section of the Mandler-Sorason test that deals with group test situations. The sports oriented test anxiety scores [TAQ (S)] were obtained from the test devised by Daugert[3] which was modeled after the Mandler-Sorason test.

The end of exercise heart rates were collected during a tread-mill walk which was conducted in the following manner. All S's started walking on the mill at 4.5 mph and a 5 percent grade for two minutes. The grade was increased 2.5 to 5 percent, de-pending on the S, every two minutes till the S fatigued. The end of exercise heart rate was recorded for the last fifteen seconds of the last minute of the walk.

## Results

As a result of the nonsignificant correlation ($r = -.08$: $p > .25$) between n Ach (T) and n Ach (S) these scored were treated separately. As a result of a significant positive correlation ($r = .55$: $p < .005$) between TAQ (T) and TAQ (S) the total score was used as a single measure of anxiety.

The means, standard deviations and medians were calculated for psychological and physical variables (Table 21-I). A chi square statistic was used to analyze the distributions of fre-quencies of those who scored above and below the median score of each variable. The results are shown in Table 21-II. The distribution of groups based on psychological variables did not differ significantly on the six hundred yard run. There were significant differences on the lay ups and end of exercise heart rate for the TAQ (Tot).

TABLE 21-I
MEANS, STANDARD DEVIATIONS AND MEDIANS FOR
PSYCHOLOGICAL AND PHYSICAL VARIABLES

| Variable | X̄ | S.D. | Median |
|---|---|---|---|
| Achievement Motive (Traditional) | 2.6 | 1.97 | 2.0 |
| Achievement Motive (Sport) | 2.2 | 1.92 | 2.0 |
| Test Anxiety (Traditional and Sport) | 69.5 | 17.62 | 70 |
| 600-yard Run | 106.65 | 21.84 | 106 |
| Lay-up Test | 21.63 | 7.12 | 22 |
| End of Exercise Heart Rate | 193.6 | 12.23 | 195 |

## Discussion

The traditional method of assessing need achievement did not show any predictive ability for the results of the performance on the three physical tasks. The assessment made with the

TABLE 21-II

CHI SQUARE* ANALYSIS OF PERFORMANCE ON SPORT RELATED PHYSICAL TASKS OF SUBJECTS ON MEDIAN SPLITS OF PSYCHOLOGICAL VARIABLES

| | | Lay-ups | | 600-yard Run | | Exercise Heart Rate | |
|---|---|---|---|---|---|---|---|
| | | Good | Poor | Good | Poor | High | Low |
| n Ach | H | 11 | 10 | 12 | 9 | 7 | 10 |
| (T) | L | 9 | 10 | 10 | 9 | 12 | 6 |
| | | $X^2$ = | 0.00 | $X^2$ = | 0.00 | $X^2$ = | 1.38 |
| n Ach | H | 11 | 8 | 8 | 11 | 12 | 4 |
| (S) | L | 9 | 12 | 14 | 7 | 7 | 12 |
| | | $X^2$ = | 0.40 | $X^2$ = | 1.54 | $X^2$ = | 3.67 |
| TAQ | H | 13 | 6 | 11 | 8 | 14 | 5 |
| (Total) | L | 7 | 14 | 11 | 10 | 5 | 11 |
| | | $X^2$ = | 4.91 | $X^2$ = | 0.00 | $X^2$ = | 4.71 |
| | | p = | .10 | | .05 | | .01 |
| | | 1df | 2.71 | | 3.84 | | 6.63 |

* Chi Square with correction for continuity from Siegel, S.: *Nonparametric Statistics.* New York, McGraw-Hill Company, 1956, p. 107.

sport-oriented pictures showed results which were more predictive than the results from the traditional pictures. The results of the lay-up test and the end of exercise heart rate were in the expected direction. The results of the six hundred yard run were in the opposite direction. The lap times for the six hundred yard run may hold the answer for this. Because of the length of the run the motivation factor may be obscured by the endurance factor. Those who scored high on n Ach (S) may have started too fast exhausting themselves before the end of the run thus causing poor times. Those who scored low on n Ach (S) who were not motivated to perform well may have started out at a moderate pace and maintained it throughout the run and thereby turned in better times. A run of a different distance, either shorter (300 yards) or longer (880 yards), may have been able to separate these two factors better.

The end of exercise heart rate was the variable best predicted by the achievement motive. The end of exercise heart rate is an indication of a person's willingness to push himself physically. The measure is not related to the work load except in relation to a person's fitness level. Both fit and unfit persons are capable of reaching high end of exercise heart rates but the unfit would reach it at a lower work load than would a fit person.

There are indications here that an assessment of an individual's need achievement motive by sport-oriented stimulus pictures may also denote an individual's willingness to put out physically.

Because of the significant correlation between the two tests of anxiety an analysis based on the total score was performed. The results showed statistically significant differences on the lay up test and the end of exercise heart rate.

The inability to predict the six hundred yard run results was discussed above. The better performance by the more anxious group may be due to nervous reactions caused by the anxiety. Anxiety, a form of fear, elicits a sympathetic nervous reaction in the body which is the same nervous reaction elicited by physical activity.[8] Thus the individuals assessed as being more anxious about performance of a physical task may be better prepared for the activity than the less anxious individual.

From these results one would expect that those individuals who were high on the sport-oriented need achievement score and high on the total anxiety score would out-perform the other groups and that those individuals low on both scores would perform least well. This was the case for the lay up test and the end of exercise heart rate. (Table 21-III)

TABLE 21-III

PERFORMANCE MEANS OF THE FOUR GROUPS BASED ON THE
SPORT ORIENTED NEED ACHIEVEMENT AND THEIR
TOTAL TEST ANXIETY

| n Ach (S) | TAQ (Total) | Lay-up Test | End of Exercise Heart Rate |
|---|---|---|---|
| | | $\overline{X}$ | $\overline{X}$ |
| High | High | 26.0 | 198.7 |
| Low | High | 25.3 | 192.5 |
| High | Low | 21.5 | 196.4 |
| Low | Low | 17.7 | 187.6 |

On the basis of the data presented it was concluded that:

1. the theory of achievement motivation does have application to performance of physical activity but that the stimulus used in the assessment of the motive must be of a kind that corresponds to the competitive interest of physical activity;

2. anxiety as measured in the study plays a different role in physical tasks than that which it plays relative to mental and paper and pencil tasks.

# References

1. Atkinson, J.W. (Ed): *Motives in Fantasy, Action and Society: A Method of Assessment and Study.* New York, Van Nostrand, 1958.
2. Atkinson, J.W., and Feather, N.T. (Eds.): *A Theory of Achievement Motivation.* New York, Wiley, 1966.
3. Daugert, P.J.: The relationship of anxiety and the need for achievement to the learning of swimming. Unpublished doctoral dissertation, Ann Arbor, University of Michigan, 1966.
4. Faulkner, J.A.: *The Effectiveness of University Physical Education Programs for Men.* Ann Arbor, Michigan, Office of Research Administration, University of Michigan, 1968.
5. Mathews, D.K.: *Measurement in Physical Education,* 2nd ed. Philadelphia, Saunders, 1963.
6. McClelland, D.C., Atkinson, J.W., Clark, Russel, and Lowell, E.L.: *The Achievement Motive.* New York, Appleton-Century-Crofts, 1953.
7. Rosenstien, A.J.: The specificity of the achievement motive and the motivation effects of Picture Cues. Unpublished honors thesis, Ann Arbor, University of Michigan, 1952.
8. Winton, F.R., and Bayliss, L.E.: *Human Physiology,* 5th ed. Boston, Little, Brown and Company, 1962.

# Chapter 22

# Causes and Consequences of Differential Leisure Participation Among Females in Halifax, Nova Scotia

DAVID H. ELLIOTT
JANET E. HOWELL

The present research arises from concern with the general problem of causes and consequences of differential uses of leisure time among Canadians. The problem of leisure in an era of large-scale social, technological, and economic change is rapidly becoming apparent to social scientists as well as to governmental and private agencies. Some of the issues which are involved within the general area of leisure in Canada were reported in *The Proceedings of the Montmorency Conference on Leisure*[5] conducted in 1969.

Our specific concern lies in examining the effects of leisure participation upon mental health—particularly in participation as a mediating variable between socioeconomic status and mental health. Our research is guided by the following model, presented in diagrammatic form in Figure 22–1:

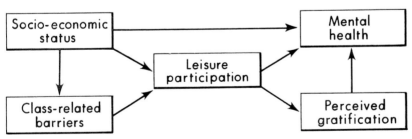

Figure 22–1. A model demonstrating the effects of leisure participation in mental health.

According to this model, class differences in mental health are hypothesized to result in part from class differences in leisure participation. Variation in leisure participation among various socioeconomic strata are predicted to reflect, in part, class-related barriers to participation such as cost. Leisure participation is predicted to be linked to mental health through such mediating variables as self-gratification resulting from profitable use of leisure time.[1]

Our choice of variables for inclusion in the model is influenced by previous studies. Class-related differences in reporting of psychoneurotic symptoms have been previously reported with the general finding that the upper classes are more "healthy" than those in the lower classes.[4,8,10] Participation in various types of leisure activities, including sports, have been reported to reflect socioeconomic status.[2,3,9,11] There is some evidence that a relationship exists between leisure-time use and mental health.[6,7]

This research represents two major departures from previous work. We are just attempting to order our variables to provide a view of the relationship between socioeconomic status and mental health. Secondly, we are focusing upon a subject population previously quite neglected in the field of leisure research. Although young wives and mothers constitute a very large proportion of the total Canadian population, they have been almost totally excluded from reported studies of leisure.

## Methods and Materials

The data reported were obtained as part of a larger study from a sample of 556 married women between the ages of twenty and forty-five residing in Halifax, Nova Scotia. The larger study is entitled "An Analysis of Actual and Desired Utilization of Leisure and Recreational Opportunities in Halifax, Nova Scotia," sponsored by the National Council of the YMCA of Canada, funded by the Federal Department of Health and Welfare, Fitness and Amateur Sport Division, and is under the direction of D.H. Elliott. Quota sampling procedures were used with the city stratified on the basis of census tracts.

Self-administered questionnaires were used for the collection of data. The questionnaires were pretested for reliability and validity and were precoded for convenient conversion to machine-readable form.

## Results

Table 22-I presents the zero-order relationship between socio-economic status and mental health index. The basic finding is a common one. There is a statistically significant linear association between class and mental health, with the lower classes

TABLE 22-I

THE RELATIONSHIP BETWEEN SOCIOECONOMIC STATUS
AND MENTAL HEALTH

| *Mental Health* *Score* | | *I* *(High)* | *II* | Socioeconomic Status *III* | *IV* | *V* *(Low)* |
|---|---|---|---|---|---|---|
| 1 (Low) | | 10 | 24 | 25 | 30 | 52 |
| 2 | | 38 | 27 | 33 | 33 | 25 |
| 3 | | 27 | 21 | 19 | 23 | 9 |
| 4 (High) | | 25 | 28 | 23 | 17 | 14 |
| | *Total* (%) | 72 | 95 | 152 | 136 | 99 |
| | (N) | 100 | 100 | 100 | 100 | 100 |

$X^2 = 47.75$     df $= 12$     p $= .001$

being consistently less healthy than the upper classes. Only 10 percent of Class I women received low mental health scores, compared with 52 percent of those in Class V.

The expected relationship between socioeconomic status and mental health was confirmed. Our major concern, however, was not with the relationship *per se*. Rather, our focus is upon lesiure participation as it intervenes in the relationship between class and mental health.

Explication of the linkages proposed in our model leads to an examination of the relationships between socioeconomic status, leisure participation and mental health. Leisure participation is a multidimensional phenomenon. Limitation of time and space forbid consideration of all its facets. Consequently, we shall here consider only participation in sports activities.

Table 22-II presents the relationship between a sports partici-

TABLE 22-II
THE RELATIONSHIP BETWEEN SPORTS PARTICIPATION
AND MENTAL HEALTH SCORE

| Mental Health Score | | Number of Sports | | | |
|---|---|---|---|---|---|
| | | 0 | 1 | 2 | 3 | 4+ |
| 1 (Low) | | 0 | 1 | 2 | 3 | 4+ |
| 2 | | 34 | 27 | 24 | 16 | 22 |
| 3 | | 23 | 38 | 34 | 34 | 25 |
| 4 (High) | | 27 | 18 | 17 | 23 | 21 |
| | | 16 | 16 | 25 | 27 | 32 |
| | Total % | 100 | 100 | 100 | 100 | 100 |
| | (N) | (88) | (91) | (145) | (106) | (133) |

$$X^2 = 26.18, \qquad df = 12, \qquad p = .05$$

pation scale and mental health. The table indicates that mental health tends to vary with sports participation among women in our sample. For example, 34 percent of those who do not participate are classified as "low" on the mental health dimension, compared with 22 percent of those participating in four or more activities. The table provides some basis for viewing leisure participation as a potential mediator between class and mental health. For participation to intervene between class and mental health, it must be shown that participation is to some degree class-determined.

Table 22-III indicates that there is a significant association between class and sports participation. Those in upper classes are much more likely to participate and to participate in more activities than those in the lower strata.

Since all the above zero-order relationships were found to be statistically significant and in the expected direction, we thus are able to support the hypothesis that leisure participation may

TABLE 22-III
THE RELATIONSHIP BETWEEN SOCIOECONOMIC STATUS
AND SPORTS PARTICIPATION

| Number of Sports | | (High) I | II | III | (Low) IV | V |
|---|---|---|---|---|---|---|
| 0 | | 2 | 8 | 18 | 20 | 21 |
| 1 | | 11 | 15 | 13 | 20 | 21 |
| 2 | | 20 | 24 | 27 | 34 | 22 |
| 3 | | 26 | 21 | 16 | 16 | 22 |
| 4+ | | 44 | 32 | 26 | 10 | 14 |
| | Total (%) | 100 | 100 | 100 | 100 | 100 |
| | (N) | (72) | (95) | (152) | (136) | (99) |

$$X^2 = 52.8, \qquad df = 16, \qquad p = .001$$

mediate the relationship between class and mental health. Before arguing conclusively that such is the case, however, an additional table should be considered.

Table 22-IV presents the conjoint effect of socioeconomic status and sports participation upon mental health. It is apparent that the two-predictor variables operate independently, and to a large extent cumulatively, to influence mental health. For all classes, except V, women who participate in sports have a significantly lower rate of mental symptoms than those who do not participate. Within each participation level, however, class differences in health remain. Women from Class IV who partici-

TABLE 22-IV

CONJOINT EFFECT OF SOCIOECONOMIC STATUS AND NUMBER OF SPORTS ON MENTAL HEALTH (PERCENT LOW MENTAL HEALTH SCORE)

| Number of Sports | Socioeconomic Status | | | | | | | | | |
|---|---|---|---|---|---|---|---|---|---|---|
| | I | | II | | III | | IV | | V | |
| | % | (N) | % | (N) | % | (N) | % | (N) | % | (N) |
| 0 | * | (2) | 37 | (8) | 57 | (28) | 34 | (23) | 47 | (21) |
| 1–3 | 14 | (41) | 23 | (59) | 23 | (85) | 23 | (100) | 51 | (64) |
| 4+ | 3 | (29) | 23 | (30) | 8 | (37) | 28 | (14) | 57 | (14) |

* Percentage not calculated due to small base

pate in four or more activities have a lower proportion of symptom occurrence than women in Class II who participate in no activities, for example.

The previous analysis indicated that an association which existed between class and sports participation helped to explain the link between class and mental health. However, no attempt was made to explain the relationship between class and participation. We shall now attempt to explain this relationship through use of an additional variable—perceived cost of participation as a barrier to participation.

Table 22-V indicates that perceived cost of leisure participation is strongly influenced by socioeconomic status. None of the Class I women perceive cost as a barrier compared with 45 and 44 percent respectively for women from Class III and V. It will be noted from the table, however, that fewer women from Class V consider cost a major barrier than do those from Class IV.

In Table 22-VI data are presented which show that those who perceive cost to be a barrier to leisure participation do, in fact,

TABLE 22-V
THE RELATIONSHIP BETWEEN SOCIOECONOMIC STATUS AND COST
AS A BARRIER TO SPORTS PARTICIPATION

| Cost as a Barrier | Socioeconomic Status | | | | |
|---|---|---|---|---|---|
| | I | II | III | IV | V |
| No | 100 | 64 | 55 | 56 | 66 |
| Yes | 0 | 36 | 45 | 44 | 34 |
| Total (%) | 100 | 100 | 100 | 100 | 100 |
| (N) | (72) | (95) | (152) | (136) | (99) |

$X^2 = 43.88$, df = 4, p = .001

TABLE 22-VI
THE RELATIONSHIP BETWEEN COST AS A BARRIER
AND SPORTS PARTICIPATION

| Number of Sports | Cost as a Barrier | |
|---|---|---|
| | Yes | No |
| 0 | 17 | 8 |
| 1–3 | 68 | 60 |
| 4+ | 15 | 32 |
| Total (%) | 100 | 100 |
| (N) | (244) | (256) |

$X^2 = 22.6$, df = 2, p = .001

participate in fewer sports than those who consider cost to be unimportant.

Turning to Table 22-VII we see the combined effect of class membership and perceived cost upon sports participation. The data indicate that class differences in participation occur in a linear manner only for those for whom cost is not mentioned as a problem. In all social classes except V, however, those who perceive cost as a barrier participate less than those who do not consider cost a problem.

The following analysis attempts to delineate one way in which leisure participation (sports, in this case) may affect mental

TABLE 22-VII
THE CONJOINT EFFECT OF SOCIOECONOMIC STATUS AND COST AS
A BARRIER TO PARTICIPATION ON ACTUAL SPORTS PARTICIPATION
(PERCENT PARTICIPATING IN FOUR OR MORE SPORTS)

| Cost as a Barrier | Socioeconomic Status | | | | | | | | | |
|---|---|---|---|---|---|---|---|---|---|---|
| | I | | II | | III | | IV | | V | |
| | % | (N) | % | (N) | % | (N) | % | (N) | % | (N) |
| No | 46 | (58) | 36 | (58) | 32 | (77) | 13 | (46) | 14 | (21) |
| Yes | 5 | (19) | 29 | (24) | 20 | (62) | 8 | (78) | 14 | (71) |

health. Boredom may represent a state in which free time is seen as being nonproductive or nongratifying by the individual. Perhaps one may not be able to be mentally healthy without believing that his time, both work-time and free-time, are profitably used.

Table 22-VIII presents the relationship between sports participation and boredom. It is evident from the table that the

TABLE 22-VIII
THE RELATIONSHIP BETWEEN SPORTS PARTICIPATION
AND BOREDOM

| Bored | Number of Sports | | |
| | 0 | 1,2,3 | 4+ |
| --- | --- | --- | --- |
| No | 28 | 40 | 50 |
| Yes | 72 | 60 | 50 |
| Total (%) | 100 | 100 | 100 |
| (N) | (83) | (335) | (132) |

$X^2 = 9.83$, df = 2, p = .01

probability of being bored decreases as a function of the number of activities in which our sample is engaged. Thus, 72 percent of those who participate in no sports activities are often bored, compared with 50 percent of those who engage in four or more activities.

Table 22-IX contains data demonstrating an exceedingly strong relationship between boredom and mental health. Fifty-seven

TABLE 22-IX
THE RELATIONSHIP BETWEEN BOREDOM
AND MENTAL HEALTH SCORE

| Mental Health Score | Boredom | |
| | No | Yes |
| --- | --- | --- |
| 1 (Low) | 11 | 57 |
| 2 | 43 | 1 |
| 3 | 15 | 27 |
| 4 (High) | 30 | 15 |
| Total (%) | 100 | 100 |
| (N) | (278) | (211) |

$X^2 = 189$, df = 3, p = .001

percent of those who are bored exhibit low mental health scores compared with only 11 percent of those who are not often in a state of boredom. Similarly, 30 percent of those who are not bored score high on the mental health dimension, while only

15 percent of those who are bored are classified as having a high degree of mental health. We are thus able to conclude that boredom may be a highly important determinant of poor mental health.

Finally, it is important to consider the combined effect of sports participation and boredom upon mental health. Boredom and sports participation exert both an independent and cumulative effect upon mental health. For example, only 7 percent of those who are not bored and who participate in four or more sports are mentally unhealthy as compared with 50 percent of those who are bored and who do not participate in any sports activities.

TABLE 22-X

THE CONJOINT EFFECT OF SPORTS PARTICIPATION
AND BOREDOM ON MENTAL HEALTH SCORE
(PERCENT LOW MENTAL HEALTH SCORE)

| | *Number of Sports* | | | | | |
|---|---|---|---|---|---|---|
| | *0* | | *1–3* | | *4+* | |
| *Bored* | % | (*N*) | % | (*N*) | % | (*N*) |
| Yes | 50 | (56) | 35 | (210) | 30 | (60) |
| No | 29 | (27) | 16 | (124) | 7 | (57) |

**Discussion**

Our study demonstrates that participation in sports is a significant factor in the mental health of a sample of Halifax women. Much, however, remains to be done to gain a fuller understanding of the role of leisure in this regard.

Since our data represent only one point in time, we are not able to determine precise causal sequences. To what extent does sports participation act in a primary capacity to *prevent* the occurrence of psychoneurotic symptoms? Alternatively, how much of the effect of participation is secondary of *therapeutic* acting to reduce symptoms which have previously occurred? Our guess is that sports participation operates at both the primary and the secondary level. However, a thorough test of this hypothesis would require data based upon multiple points in time.

Specific policy implications should await a more thorough and comprehensive analysis. However, since mental health in contemporary society presents an immediate problem, it is obvious that detailed research into the relationship between leisure and mental health should begin at once.

## References

1. Brightbill, C.: *The Challenge of Leisure*. New Jersey, Prentice-Hall, 1960.
2. Eisenstadt, S.: *Explorations in Entrepreneurial History*. Winter Supplement, 1956.
3. Hollingshead, A.B.: *Elmtown's Youth: The Impact of Social Classes on Adolescents*. New York, Wiley, 1959.
4. Langer, S., and Michael, S.: *Life Stress and Mental Health*. New York, Collier-MacMillan, 1963.
5. *Leisure in Canada*. The Montmorency Conference on Leisure. Canada, The Fitness and Amateur Sport Directorate, Department of National Health and Welfare, 1969.
6. Merritt, M.A.: The relationship of selected physical, mental, emotional, and social factors to the recreational preferences of college women. Unpublished doctoral dissertation, Ames, State University of Iowa, 1961.
7. Moore, R.A.: *Sports and Mental Health*. Springfield, Thomas, 1966.
8. Pasamanick, B. *et al.: Mental Health of the Poor*. Riessman, Cohen, Pearl (Eds.). New York, Free Press, 1964.
9. Reich, C.M.: *Socio-economic Factors Related to Household Participation in Community Recreation*. University Park, Pennsylvania State University, 1965.
10. Srole, L., and Langer, T.: *The Sociology of Mental Disorders*, Weinberg, S.K., (Ed.). Chicago, Aldine, 1967.
11. Vaz, E.W.: *The Canadian Review of Sociology and Anthropology* 2, No. 1, 1965.

# Chapter 23

# The Culture of Young Hockey Players:
# Some Initial Observations

EDMUND W. VAZ

**B**ecause young hockey players undergo a recurrent set of relatively common experiences there develops an occupational culture, a system of values, rules and attitudes that helps guide the behavior of players. Although the value system of the larger community tends to subsume the "official" rhetoric of the Minor Hockey League, the informal values, attitudes and customs of the League fit more easily into the general value system of the lower socioeconomic strata. Moreover, boys who remain in Allstar Minor League Hockey likely come from lower socioeconomic levels; this facilitates their adaptation to the role of hockey player, and the acceptance of its values, attitudes and practices.

Older Allstar players (seventeen to nineteen years) often face a conflict between academic and hockey obligations. Problematic academic success, the improbability of a university education, the lack of clear occupational goals, plus the increasing likelihood of being selected for the Junior professional ranks make a professional hockey career appear meaningfully realistic for these boys.

We suggest that physically aggressive behavior is normative, institutionalized behavior, and is learned during the formal and informal socialization of young hockey players. This kind of behavior becomes an integral part of the role obligations of older Allstar players. Intense competition, the injunction to use in-

*Note:* This study was aided by a research grant from the Canada Council for which I am grateful. I am also indebted to Mr. Barry Boddy, my assistant, who helped collect much of the material.

creasingly aggressive means, and the strong motivation to be chosen for the Junior professional ranks are structural conditions which help generate, and differentially account for physical aggression in the league, i.e. among players on higher level teams. These conditions are less applicable to younger boys.

This is a working paper based on my first impressions of data collected during the first stage of a research project among boys aged 8 to 20 engaged in Minor League Hockey* in a medium-sized town in Ontario. Our interest is in the occupational culture of young players, their socioeconomic status, the process of their professionalization, with special consideration given the use of illegal tactics and physical aggression in their role as hockey player. This paper will touch on a few of these points.

### Occupational Culture

Most groups that play together and work together develop a common set of norms (both formal and informal) that helps guide the behavior of their members. There emerges also a set of relatively common values and sentiments that underlies group norms, strengthens group solidarity, and often helps members overcome their everyday occupational anxieties and problems. This is the occupational culture—the group heritage that is transmitted to members. And research has revealed the occupational cultures of boxers, medical doctors, pickpockets, professors, even pot smokers. There is also the occupational culture of young hockey players.

Part of the culture of an occupation is its charter, the more or less formal statement or rhetoric of its objectives and ideals. This resembles an official version of meanings directed towards

---

* Three methods were used to collect the data for this project. First, a portable tape recorder was used throughout one season to gather material in the dressing rooms of teams at all levels in the Minor Hockey League. This involved visiting teams in their dressing rooms before a game, between periods and after a game. Second, a series of partially structured interviews was conducted with players from the Minor and Junior professional leagues. Each interview lasted approximately 1½ hours. Junior professional players were paid five dollars per interview. Third, a questionnaire was designed and data were collected from all players enrolled in the Minor Hockey League.

the representation of a specific image or impression of the group and what transpires within it, and is necessarily couched in abstract terms. It relates the group to the general values of the total community in which it operates, and in turn the group receives the blessings of the community.

In general the rhetoric of Minor League Hockey tends to emphasize the following objectives: to provide exercise, health and recreation for young people; to develop respect for the spirit and letter of the law, to develop sportsmanship and fair play; to develop the qualities of self-discipline and loyalty, and also to develop emotional maturity, social competence and moral character in young boys. This is an imposing list, and any community concerned about its young people would find it hard to reject a group that espouses and publicizes these virtues.

But we know that things are seldom what they seem. Good intentions and purposes are one thing, what transpires in the dressing rooms and on the ice is something else. In the course of reaching objectives and realizing goals social change occurs: original intentions are forgotten, meanings are transformed, short-term goals subvert long-term objectives, strategy replaces ideals. For example, the conceptions of sportsmanship and fair play have different meanings for different age groups. Youngsters think of it as shaking hands after the game and being a good loser. Among older experienced boys on the higher level teams the practice of shaking hands often leads to violence.* Similarly the qualities of sportsmanship and fair play are differentially emphasized in the system. Once boys reach the Bantam level (thirteen or fourteen years) these virtues are nearly dead letters.

Similarly, at the higher levels the value of success, i.e. winning the game, rapidly takes precedence over other considerations among coaches and managers as well as players. Little attention is paid to developing respect for the "spirit and letter" of the normative rules of the game. In fact, at an early age youngsters learn the institutionalized means of violating certain rules, and this becomes routine practice. They learn that there are "good"

---

* In more than one instance the practice of shaking hands after the game had to be discontinued because of the regular outbreaks of violence among players.

and "bad" penalties; the former are tolerated even encouraged, the latter are deplored.

Although the values of the larger community tend to subsume the purposes and ideals of Minor League Hockey, in fact what occurs in the dressing rooms and on the ice, and the informal codes and tactics by which players are controlled and the game conducted, reflect a narrower perspective. Many of the attitudes and values common to Minor League Hockey seem to fit neatly into the general value system of the *lower socioeconomic strata*. We know that there is a relationship between body-contact sports and socioeconomic levels; body-contact sports are correlated with the lower socioeconomic strata.[1] Within Minor League Hockey body contact is a much proclaimed and highly cherished virtue of the sport; it is alleged that to eliminate or seriously reduce the amount of body contact would irreparably damage the sport of hockey.

One of the most closely guarded privileges of the professions is their right to determine the proper training and education for entry into a profession, i.e. before full professional status is granted. Whenever, and in whatever manner, the professional education and training is acquired it may be viewed also as part of the recruit's socialization. Learning the expectations and obligations of the role of hockey player is the process of socialization, and it is an integral part of learning the culture of the occupation. A major function of the socialization of Allstar hockey players in the Minor Hockey League is their preparation for the higher professional ranks. And the standards according to which this training takes place reflect the considerable influence of the higher professional groups on the socialization of young players.

An important subject matter of rules is establishing the criteria for recognizing a true fellow worker, or in this case, a true hockey player. Although technical skills and competence (especially skating and shooting) are necessary features of the role of hockey players they are not sufficient. Justification for the violation of formal rules, such as tripping, elbowing, fighting, use of one's stick in a fight, besides one's attitudes towards courage, toughness, the ability to endure pain, among others, are vital aspects in recognizing the developing professional hockey player. These are not technical skills, but qualities that mirror the internalization of cherished values and the success of the professionalization process.

If the middle-class ethic tends to value the cultivation of patience, the inhibition of spontaneity, self-control and the regulation of physical aggression, then the working class tends to emphasize the spontaneity of behavior; it praises courage, stamina, physical strength and resiliency, and rewards those who "never back down from a fight." Toughness is considered a virtue, and within the working class fighting is often recognized as a moral and legitimate activity in settling disputes. This suggests that the working class both supports the sport of hockey and is supported by it through the relatively common attitudes and general system of values that they share. This overlap in values between the working class and hockey suggests that hockey is likely considered a prestigious occupation and is acceptable to both working-class boys and their fathers. This differential evaluation of occupations will likely influence some individuals to select hockey as a career.

### Socioeconomic Status

All socioeconomic strata are likely represented among the youngest age groups that volunteer to play Minor League Hockey. Although the majority of boys will come from the lower socioeconomic levels, the sons of professionals will also be found. But I believe that the data will show that the majority of boys who *remain* in Allstar Minor League Hockey until seventeen or eighteen years come largely from the working and lower middle classes. Boys from the higher socioeconomic levels drop out of hockey. This implies that the National Hockey League is comprised largely of players from working-class levels.

We know that there exists a strong relationship between the years a boy remains in school and his family's socioeconomic status; sons of the most favored families stay in school longer and more often attend university. Children of less favored families drop out of school earlier, and fewer enroll in university.[2] It may be that as a career hockey becomes a meaningful occupational choice to those boys who contemplate dropping out of high school, or who are doing poorly in school and/or who do not envisage a university career—boys generally from the lower socioeconomic strata. Furthermore, as a career hockey will likely fall within the range of preferred occupational choices of working-class boys, but not those from the higher socioeconomic strata.

An area of particular interest is to study the variables that influence a boy's decision to select hockey as a career. Although a number of variables will operate, such as parental influence (which is apt to be encouraging), a boy's hockey "talent," family tradition, and available alternative work opportunities, there are a number of structural features that strongly corral working-class boys toward a professional hockey career.

By sixteen or seventeen years of age a boy who remains in Allstar hockey has reached the Midget level of the league where the competition becomes intense. It is precisely at this level that boys are scouted and evaluated for advancement to the Junior professional ranks. At this point they identify strongly with their team and are strongly motivated to play in the higher ranks, but the increasingly heavy emphasis on size, toughness, physical strength, aggressiveness and the ability to withstand pain makes conformity to role obligations especially difficult to achieve. Their efforts to conform to these expectations, the intense competition, the risk of being "dropped" from the team, and their desire to reach the Junior professional* ranks comprise a major structural source of anxiety.

At the same time these boys are still in high school where the work is becoming difficult, and successful examination results critical for academic promotion. The conflict of academic expectations and increasingly stringent hockey obligations is a further structural source of strain.† Under these circumstances

---

* The term professional is used since players on Junior A and B teams are paid for their services.

† When seemingly distinct although interrelated groups create conflicting demands on their joint members, sometimes tiny albeit deviant efforts are made by one group to help alleviate the strain. In this case coaches and managers sometimes attempt to get high school examinations postponed or special

many boys will experience academic problems; in any case (and this is important) few boys will envisage a university education. Yet they have now reached a point where they must at least begin to consider their future careers. But academic success is problematic, a university education unlikely, and many will not have any clearcut occupational goal. Moreover, at this time they are continuously preoccupied with hockey and faced with the possibility of being chosen for Junior professional teams. It is at this juncture that hockey as an occupational career will appear more meaningful and attractive to them, precisely because it has become a realistic possibility. Once they are selected for the Junior professional teams their chances of playing in the higher professional ranks are greatly enhanced.‡

## Fighting and Physical Aggression

Where fighting is found to be a relatively recurrent activity,§ differentially distributed in the system, and assumes much the same form, the sociologist will suspect that it is attributable to some structural condition of the system itself. Explanations that focus on personality defects, faulty control systems or the debilitating childhood experiences of individuals are apt to be by-passed.

conditions arranged for their players. The status of athletics is so high and its influence so pervasive in the high schools that independent of outside pressure players are often given special treatment, consideration and privileges by teachers. This helps players remain in school, play on the team, and also helps reduce strain. In any case at this level few Allstar players are apt to sacrifice hockey for school obligations.

‡ With the slowly increasing number of athletic scholarships a trickle of boys are able to play hockey while attending university. This provides another though longer route towards the professional ranks. One question is: to what extent does playing hockey subvert their desire to complete their education once in university? Is it the university dropout who pursues a professional hockey career? Any large increase in the number of players who proceed to the National Hockey League via the university route must ultimately mean a shorter career for them since they begin later, the National Hockey League schedule is getting longer, and the game has become more physically demanding.

§ It is generally agreed throughout the league that there is more physical aggression at the Midget and Junior professional levels than among the lower level teams.

Sports have traditionally been considered a means of controlling violence. Yet the "routinization of violence" has never been complete. Violence has persistently erupted in the form of rough play and dirty tactics. But this behavior is not necessarily an uncontrolled, spontaneous outburst of physical aggression. Fighting, rough play, and dirty tactics may be normative, expected forms of conduct. I suggest that the larger amount of physical aggression, especially fighting, that occurs at the Midget and Junior professional levels is normative, institutionalized behavior; it is learned during the socialization of the youngster, and it is part of the role expectations of the player. Under certain conditions failure to fight is variously sanctioned by coaches and players. The bulk of fighting can be accounted for according to structually produced strains within the system itself.

If boys are to succeed in professional hockey they are expected to demonstrate hockey "potential" no later than the Bantam level (thirteen or fourteen years).* It is at this level that the criteria for player evaluation gradually undergo change. There is an increased emphasis on body contact ("hitting"); players must be continuously aggressive; physical size becomes a major factor in the selection of players ("a good big man is always better than a good small man"); there is the expectation that a boy "play with pain," and still greater emphasis is placed on winning the game. The ideals of sportsmanship and fair play are soon ignored.*

The influence of the mass media, the selection of professionals as role models, and the formal teaching of coaches are major sources of learning in the socialization of the developing player. As boys progress from the Bantam to Midget ranks (fifteen to seventeen years) the cultural value of winning increases even more. Less attention is paid to the legitimate rules of success. At the Midget level teaching concentrates on the technical aspects of "playing the man" and the subtler methods of "hitting"

---

* Some boys develop more slowly than others and scouts and coaches are alert for "late starters."
This reflects the influence of the higher professional leagues. These criteria are used by professional scouts and mirror the skills, attitudes and values desired by professional teams.

the opposing player and "taking him out." It is perhaps no exaggeration to say that the implicit objective is to put the opposing star player out of action without doing him serious injury. Illegal tactics and "tricks" of the game are both encouraged and taught; rough play and physically aggressive performance are strongly encouraged, and sometimes players are taught the techniques of fighting. Minimal† consideration is given the formal normative rules of the game, and the conceptions of sportsmanship and fair play are forgotten. Evaluation of individual performances (whether deviant or not) is according to their contribution to the ultimate success of the team. Of course certain rule violations are normative, expected. Under such conditions playing the game according to the "spirit and letter of the law" seems meaningless.‡ By the time boys reach the Midget and Junior professional levels dominant role expectations of the hockey player include toughness, aggressiveness, physical strength and size, and the ability to endure pain.§ Gradually the team is molded into a tough fighting unit prepared for violence whose primary objective is to win hockey games.*

Simultaneously, competition intensifies for selection to the Junior professional ranks, and the boys are made patently aware of the spartan criteria for advancement. The obligation to "produce," i.e. to perform in an unrelentingly, physically aggressive manner becomes normative, routine, and substandard

---

† So common is fighting and rough play that the role of "policeman" is common knowledge in the league and is employed by coaches. A "policeman" on a team is a player who is recognized as being especially tough and able to "handle himself." The "policeman" is sometimes used by coaches to "get" an opposing player who is especially rough or "dirty."

‡ The coaches themselves are notorious for violating at least the "spirit of the law." The seemingly innumerable methods they employ to prolong the game or otherwise interfere with the smooth conduct of the game in order to benefit their teams are hardly commendable, nor does it set a good example for youngsters.

§ This does not deny the considerable amount of body contact that occurs among the younger aged boys. Hard body contact is strongly encouraged at the very early stages of development throughout the league.

* Coaches and managers of higher level teams pay lip service only to the value of education for their players. At game time hockey comes first. Players who opt for homework during examination time lose favor, and are sometimes "benched."

performance is not tolerated. The sanctions of being "dropped" from the team or "benched" become a reality. As competition intensifies so does the structurally generated pressure in attempting to meet these difficult standards.

The major structural conditions which generate the amount and differential distribution of fighting and violent behavior among players in the league, i.e. at the Midget and Junior professional levels, comprise (a) the strong motivation of these players to advance to higher level teams (and thereby improve their opportunities for a professional hockey career),† (b) the considerable competition for a limited number of positions on Junior professional teams, and (c) the informal injunction to employ increasingly aggressive and rough means in the performance of their role. Because these boys are highly motivated to learn and incorporate the appropriate attitudes, sentiments and behavior of the role, they are thereby constrained to conform to the demands of the role they admire and wish others to identify them with. These attitudes and sentiments, and their role performance coincide with those groups that comprise their reference groups and with others to whom they look for encouragement and validity for their conduct.

The violation of a rule depends as much on the occurrence of an act as on the existence of the rule. Any explanation of rule violation (which includes fighting) in the game of hockey must consider the particular set of rules that governs the contest. A change in the rules may not only discourage deviance (e.g. physical aggression), but indeed create it or, as in this instance, foster conditions especially conductive to physical violence. A change in rules in a contest will often transform the course of the game, and affect teams to adapt their game strategies and tactics.

Introduction of the red line which divides the ice surface into opposing zones has forced teams to employ new game tactics and strategies. This has led to an increase in physical aggression. The strategy of "shooting it in," i.e. shooting the puck from the red line into the corner of the opposing team's zone has rendered

---

† We have already noted that at this level boys will give greater consideration to pursuing hockey as a professional career.

each of the corners of the ice a veritable "no man's land." This kind of game strategy has greatly increased violent body contact between opposing players and also contributed to violation of the rules. Some players participate in fear of having to engage in corner activity. Indeed, so crucial is the quality of toughness to the game that a player's ability in the corners is often a significant criterion in judging his determination, courage and professional potential. Coaching of younger players (eight to twelve years) usually focuses on the rudiments of hockey, and game strategies are less often employed among younger aged teams. Hence corner activity is less feared among younger players.

We can now ask the question, why is there much less fighting and physical aggression among players (aged eight to twelve) on the lower level teams? If we are correct the major variables that help account for fighting and violence among higher level teams should be less important to these youngsters.

As a career hockey has little real meaning for younger aged boys. Unlike older boys their futures do not yet require serious consideration nor decision making. Although they aspire to play hockey professionally their ambitions are "fantasy choices," rational considerations are not yet involved in their selections. They are not yet seriously oriented towards the Junior professional ranks and there is less competition for advancement.

At this age conflict between academic expectations and hockey obligations is minimal; school work is easier, examinations less important and hockey obligations less demanding. These boys are too young to be scouted and evaluated for their professional potential which eliminates another source of pressure. While they are strongly motivated to play Allstar hockey, conformity to role expectations does not as often require toughness, physical aggressiveness, nor courage. These are not yet major role obligations, which greatly reduces the amount and quality of violence in their performances. Youngsters receive little or no instruction in fighting, in fact fighting is strongly discouraged at the younger age levels. Although some illegal tactics are already institutionalized, these kids generally believe in the normative rules of the game and in the "official" virtues of sportsmanship and fair play. This is reflected in the formal practice of shaking hands with opposing players at the end of each game—and these youngsters believe that this practice is an important sign of sportsmanship. Finally, fighting and physical aggression accomplish little for these youngsters; it gets them a bad name; it interferes with their performance since it is not expected of them and it jeopardizes the good name and ideology of the league. Briefly, there are few structured sources of pressure towards fighting and violence; their training strongly discourages violence and there is little common motivation for this kind of conduct. Fighters are not rewarded at this level.

### Functions of Institutionalized Physical Aggression Among Young Hockey Players

If deviance is not contained it always becomes a threat to the organization of the system in which it occurs. At the same time under certain conditions institutionalized deviance may contribute to the vitality and operation of the system. At the higher levels of Minor League Hockey physical aggression becomes a criterion according to which rewards are distributed to those who uphold its values and attitudes, and who conform to role obligations. The player whose role performance personifies highly desired professional values and attitudes, and who conforms to behavioral expectations will rank high in the scale of evaluation.

Again physical aggressiveness reflects the success of the socialization process, i.e. the professionalization of young players for Junior professional and higher professional ranks. Players who "have guts," who "never back down from a fight," who never "give up," and who are otherwise consistently aggressive are breathing examples of the success of the prevailing system and its values and definitions of the game.

Given the accumulation of pressure, strain and discontent from daily participation in the legitimate order of the system, e.g. practices, games, (playoffs), the spartan requirements of training, school obligations, and other formal and informal controls, a certain amount of deviance (physical aggression) which is not rigorously repressed may serve to release tension. This acts as a safety valve and helps drain some of the strain and discontent off the legitimate order. The tactics used by referees in handling fights suggest this. Combatants are permitted to "fight it out." This helps insure that they will not wish to renew hostilities. In such instances the function of the referees is to prevent the interference of others and thereby control the spread of violence.

The collective meanings and definitions of young hockey players are reflected in the norms, attitudes and practices which govern their work performance. The "official" rhetoric of the Minor Hockey League does not always coincide with what transpires among its members. Although the value system of the larger community likely subsumes the official objectives and ideals of Minor League Hockey, the everyday working values, attitudes and customs of the group coincide more closely with working-class values.

It was suggested that Allstar players who remain in Minor League Hockey come from the lower socioeconomic levels of the community. This facilitates their adaptation to role obligations and their preparation for the Junior professional ranks. Once they reach a certain level in Minor League Hockey, structural conditions influence many of these boys to pursue a professional hockey career.

The principal conditions that generate fighting and physical aggression among players on higher level teams are (a) the strong motivation of players to be selected for Junior professional ranks, (b) the intense competition for a limited number of positions on Junior professional teams, and (c) the informal obligation to employ increasing aggressive, sometimes violent means in the performance of their roles. It was noted also that changes in the rules governing conduct of the game created conditions conducive to physical aggression.

## References

1. Loy, John W., Jr.: The study of sport and social mobility. In *Aspects of Contemporary Sport Sociology*, Gerald S. Kenyon, (Ed.). University of Wisconsin, The Athletic Institute, 1969.
2. Porter, John: *The Vertical Mosaic*. Ontario, University of Toronto Press, p. 165, 1965.

# Chapter 24

# The Effects of Ordinal Position and Sibling's Sex on Males' Sport Participation

Daniel M. Landers

## Abstract

The effect of sibling sex on males' subsequent sport participation was determined. Sibling's sex information was obtained from over 1500 junior high school boys and 344 high school baseball players. Ss participation in sports was derived from coaches records. 394 junior high school athletes and nonathletes and 115 high school varsity baseball players from one- and two-child families were compared for their frequencies in the five ordinal position-sibling-sex categories for males. Results showed no significant differences between junior high school athletes' and nonathletes' frequencies within the five family position categories. However, males with an older sister participated in more varsity sports at the junior high school level and were overrepresented among high school varsity baseball players.

The relationship between the distribution of rewards and punishments associated with children in the same family and various personality and behavioral variables has been a major concern among social scientists. It is often maintained that children in the same family tend to acquire each other's characteristics. Brim[1] formulated what later investigators[3,5] have referred to as the sibling-similarity hypothesis. This hypothesis holds that, because of various socializing experiences in the family, opposite sex siblings tend to display more of the per-

Note: This investigation was supported in part by a research grant to the Motor Performance and Play Research Laboratory via the Adler Zone Center by the Department of Mental Health of the State of Illinois and by United States Public Health Grant No. MH-07346 from the National Institute of Mental Health.

sonality and behavioral characteristics of their opposite sex sibling, particularly younger siblings since they tend to model the older, more powerful sibling.

There have been recent attempts to test this hypothesis using various psychological femininity and sports participation scales. Since sport participation is positively associated with the masculine sex role in American society[6,10] it would follow from the sibling-similarity hypothesis that males or females with a brother would acquire more masculine personalities and behaviors and therefore participate more in sport and physical activities.

In general, the available literature is inconclusive with regard to the sibling-sex variable. The majority of the studies[1,8,9,11] have found support for the sibling-similarity hypothesis for females' responses to various vocational and psychological femininity scales. Other studies,[2,12] however, have confirmed the sibling-similarity hypothesis for males but not for females. Sutton-Smith and Rosenberg[13] also found that male and female college students with a male sibling reported significantly more past participation in games of physical skill plus strategy and games of pure physical skill. Further support has been reported by Landers[3] who found second-born females with an older brother (MF2)* were overrepresented among women physical education majors as opposed to women education majors.

Other evidence obtained from males has not supported the sibling-similarity hypothesis. Leventhal[4,5] using 1,152 male college students with one sibling, found that FM2's reported higher psychological masculinity and interest in outdoor activities as well as higher motor fitness scores and aquatic classifications than MM2's. Based upon his finding, Leventhal[5] proposed a sibling-opposites hypothesis to account for sibling influences in the above activities. Leventhal further suggests that an older female sibling may serve as a negative model and thereby motivate the younger male to adopt a response pattern opposite

---

* The number indicates ordinal position and always follows the subject of discussion; the "F" (female) or "M" (male) not followed by a number indicates the sex and position of the subject's sibling. For example, an M1F is a first-born male with a younger sister while an MM2 is a second-born male with an older brother.

that of his sister. This interpretation is also consistent with other findings that preadolescent boys with two sisters express more psychological masculinity than a boy with one sister[8] and that fathers with two daughters display greater psychological masculinity than a father with a daughter and a son.[9]

The veracity of the sibling-opposites or sibling-similarity hypothesis for explaining differences in sport participation has yet to be determined. The various self-report personality and past sport participation scales as well as motor fitness scores provide only indirect information relative to actual sport participation. What is needed are more unobtrusive indicators, other than motor fitness scores, of sport team membership. The purpose of the present study, therefore, is to examine the frequencies of male athletes from one- and two-child families who appeared on coaches' athletic rosters. In addition, since sibling effects have been shown to differ at different age periods,[12] family position frequencies of athletes from two different age groups were examined.

## Methods and Materials

During the 1969–70 school year, a short questionnaire was administered to boys physical education classes in four junior high schools in Champaign-Urbana. Information regarding S's age, the age and sex of each sibling as well as the number of varsity sport teams in which S competed while in junior high school were solicited from 1,691 seventh, eighth and ninth grade males. Coaches from each school were used to verify each S's responses regarding competitive sport participation. Competitive sports included football, cross-country, basketball, wrestling, and track. Athletes included 597 students who competed on one or more varsity or junior varsity sport teams. The athletic group was then compared to 1,094 students who had not competed on a sport team. In order to investigate sibling influence, 135 athletes and 259 nonathletes from one- and two-child families were obtained from the larger sample and were compared on their frequencies within the five one- and two-child family position categories.

In addition to the junior high school students, sibling information was obtained from 344 varsity baseball players representing twenty-nine teams primarily in the suburban Chicago area* From this sample 115 players came from one- and two-child families and were compared for their frequencies in each of the five family position categories. Tests of independence for the frequencies of athletes in each of the family position categories were made by using one and two sample chi square tests.

## Results

The results of the chi square analysis between junior high school athletes' and nonathletes' frequencies within the five one- and two-child family position categories is summarized in Table 24-I. This analysis showed that the two groups did not differ significantly from one another ($X^2 = 3.07$, $df = 4$, $p > .05$).

TABLE 24-I

FREQUENCY OF ORDINAL POSITION-SIBLING-SEX COMBINATIONS FOR JUNIOR HIGH SCHOOL ATHLETES AND NONATHELTES

|  | M1 | M1M | M1F | MM2 | FM2 | Total |
|---|---|---|---|---|---|---|
| Athletes | 23 | 19 | 32 | 30 | 31 | 135 |
| Nonathletes | 33 | 50 | 67 | 51 | 58 | 259 |
| Total | 56 | 69 | 99 | 81 | 89 | 394 |

$X^2 = 3.07$, df = 4, p > .05

Since many of the Ss indicated playing on more than one sport team, a one sample chi square test was applied to the number of sports competed in by Ss in each family position category. The results of the chi square analysis, which are summarized in Table 24-II, show that FM2's competed in significantly ($X^2 = 10.45$, $df = 4$, $p < .05$) greater number of sports than M1's and M1M's.

TABLE 24-II

TOTAL NUMBER OF SPORT TEAMS MADE BY JUNIOR HIGH SCHOOL ATHLETES AS A FUNCTION OF THE VARIOUS ORDINAL POSITION-SIBLING-SEX COMBINATIONS IN ONE- AND TWO-CHILD FAMILIES

| Family Positions | M1 | M1M | M1F | MM2 | FM2 |
|---|---|---|---|---|---|
| Sport Frequency | 32 | 38 | 47 | 48 | 60 |

$X^2 = 10.45$, df = 4, p < .05

* Appreciation is extended to Thomas F. Crum who collected the data for this analysis.

The frequencies of high school baseball players in the various one- and two-child family position categories are summarized in Table 24-III. The resulting chi square was significant ($X^2 = 15.91$, $df = 4$, $p < .01$). A similar trend as in the preceding analysis was observed with FM2's being overrepresented among high school baseball players and M1's and M1M's underrepresented.

TABLE 24-III

FREQUENCY OF HIGH SCHOOL BASEBALL PLAYERS IN THE ONE-
AND TWO-CHILD FAMILY POSITION CATEGORIES

| Family Positions | M1 | M1M | M1F | MM2 | FM2 |
|---|---|---|---|---|---|
| Frequency of Subjects | 14 | 14 | 25 | 25 | 37 |

$X^2 = 15.91$, df = 4, p < .01

## Discussion

The finding of the present study that FM2's are overrepresented among high school baseball players and compete in more varsity and junior varsity sports while in junior high school supports the sibling-opposites rather than sibling-similarity hypothesis. The underrepresentation of the M1's and to a lesser extent the M1M's may only be a reflection of their smaller numbers in the junior high school sample. The number of FM2's among junior high school athletes, however, were the number expected for the sample size and therefore the greater number of sports in which they competed was not due to any initial overrepresentation among FM2 athletes. The similarity of these findings and those of high school baseball players further strengthens the validity of the observed differences.

At least three processes occurring in the sex-role development of children have been suggested to account for the acquiring of characteristics and behaviors assumed to be opposite that of one's sibling. Leventhal[5] suggests that the sibling may serve as a negative model who possesses traits which the younger child is motivated to avoid acquiring. Leventhal[5] states that:

> To whatever extent the boy does acquire his older sister's feminine response patterns, he will probably find himself disapproved by parents and peers. Consequently, he will be motivated to eschew and to avoid further acquisition of his sister's response

patterns. On trait dimensions for which such processes operate (e.g. sport participation), boys with an older sister are likely to adopt a highly masculine response pattern.

Rosenberg and Sutton-Smith[9] suggest that such a counter-active response can be interpreted in clinical terms as a reaction to a sense of sex-role inadequacy by a compensatory heightening of their own sex-role characteristics. The processes underlying the sibling-opposites hypothesis can also be interpreted in structural or normative terms as an attempt to reestablish a sex-role balance in a family whose structure might facilitate deviation towards one or the other sex-role polarity.[7]

Although the present study is suggestive of sibling influences regarding sport participation, the nature of these differences is far from clear. More in-depth studies including all family members of athletes are needed so that the interactive effects between siblings as well as siblings and parents can be determined. The varying effects of ordinal position-sibling-sex combinations on males' sport participation and the socialization processes bringing about observed differences cannot be known until studies are designed which take into account a multiplicity of family effects upon children.

## References

1. Brim, O.G.: *Sociometry.* 21:1, 1958.
2. Koch, H.: *J. Genet. Psychol.* 88:231, 1956.
3. Landers, D.M.: *J. Soc. Psychol.* 80:247, 1970.
4. Leventhal, G.S.: Sex of sibling as a predictor of personality characteristics. Paper presented at the Southeastern Psychological Association, Atlanta, 1965.
5. Leventhal, G.S.: Some effects of having a brother or sister. Paper presented at the meeting of the American Psychological Association, San Francisco, August, 1968.
6. Moss, H.A., and Kagan, J.: *J. Abnorm. Soc. Psychol.* 62:504, 1961.
7. Parsons, T., and Bales, R.F.: *Family, Socialization and Interaction Process.* Glencoe, Free Press, 1955.
8. Rosenberg, B.G., and Sutton-Smith, B.: *Genet. Psychol. Monogr.* 70: 297, 1964.
9. Rosenberg, B.G., and Sutton-Smith, B.: *J. Pers. Soc. Psychol.* 8:117, 1968.

10. Sutton-Smith, B., Rosenberg, B.G., and Morgan, E.E.: *Child Develp.* 34:119, 1963.
11. Sutton-Smith, B., Roberts, J.M., and Rosenberg, B.G.: *Merrill-Palmer Quarterly.* 10:25, 1964.
12. Sutton-Smith, B., and Rosenberg, B.G.: *J. Genet. Psychol.* 107:61, 1965.
13. Sutton-Smith, B., and Rosenberg, B.G.: *The Sibling.* New York, Holt, Rinehart and Winston, 1970.

# Chapter 25

# A Field Experimental Study of Attitude Change in Four Biracial Small Sport Groups

Thomas D. McIntyre

When one examines contemporary American society it is readily apparent that differences among groups and individuals are often the sources of conflicts and tensions. Many of these tensions have been with us for years; others are of more recent vintage. Conflicts as a result of tensions and group differences existed on many fronts during the decade of the 1960's. Technological advancements in communications and transportation have functioned to make more people aware of cultural differences and conflicts. Human groupings must inevitably have traffic with one another, whether they like it or not. Thus, one of the most fundamental and challenging problems in the modern world is that of "intergroup relations." The present study was an attempt to investigate human relations in the small biracial sport group.

This study is significant both from a theoretical and an applied standpoint. Sociological and social-psychological theory was tested utilizing the social institution, sport, as the stimulus. This study serves to extend sociological and social psychological theory to small biracial sport groups. From an applied standpoint, the study of intergroup relations is an intriguing enterprise, especially in view of existing assumptions about the value of sport in changing intergroup hostilities.

The early approach reported in Allport[1] and Murphy et al.[5] to attitudes was mainly descriptive and correlational. Such research could cast little light upon the specific conditions under which attitudes are formed and modified. It could not link the psychology of attitudes clearly with more general explanatory principles.

More recently, studies of attitude change have proliferated. There seems to be a general consensus that attitudes: (a) may be explicit or implicit, (b) are formed through experience, that is learned, (c) are relatively stable, but can be changed through different experiences, (d) may be evoked either by perceptual signs or linguistic signs, (e) are predispositions to respond evaluatively to these signs, and (f) may range anywhere from extremely favorable to extremely unfavorable.

The literature, represented by the work of Sherif and Sherif,[8] Allport,[2] Pettigrew,[6] Williams,[10] and Klineberg[3] lend support to the conclusion that contact can create both harmony and tension.

The purpose of the study was to investigate and measure the amount of attitude change of black and white subjects on the issue of ethnicity.

## Methods and Procedures

The Metropolitan Center of Rochester, New York served as the physical setting for this research. Flag football functioned as the social stimulus setting for twenty-three black boys (mean age 162.7 months) with twenty-three white boys (mean age 148.1 months. The black boys were drawn from an urban school with a 74.2 percent nonwhite ethnic composition; in contrast, the white boys in the experimental group came from a suburban school composed of 99.2 percent white students. These forty-six *S's* were given three skills tests in an effort to form four biracial teams that would be equally matched. The experimental treatment, i.e. contact in a sport stimulus setting, was conducted for twenty sessions over a five-week period. Upon completion of the experimental treatment, a control group was randomly chosen from each school. The seventh grade boys in this group consisted of twenty-three black boys from the urban school and a comparable number of white boys from the suburban school. The Own Categories technique was used to assess attitudes on the issue ethnicity. Analysis of these data involved three aspects:

(a) the number of categories used, (b) the extent of latitude of acceptance, noncommitment, and rejection, and (c) evaluation of attitude statements. Instructions for sorting statements can be found in Appendix B.

## Results

Since the present experiment concerned categorizations by subjects representing two distinct ethnic groups, analysis compared across and within ethnic groups. The stimuli (Appendix A) sorted by the subjects represented a range of variation, on the dimension ethnicity, from highly favorable to most unfavorable for both black and white subjects. Subjects' ego-involvement and attitudinal change on this issue were examined by analyzing the number of categories used and the relative widths of the latitudes of acceptance, rejection, and noncommitment. The number of categories employed by black and white subjects under experimental and control conditions are presented in Table 25-I.

The mean number of categories used by each group are presented in Tables 25-IX, 25-X, 25-XI, 25-XII. Results were not significant when comparing the black experimental group (mean = 3.09) with the black control group (mean = 3.22). This indicated that the experimental treatment had no effect on black subjects in the comparison of number of categories used. White experimental subjects used an average of 4.41 categories compared to 4.04 by the white control group. Again, these data do not differ significantly ($p < .05$).

TABLE 25-I
NUMBER OF CATEGORIES USED BY SUBJECTS
WITHIN THE FOUR GROUPS

| | | Number of Categories Used | | | | | | |
|---|---|---|---|---|---|---|---|---|
| Group | N | 2 | 3 | 4 | 5 | 6 | 7 | 8 |
| Black Experimental | 23 | 3 | 16 | 3 | 1 | | | |
| Black Control | 23 | 2 | 19 | | 1 | | | 1 |
| White Experimental | 22 | | 2 | 11 | 7 | 2 | | |
| White Control | 23 | 1 | 4 | 13 | 3 | 2 | | |
| Total (all Ss) | 91 | | | | | | | |

The Mann-Whitney $U$ test was applied to determine whether the four groups of subjects used a significantly different number of categories in sorting the forty attitude statements. These results are presented in Table 25-II.

Results were highly significant ($p<.001$) when comparisons were made between black and white experimental groups and black and white control groups. These differences indicated a higher commitment and stronger involvement for blacks on the ethnicity issue than for whites. This might have been expected since the black subjects in this study lived in a urban ghetto, while on the other hand white subjects were drawn from suburbia.

TABLE 25-II

**VALUES OF THE MANN-WHITNEY $U$ TEST TRANSFORMED TO Z FOR NUMBER OF CATEGORIES USED IN SORTING ATTITUDE STATEMENTS**

| Groups Compared | U | z |
|---|---|---|
| Black Experimental (N = 23) to Black Control (N = 23) | 257.5 | −0.21 |
| White Experimental (N = 22) to White Control (N = 23) | 178.5 | −1.85 |
| Black Experimental to White Experimental | 449.5 | 4.70[a] |
| Black Control to White Control | 428.5 | 3.90[a] |

[a] Significant at the .001 level (one-tailed test)

Latitudes of acceptance, rejection, and noncommitment are graphically represented in Figures 25–1, 25–2, 25–3, and 25–4. These graphs convey the extent of differences in mean number of statements accepted, rejected and not evaluated (noncommitment) for each of the four groups. For the most part there were no striking disparities with regard to the relative sizes of their latitudes. Attitudinal theory indicated that highly involved persons have a broader latitude of rejection than persons less concerned, and that they remain noncommittal toward fewer positions. Also, the highly involved person's latitude of acceptance is generally narrower than his less involved counterpart.

Mann Whitney $U$ tests were applied to determine whether the relative sizes of attitudinal latitudes of subjects were

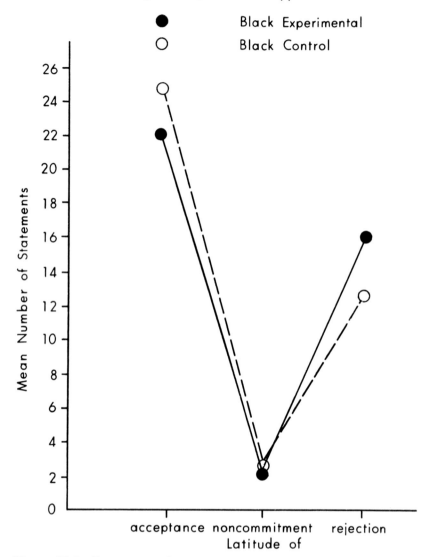

Figure 25–1. Comparison of mean size of attitudinal latitudes of black experimental subjects to black control subjects.

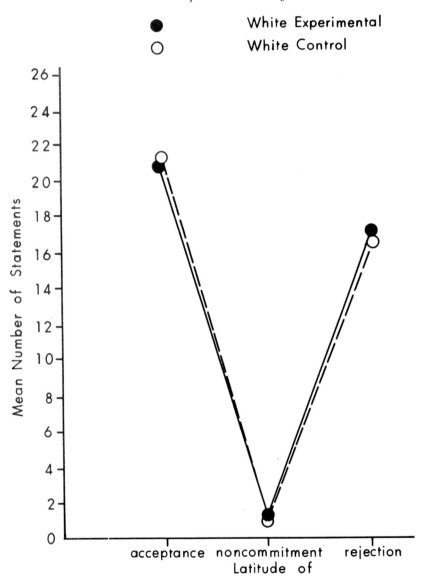

Figure 25–2. Comparison of mean size of attitudinal latitudes of white experimental subjects to white control subjects.

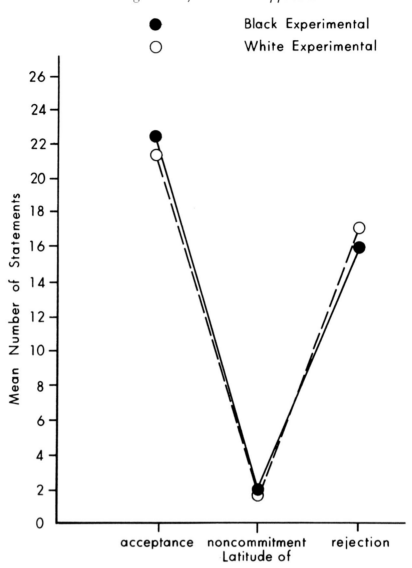

Figure 25–3. Comparison of mean size of attitudinal latitudes of black experimental subjects to white experimental subjects.

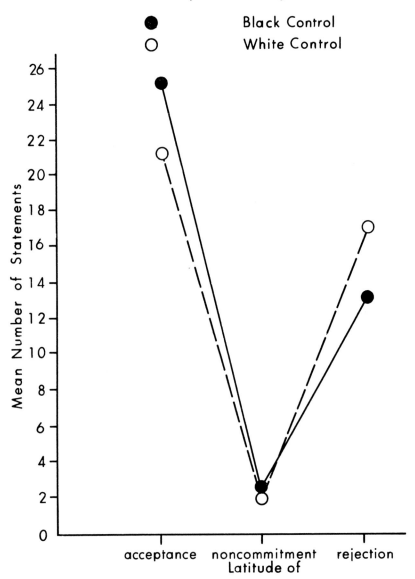

Figure 25–4. Comparison of mean size of attitudinal latitudes of black control subjects to white control subjects.

significantly different. These results are presented in Tables
25-III, 25-IV, and 25-V. Significance was attained (p<.05)
when a comparison was made of the latitude of acceptance for

TABLE 25-III

VALUES OF THE MANN-WHITNEY $U$ STATISTIC TRANSFORMED TO
$z$ FOR NUMBER OF ATTITUDE STATEMENTS SORTED IN THE
LATITUDE OF ACCEPTANCE

| Groups Compared | $U$ | $z$ |
|---|---|---|
| Black Experimental (N = 23) to Black Control (N = 23) | 325.0 | 1.33 |
| White Experimental (N = 22) to White Control (N = 23) | 245.0 | −0.18 |
| Black Experimental (N = 23) to White Experimental (N = 22) | 225.0 | −0.64 |
| Black Control (N = 23) to White Control (N = 23) | 356.0 | 2.02[a] |

[a] Significant at the .05 level (one-tailed test)

TABLE 25-IV

VALUES OF THE MANN-WHITNEY $U$ STATISTIC TRANSFORMED TO
$z$ FOR NUMBER OF ATTITUDE STATEMENTS SORTED IN THE
LATITUDE OF NONCOMMITMENT

| Groups Compared | $U$ | $z$ |
|---|---|---|
| Black Experimental (N = 23) to Black Control (N = 23) | 22.0 | .14[a] |
| White Experimental (N = 22) to White Control (N = 23) | 25.5 | .20[a] |
| Black Experimental (N = 23) to White Experimental (N = 22) | 34.0 | 1.30[a] |
| Black Control (N = 23) to White Control (N = 23) | 20.5 | −.07[a] |

[a] All z values nonsignificant

TABLE 25-V

VALUES OF THE MANN-WHITNEY $U$ STATISTIC TRANSFORMED TO
$z$ FOR NUMBER OF ATTITUDE STATEMENTS SORTED IN THE
LATITUDE OF REJECTION

| Groups Compared | $U$ | $z$ |
|---|---|---|
| Black Experimental (N = 23) to Black Control (N = 23) | 197.5 | −1.48 |
| White Experimental (N = 22) to White Control (N = 23) | 255.5 | .06 |
| Black Experimental (N = 23) to White Experimental (N = 22) | 300.5 | 1.08 |
| Black Control (N = 23) to White Control (N = 23) | 138.0 | −2.79[a] |

[a] Significant at the .01 level (one-tailed test)

black and white controls. Black controls accepted an average of 24.96 statements compared to an average of 21.74 statements accepted by white controls. All comparisons made of the widths of latitudes of noncommitment were nonsignificant. Significance was again attained ($p < .01$) when comparing latitudes of rejection for black and white control groups. Black controls rejected an average of 12.96 statements compared to an average of 16.61 statements for white controls. These results indicated that strong differences existed in how the two control groups perceived the ethnicity issue.

White controls had a significantly broader latitude of rejection and a significantly narrower latitude of acceptance than did black controls. The assumption must be made that on the issue examined, white controls were more highly ego-involved than were black controls. Statistical treatment of the latitudes of control subjects indicated white controls more strongly committed than were black controls. Since significance was not attained when comparing experimental groups, it seems logical to assume the experimental treatment had a more positive effect upon white subjects than upon black experimental subjects who also used significantly fewer categories ($p < .001$) in sorting the forty attitude statements.

This differential effect of the experimental treatment upon the contrasting ethnic groups can possibly be explained by lack of equivalence in age and skill. As previously indicated black experimental subjects had a mean age 14.6 months greater than their white counterparts. That fact, coupled with athletic skill differential may well explain why contact in sport had a differential effect upon the two groups.

The latitudes of acceptance, rejection, and noncommitment of the four groups provide a more adequate measure of attitude than does number of categories though not as sensitive a measure as consideration of the actual content of those categories. An analysis of each statement was carried out to determine which items had been accepted, which rejected, and which placed into latitudes of noncommitment for each group.

Over the total sample twenty-one statements (52.5 percent) were sorted with 70 percent or better consensus among ninety-one subjects. The 70 percent level was arbitrarily chosen. Statements 1–5, 8, 9, 13, 14, 18–20, 23, 24, and 29 were accepted while the criteria for responses to these statements were further analyzed. Statements 15, 16, 25, 27, 34, and 38 were rejected with 70 percent or better consensus by all subjects (see Appendix A).

Four statements were sorted significantly different when a comparison was made between black experimental and black control groups. These four statements and the resultant chi squares are presented in Table 25-VI.

The first two statements sorted significantly different by black experimental and black control subjects indicated that black experimental subjects were not willing to use skin color as a criterion for selecting someone to depend upon. This would appear to indicate that the biracial contact in sport produced a positive effect upon black experimental subjects. But, analysis of the other two statements sorted significantly different results

TABLE 25-VI

COMPARISON OF BLACK EXPERIMENTAL AND BLACK CONTROL
SUBJECTS' RESPONSES ON SIGNIFICANT ATTITUDE STATEMENTS

If a black person and a white person seem to be able to do something well it is best to trust the *White* if you must really depend on someone.

| Group | Accept | Reject |
|---|---|---|
| Black Experimental | 5 | 18 |
| Black Control | 11 | 11 |
| $X^2 = 3.92$ | d.f. $= 1$ | p   .05 |

If a black person and a white person both seem to be able to do something well it is best to trust the *Black* if you must really depend on someone.

| Group | Accept | Reject |
|---|---|---|
| Black Experimental | 4 | 18 |
| Black Control | 14 | 8 |
| $X^2 = 9.40$ | d.f. $= 1$ | p   .01 |

People of different races will get along better if they visit each other and share things.

| Group | Accept | Reject |
|---|---|---|
| Black Experimental | 13 | 9 |
| Black Control | 20 | 2 |
| $X^2 = 5.94$ | d.f. $= 1$ | p   .02 |

The practice of dividing men into groups based upon the color of skin is not fair.

| Group | Accept | Reject |
|---|---|---|
| Black Experimental | 12 | 11 |
| Black Control | 18 | 4 |
| $X^2 = 4.85$ | d.f. $= 1$ | p   .05 |

Total number of group responses is not always twenty-three because noncommitment responses are not presented in a contradictory conclusion. Analysis of these statements implies that black experimental subjects seemed more reluctant to mix; they did accept the salience of color as a basis for division.

Only two attitude statements were sorted significantly different by white experimental and white control subjects. One would expect to find two statements sorted differently by chance alone, so very little value can be attached to these data and, hence, are not included.

A comparison of black experimental to white experimental subjects (see Table 25-VII) produced four attitude statements sorted significantly different. Black subjects surprisingly, indicated that prejudice was not a social problem in the Rochester area. White subjects accepted the polar position ($p < .01$). These results are difficult to explain when one considers the amount of racial tension in the Rochester schools particularly during the period that this study was being conducted. The

TABLE 25-VII

COMPARISON OF BLACK EXPERIMENTAL AND WHITE
EXPERIMENTAL SUBJECTS' RESPONSES ON
SIGNIFICANT ATTITUDE STATEMENTS

Prejudice is not a social problem in the Rochester area.

| Group | Accept | Reject |
|---|---|---|
| Black Experimental | 13 | 8 |
| White Experimental | 4 | 16 |
| $X^2 = 7.41$ | d.f. $= 1$ | p  .01 |

The practice of dividing men into groups based upon the color of skin is not fair.

| Group | Accept | Reject |
|---|---|---|
| Black Experimental | 12 | 11 |
| White Experimental | 19 | 4 |
| $X^2 = 4.85$ | d.f. $= 1$ | p  .05 |

White officials, in sport, seem to favor the white players.

| Group | Accept | Reject |
|---|---|---|
| Black Experimental | 10 | 12 |
| White Experimental | 1 | 22 |
| $X^2 = 10.29$ | d.f. $= 1$ | p  .01 |

Some groups of people are naturally inferior and should be treated in like manner.

| Group | Accept | Reject |
|---|---|---|
| Black Experimental | 13 | 9 |
| White Experimental | 6 | 16 |
| $X^2 = 4.54$ | d.f. $= 1$ | p  .05 |

Total number of group responses is not always twenty-three because noncommitment responses are not presented second statement dealt with the practice of dividing people into groups based upon the color of skin. Black subjects split their responses about equally on this statement, while whites took a more liberal stand ($p<.05$), nineteen accepting division by color as unfair. Ten black experimental subjects accepted the statement that white sport officials seem to favor the white players while in contrast only one white subject took this stand ($p<.01$). There results were not supported by the observational data. Two games were always in progress throughout the duration of the project; a black and a white official alternated working these games. Verbal abuse by the players was consistent throughout the project regardless of the official's skin color. On the final statement the white subjects again took a more liberal stand rejecting that some groups of people are naturally inferior and should be treated in like manner ($p<.05$). The black subjects' responses to this statement may have resulted from their contact with whites in this project since, for the most part, they were more skillful at flag football.

Seven statements were sorted significantly different by black and white control subjects (see Table 25-VIII). An overall analysis of these statements seems to indicate that black control subjects were more willing to make judgments using color as the criterion. On the two statements dealing with getting good grades in school black subjects selected about equally that white boys/or black boys seem to do better while white subjects, for the most part, rejected color as an adequate measure of grades in school ($p<.05$). Twenty-two white controls accepted the statement that "facts and understanding and a desire to do away with prejudice can lead to social change" in contrast to fifteen black controls ($p<.02$). This seems to suggest that white control subjects were more willing to accept the potential for improving intergroup relations while seven of the black controls perceived the situation quite hopeless. It's surprising that black subjects split their choices equally on the statement "social conditions for whites and blacks are equal in America." One plausible explanation is that these boys were still quite young and possibly not entirely aware of the many subtle (some not so subtle) social inequities in American society. They are

TABLE 25-VIII
COMPARISON OF BLACK CONTROL AND WHITE CONTROL
SUBJECTS' RESPONSES SIGNIFICANT ATTITUDE STATEMENTS

Black and whites are different in natural ability.

| Group | Accept | Reject |
|---|---|---|
| Black Control | 13 | 10 |
| White Control | 6 | 16 |
| $X^2 = 3.94$ | d.f. = 1 | p  .05 |

Facts and understanding and a desire to do away with prejudice can lead to social change.

| Group | Accept | Reject |
|---|---|---|
| Black Control | 15 | 7 |
| White Control | 22 | 0 |
| $X^2$ (with Yates' Correction) = 6.12 | d.f. = 1 | p  .02 |

If a black person and a white person both seem to be able to do something well it is best to trust the *White* if you must really depend on someone.

| Group | Accept | Reject |
|---|---|---|
| Black Control | 11 | 11 |
| White Control | 2 | 21 |
| $X^2 = 9.34$ | d.f. = 1 | p  .01 |

When it comes to getting good grades in school *Black* boys always seem to do better.

| Group | Accept | Reject |
|---|---|---|
| Black Control | 11 | 12 |
| White Control | 3 | 17 |
| $X^2 = 5.25$ | d.f. = 1 | p  .01 |

When it comes to getting good grades in school *White* boys always seem to do better.

| Group | Accept | Reject |
|---|---|---|
| Black Control | 11 | 11 |
| White Control | 4 | 19 |
| $X^2 = 5.38$ | d.f. = 1 | p  .05 |

Social conditions for whites and blacks are equal in America.

| Group | Accept | Reject |
|---|---|---|
| Black Control | 11 | 11 |
| White Control | 4 | 18 |
| $X^2 = 4.96$ | d.f. = 1 | p  .05 |

Some groups of people are naturally inferior and should be treated in like manner.

| Group | Accept | Reject |
|---|---|---|
| Black Control | 9 | 13 |
| White Control | 3 | 19 |
| $X^2 = 4.13$ | d.f. = 1 | p  .05 |

Total number of group responses is not always twenty-three because noncommitment responses are not presented

probably aware of the disproportionate number of black entertainers and professional athletes in our culture and equate this fact with equal social conditions. The last statement that "some groups of people are naturally inferior and should be treated

## TABLE 25-IX
## OWN CATEGORIES RESPONSES TO ATTITUDE STATEMENTS
### WHITE EXPERIMENTAL GROUP

| | | Number of Statements in | | |
|---|---|---|---|---|
| Case # | Number of Categories | Latitude of Acceptance | Latitude of Noncommitment | Latitude of Rejection |
| 1 | 6 | 21 | 6 | 13 |
| 2 | 4 | 22 | 2 | 16 |
| 3 | 3 | 19 | 8 | 13 |
| 4 | 4 | 22 | 0 | 18 |
| 5 | 4 | 24 | 0 | 16 |
| 6 | 4 | 14 | 0 | 26 |
| 7 | 4 | 18 | 0 | 22 |
| 8 | 4 | 25 | 0 | 15 |
| 9 | 4 | 22 | 0 | 18 |
| 10 | 4 | 23 | 0 | 17 |
| 11 | 5 | 22 | 7 | 11 |
| 12 | 4 | 17 | 0 | 23 |
| 13 | 4 | 23 | 0 | 17 |
| 14 | 4 | 18 | 0 | 22 |
| 15 | 5 | 14 | 5 | 21 |
| 16 | 5 | 21 | 5 | 14 |
| 17 | 5 | 21 | 0 | 19 |
| 18 | 5 | 20 | 3 | 17 |
| 19 | 5 | 24 | 2 | 14 |
| 20 | 3 | 27 | 0 | 13 |
| 21 | 5 | 25 | 0 | 15 |
| 22 | 6 | 28 | 0 | 12 |
| Mean | 4.41 | 21.36 | 1.73 | 16.91 |
| S D. | 0.80 | 3.66 | 2.68 | 3.94 |

## TABLE 25-X
## OWN CATEGORIES RESPONSES TO ATTITUDE STATEMENTS
### BLACK CONTROL GROUP

| | | Number of Statements in | | |
|---|---|---|---|---|
| Case # | Number of Categories | Latitude of Acceptance | Latitude of Noncommitment | Latitude of Rejection |
| 1 | 3 | 18 | 4 | 18 |
| 2 | 3 | 36 | 0 | 4 |
| 3 | 2 | 35 | 0 | 5 |
| 4 | 8 | 22 | 3 | 15 |
| 5 | 5 | 20 | 4 | 16 |
| 6 | 3 | 28 | 0 | 12 |
| 7 | 3 | 22 | 1 | 17 |
| 8 | 3 | 30 | 0 | 10 |
| 9 | 3 | 27 | 0 | 13 |
| 10 | 3 | 27 | 0 | 13 |
| 11 | 2 | 16 | 0 | 24 |
| 12 | 3 | 12 | 13 | 15 |
| 13 | 3 | 27 | 0 | 13 |
| 14 | 3 | 32 | 0 | 8 |
| 15 | 3 | 27 | 0 | 13 |
| 16 | 3 | 20 | 0 | 20 |
| 17 | 3 | 30 | 0 | 10 |
| 18 | 3 | 27 | 0 | 13 |
| 19 | 3 | 11 | 16 | 13 |
| 20 | 3 | 24 | 0 | 16 |
| 21 | 3 | 36 | 0 | 4 |
| 22 | 3 | 25 | 0 | 15 |
| 23 | 3 | 22 | 7 | 11 |
| Mean | 3.22 | 24.96 | 2.09 | 12.96 |
| S.D. | 1.17 | 6.89 | 4.35 | 4.84 |

## TABLE 25-XI
## OWN CATEGORIES RESPONSES TO ATTITUDE STATEMENTS
### WHITE CONTROL GROUP

| Case # | Number of Categories | Number of Statements in Latitude of Acceptance | Latitude of Noncommitment | Latitude of Rejection |
|---|---|---|---|---|
| 1 | 4 | 21 | 0 | 19 |
| 2 | 5 | 18 | 6 | 16 |
| 3 | 4 | 21 | 0 | 19 |
| 4 | 4 | 20 | 0 | 20 |
| 5 | 4 | 22 | 0 | 18 |
| 6 | 4 | 22 | 0 | 18 |
| 7 | 4 | 26 | 4 | 10 |
| 8 | 3 | 26 | 0 | 14 |
| 9 | 3 | 25 | 0 | 15 |
| 10 | 4 | 26 | 0 | 14 |
| 11 | 3 | 12 | 17 | 11 |
| 12 | 5 | 23 | 3 | 14 |
| 13 | 6 | 15 | 6 | 19 |
| 14 | 5 | 28 | 0 | 12 |
| 15 | 4 | 21 | 0 | 19 |
| 16 | 4 | 19 | 0 | 21 |
| 17 | 4 | 25 | 0 | 15 |
| 18 | 3 | 28 | 0 | 12 |
| 19 | 6 | 20 | 2 | 18 |
| 20 | 2 | 21 | 0 | 19 |
| 21 | 4 | 23 | 0 | 17 |
| 22 | 4 | 19 | 0 | 21 |
| 23 | 4 | 19 | 0 | 21 |
| Mean | 4.04 | 21.74 | 1.65 | 16.61 |
| S.D | 0.93 | 3.95 | 3.86 | 3.35 |

## TABLE 25-XII
## OWN CATEGORIES RESPONSES TO ATTITUDE STATEMENTS
### BLACK EXPERIMENTAL GROUP

| Case # | Number of Categories | Number of Statements in Latitude of Acceptance | Latitude of Noncommitment | Latitude of Rejection |
|---|---|---|---|---|
| 1 | 5 | 19 | 1 | 20 |
| 2 | 4 | 26 | 0 | 14 |
| 3 | 4 | 17 | 0 | 23 |
| 4 | 4 | 15 | 0 | 25 |
| 5 | 2 | 21 | 0 | 19 |
| 6 | 3 | 17 | 0 | 23 |
| 7 | 3 | 33 | 0 | 7 |
| 8 | 3 | 25 | 3 | 12 |
| 9 | 3 | 16 | 8 | 16 |
| 10 | 3 | 28 | 0 | 12 |
| 11 | 3 | 29 | 0 | 11 |
| 12 | 3 | 20 | 0 | 20 |
| 13 | 3 | 31 | 0 | 9 |
| 14 | 3 | 29 | 0 | 11 |
| 15 | 3 | 25 | 0 | 15 |
| 16 | 3 | 16 | 10 | 14 |
| 17 | 3 | 12 | 12 | 16 |
| 18 | 3 | 24 | 0 | 16 |
| 19 | 3 | 26 | 0 | 14 |
| 20 | 3 | 19 | 12 | 9 |
| 21 | 3 | 28 | 0 | 12 |
| 22 | 2 | 19 | 0 | 21 |
| 23 | 2 | 13 | 0 | 27 |
| Mean | 3.09 | 22.09 | 2.00 | 15.91 |
| S.D. | 0.67 | 6.07 | 4.10 | 5.46 |

in like manner" was rejected by nineteen white controls and accepted by nine black controls ($p<.05$). Again, whites took a more liberal stand. From the context of these data it's impossible to ascertain which groups of people the black control subjects felt were naturally inferior.

## Discussion

Effects of contact is a fundamental issue of intergroup and ethnic relations. Some writers maintain that increased contact between groups of markedly different values and origins will lead only to heightened conflict; others hold that increased contact between such groups will decrease prejudice and fear and lead to greater intergroup harmony.[2] Social science evidence supports neither extreme. Although the experimenter believed that equal status contact was extremely important, and it was noticed very early that complete equivalence of groups had not been attained, the experiment was carried out because of an overriding assumption, i.e. the type of contact that leads people to do things together was likely to result in changed attitudes. The assumption was that on athletic teams the goal is all-important, ethnicity is irrelevant.

In this experiment, the lack of complete equivalence of black and white participants in age and skill had a marked influence upon the outcome. While this is unfortunate any field study necessarily sacrifices some rigor in control for richness of data. Laboratory studies of attitude change generally effect more significant results than do field studies, but, do they measure reality or a contrived experience?

The experimental hypothesis which indicated that the latitude of acceptance for attitude statements will be wider among those individuals within groups involved in biracial interaction in sport than for those not participating in biracial sport activities was not supported. The experimental hypothesis which specified that individuals with no contact (control) will display a narrow latitude of acceptance for attitude statements and a wide latitude of rejection in comparison to the members of groups who have contact in sport groups was also not supported. Mann-Whitney

*U* tests were not significant when comparing relative widths of latitudes of acceptance and rejection for experimental and control subjects.

Although statistical significance was not attained when comparing black and white experimental groups to their respective black and white controls, the instrument proved a highly sensitive measure of ego-involvement. When experimental and control groups were compared across ethnic lines results were highly significant. This indicated that black subjects were much more highly ego-involved with the issue ethnicity than were their white counterparts. These results are consistent with the findings of Sherif, Sherif, and Nebergall[3] and LaFave and Sherif.[4]

In regard to cohesiveness and attitudes, one hypothesis specified that members in the high cohesive, interracial group would exhibit more attitude change toward out-group members than would subjects from a low cohesive group. Analysis of observational and cohesiveness questionnaire data indicated that the Oakland Raiders were the most cohesive team while the Blue Devils were the least cohesive group. The attitude data for these two groups was pooled and treated statistically without regard to ethnicity. Mann-Whitney *U* test with z transformation produced a nonsignificant z of .41 when an analysis was made of the number of categories used in sorting attitude statements. Results were also nonsignificant when a comparison was made of their latitudes of acceptance and rejection (z = 1.03 and −.87, respectively). There was no evidence that attitudes in high cohesive groups was more favorable than in less cohesive groups, therefore the hypothesis was not supported.

## References

1. Allport, G.W.: *Handbook of Social Psychology*, Murchison, C. (Ed.). Worcester, Massachusetts, Clark University Press, 1955.
2. Allport, G.W.: *The Nature of Prejudice*. Reading, Massachusetts, Addison-Wesley, 1954.
3. Klineberg, O.: *The Human Dimension in International Relations*. New York, Holt, Rinehart and Winston, 1965.
4. LaFave, L., and M. Sherif: *J Soc Psychol.* 76:75, 1968.

5. Murphy, G. *et al.*: *Experimental Social Psychology,* 2nd Ed. New York, Harper and Row, 1937.

6. Pettigrew, T.F.: *J Conflict Resolution.* 2:29, 1958.

7. Sherif, C.W., Sherif, M., and Nebergall, R.E.: *Attitude and Attitude Change: The Social Judgment-Involvement Approach.* Philadelphia, Saunders, 1965.

8. Sherif, M., and Sherif, C.W.: *Groups in Harmony and Tension.* New York, Harper and Row, 1953.

9. Siegel, S.: *Nonparametric Statistics for the Behavioral Sciences.* New York, McGraw-Hill, 1956.

10. Williams, R.M., Jr.: *Strangers Next Door.* Englewood Cliffs, New Jersey, Prentice-Hall, 1964.

# Appendix A

## FORTY STATEMENTS RELEVANT TO THE ISSUE ETHNICITY UTILIZED IN OWN CATEGORIES TECHNIQUE

1. In our modern day we need the efforts of people from every race.
2. It is not one's color that causes one to act as one does.
3. It makes very little sense to say that a man with one color skin is less able to be educated than a man with another skin color.
4. People should be accepted for what they are, not for what color skin they happen to have.
5. The ability to excel in sports like football is not at all related to the color of a man's skin.
6. A great deal of my prejudice has been formed by misunderstanding of the facts.
7. Anyone who has known black people knows why they are like they are.
8. All men are very much alike in the way their bodies are built and are closely related to each other.
9. Americans, white and black, may have to go through a time of hatred and fighting before they ever learn to live with each other in peace.
10. Anyone who has known white people knows why they are like they are.
11. Blacks and whites are different in natural ability.
12. Black officials, in sports, act in the best interests of both teams.
13. Each one of us has his own idea of what is meant by the word race.
14. Facts and understandings and a desire to do away with prejudice can lead to social change.
15. If a black person and a white person both seem to be able to do something well it is best to trust the *white* if you must really depend on someone.
16. If a black person and a white person both seem to be able to do something well it is best to trust the *black* if you must really depend on someone.
17. In a prejudiced society it is very hard to hold no prejudices of your own.
18. In all sports contests I like to win and the color of my teammates' skin is not important.
19. It is possible to break hrough prejudice and teach every man to feel, to understand, and to appreciate the ability of all men.
20. Many races, many religions, many different people, and people from many different countries can live together in understanding and peace.
21. No one is ever cured of prejudice without knowing the facts.

22. Our country is a lot better off because of the people from many different countries who live here.
23. People of all races have been rulers, scholars, farmers, artists, statesmen, and skilled workers.
24. People of different races will get along better if they visit each other and share things.
25. People of different races will *not* get along better if they visit each other and share things.
26. Prejudice is not a social problem in the Rochester area.
27. The color of one's skin can be used to determine the natural goodness or evil in a person.
28. The great majority of the white population has social, economic, and educational advantages that are not available to large numbers of black people.
29. The practice of dividing men into groups based upon the color of skin is not fair.
30. There have been periods in history during which the deeds of the black people were greater than those of the white people.
31. There is not much communication and understanding between the races whether it be white toward black or black toward white.
32. There is really no single cause for prejudice.
33. Violence seems to be the best means by which the blacks can better themselves.
34. When it comes to getting good grades in school *black* boys always seem to do better.
35. When it comes to getting good grades in school *white* boys always seem to do better.
36. When those we love and admire support prejudiced attitudes, it is not easy to differ with them.
37. White officials, in sport, seem to favor the white players.
38. Equal rights are fine, but I wouldn't want someone of a different color living right next door to me.
39. Social conditions for whites and blacks are equal in America.
40. Some groups of people are naturally inferior and should be treated in like manner.

# Appendix B

## INSTRUCTIONS FOR SORTING STATEMENTS

**Step I.** Please sort these statements into any number of stacks that seem necessary to you. You may use as many stacks as you wish, and you may put as many statements into each stack as you wish.

At one end of the stacks should be statements that you agree with very strongly and at the other end of the stacks you should put statements that do not agree with your way of thinking.

**Step II.** Now tightly place a rubber band around each stack.

**Step III.** Now that all the statements are sorted into stacks, write *"most agree"* on the pile that you agree with very strongly. Mark that stack No. 1. Mark No. 2 on the next stack and continue numbering your piles in succession down to the stack you disagree with the most. Also number that stack and write on it *"strongly disagree."*

**Step IV.** Now write *"agree"* on any other stacks that seem to agree with your way of thinking.

**Step V.** Write *"disagree"* on any other stacks that you disagree with.

# C. SPORTS MEDICINE AND KINESIOLOGY

# The Influence of Ultrasound and High Frequency Radio Waves on the Rate of Reabsorption of Experimental Hematomas

DAVID C. REID
JOHN B. REDFORD
PETER KING

Trauma, either by direct violence or by stretching and twisting strains is invariably accompanied by a degree of hemorrhage and edema. This hemorrhage may contribute to the functional impairment of the affected body part.

Little experimental work has been done with animals to demonstrate the effects of commonly used physical agents in the treatment of hematomas in tissue.[4,7,13,14] Following subcutaneous hemorrhage, the main recommendations have generally been to elevate and rest the part and to apply cold pressure bandages or ice. These methods are thought to be effective in arresting hemorrhage and preventing further tissue damage. It is also generally accepted that twenty-four to forty-eight hours after the injury, mild active exercises, heat and massage may be instituted to aid in the absorption of the extravate of blood and tissue exudate. In the clinic the forms of heat advocated usually consist of whirlpool baths, ultrasound treatments or hot moist packs. Recently there has been considerable interest in a new form of pulsed high frequency electromagnetic energy that has been said not to produce significant heating and yet has similar therapeutic effects to established agents.[15,21,31]

*Note:* The authors wish to express their thanks for the assistance given by Miss Birgitte Lund, Miss Sue Roberts, and Miss Judy Hannon.

The purpose of this study was to evaluate the influence of ultrasound and high frequency radio waves on the rate of reabsorption of experimental hematomas in rabbits' ears. The study was based on a technique described by Fenn,[7] who compared the effects of pulsed high frequency therapy with an untreated control group in the removal of experimental hematomas. The method of producing these hematomas and of studying the effects of high frequency energy are very simple and can have widespread application in experimental work using physical modalities. Fenn's study clearly demonstrated that the hematoma was removed from the treated group more rapidly than from the untreated group. However, he did not compare these effects with those produced by any other modality.

The present study was an extension of that reported by Fenn, including the effects of shortwave diathermy and ultrasound.

## Materials and Methods

Thirty New Zealand white male rabbits weighing 1,500 to 2,000 gms were housed in individual cages in a controlled environment, and were fed a standard laboratory diet.

Twenty-four hours after shaving the ears, blood was taken by cardiac puncture using an 18 gauge hypodermic needle and 0.5 cc were reinjected into the rabbit's left ear with a 1½", 24 gauge hypodermic needle. Care was taken to avoid the main arterial arch. In each case the blood was injected about 20 mm from the tip of the ear between the cartilage and the subcutaneous tissues. This was later verified by histological sections (hematoxylin and eosin stain).

The animals were divided at random into five groups including an untreated control group, a group receiving shortwave diathermy* (S.W.D.) once daily, a group receiving shortwave diathermy twice daily, a group receiving ultrasound† (U.S.)

---

* Short Wave Diathermy machine, Model 490, from Burdick Corporation. Frequency controlled, harmonic depressed, 27.120 K.C. ± .160 K.C., working on mains supply. Maximum output of 560 watts and 8.4 amps.

† Ultrasound: Using Siemans Sonostate .631 with continuous output control that goes up to 3 watts per cm² and has a treatment head of 4 cm² producing unmodulated ultrasonic frequency of 870 K.C.

once daily, and a group receiving ultrasound twice daily. The treated animals were observed over a period of twelve days.

For treatment and measurement purposes the animals were secured in a canvas holding bag with velcro fasteners. The S.W.D. was applied with two condensor plate malleable electrodes with felt spacing, using a minimal thermal dosage for twenty minutes either once or twice daily according to the group. The ultrasound was given in water in order to prevent the massage effect of the treatment head. The dosage was .8 watts/cm$^2$ for five minutes.

A record of the rate of reabsorption as indicated by the change in surface area of hematoma was obtained by photographing the rabbit's ears daily, after the treatment. The surface area was outlined and measured by means of a planimeter.[7] An apparatus was designed to hold the ear in a glass screen and render it translucent with reflected light. High speed ectochrome color film (type B135-20 at 1/30 sec.) was used at a distance of 17 cm.

A separate group of control and treated animals were sacrificed at intervals in order to obtain histological sections of the hematoma reabsorption.

The data for each condition were averaged for each rabbit over four series of three consecutive days (i.e. reduced to 4 values per rabbit per condition). The data was subjected to a two-factor analysis of variance or repeated measures. Conditions constituted level of one factor and blocks of three consecutive days constituted levels of the second factor. Since the groups ultimately involved different numbers of rabbits, an unweighted means solution was appropriate. The conditions x days interaction in the overall analysis of variance was significant ($F = 710.78$), and an analysis of simple effects was subsequently made.

## Results

The injected hematoma slowly spread in the fascial plane of the rabbit's ear. After twenty-four hours, the hematoma had spread to its maximum extent and was surrounded by a red flare about 2 mm wide. In the initial four days, there was considerable

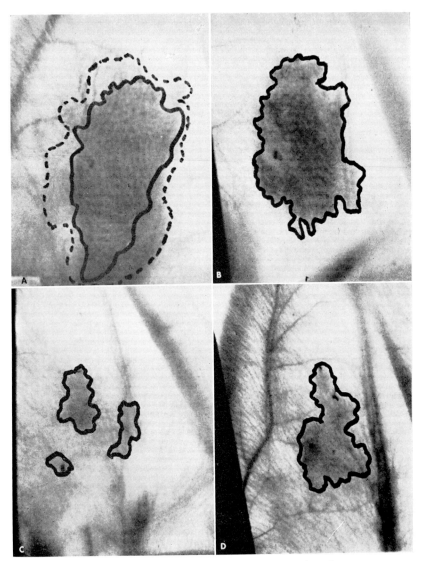

Figure 26–1. Photographs to show sequence of reabsorption.

a. S.W.D. twice daily. The continuous line indicates the hematoma on the day of injection and the dotted line indicates subsequent spread of hematoma by the second day.

b. S.W.D. twice daily, hematoma at day four.

c. S.W.D. twice daily. Hematoma at day eight. Note that there is almost complete reabsorption in this particular rabbit's ear.

d. Control rabbit receiving no treatment. This photograph indicates the state of reabsorption at day 9.

reabsorption as indicated by a change in color and reduction of the hematoma size. This was accompanied by a certain amount of hematoma migration toward the root of the ear. The extravasation followed the lines of least resistance. This made measurement of the surface area more difficult, and was a possible source of error. By ten days, very little visible sign of the hematoma remained. The site of the hematoma in all animals felt thickened to the touch.

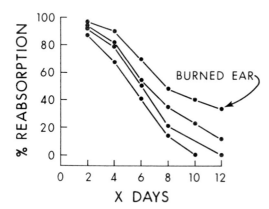

Figure 26–2. Rate of reabsorption for individual rabbits receiving ultrasound twice daily.

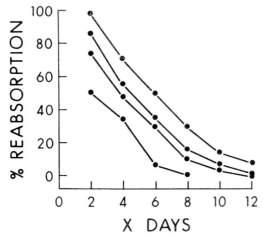

Figure 26–3. Rate of reabsorption for individual rabbits receiving shortwave diathermy twice daily.

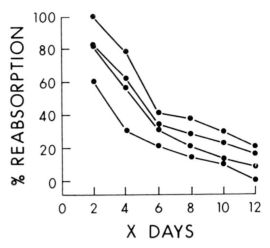

Figure 26–4. Rate of reabsorption for individual control rabbits. These received no treatment.

Differences among conditions for each of the time blocks and differences among time blocks for each of the conditions are given in Table 26-I. The Tukey (a) procedure was employed to determine specific mean differences subsequent to a significant F ratio in each of the several analyses. A .01 rejection level was adopted for the hypothesis of no mean difference. In view of the

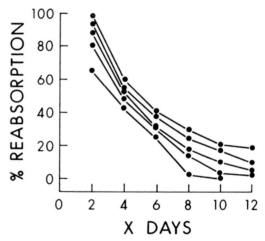

Figure 26–5. Rate of reabsorption, for individual rabbits receiving ultrasound once daily.

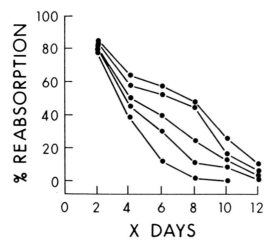

Figure 26–6. Rate of reabsorption for individual rabbits receiving short-wave diathermy once daily.

fact that the principal purpose of the study was to determine trends and since there were relatively few rabbits per group, the analysis employed may be too conservative. Whether or not the error variance could be substantially reduced by a larger number of rabbits remains to be determined.

The analysis of variance was included primarily to suggest the possibility of differences and discussion is largely limited to the graphic differences. Such discussion may suggest a logical basis for expecting differences in subsequent studies which employ a greater number of rabbits.

In order to obtain the best single smooth curve for each group of rabbits the mean points were calculated and approximated (Fig. 26–7). The data obtained from this project were then compared with data from an identical experiment using pulsed high frequency therapy* (Fig. 26–8).

## Discussion

The response to an injected hematoma will be different from that following blunt trauma, and in fact the injected blood may

* Diapulse Corporation of America, Lake Success, New York. Frequency 27.12 megacycles, crystal controlled to ± .005 megacycles.

TABLE 26-I

ANALYSIS OF MEAN DIFFERENCES AMONG TREATMENTS FOR EACH BLOCK OF THREE CONSECUTIVE DAYS AND AMONG BLOCKS OF THREE CONSECUTIVE DAYS FOR EACH TREATMENT

| Treatments | | Days 1–3 | 4–6 | 7–9 | 10–12 | MS Days | F(df 3,51)[a] | Critical Difference[b] |
|---|---|---|---|---|---|---|---|---|
| Control | M | 80.17 | 43.67 | 24.58 | 14.75 | 3332.70 | 102.36 | 13.25 |
| | SD | 13.56 | 9.72 | 7.37 | 8.41 | | | |
| S.W.D. 1X daily | M | 82.07 | 45.87 | 27.27 | 8.33 | 4943.03 | 151.82 | 11.85 |
| | SD | 1.34 | 12.03 | 16.50 | 5.88 | | | |
| S.W.D. 2X daily | M | 77.92 | 44.25 | 13.58 | 3.58 | 4497.29 | 138.13 | 13.25 |
| | SD | 12.87 | 13.05 | 10.08 | 3.90 | | | |
| U.S.　1X daily | M | 86.67 | 42.53 | 19.27 | 7.80 | 6079.02 | 186.72 | 11.85 |
| | SD | 10.25 | 4.48 | 8.26 | 7.10 | | | |
| U.S.　2X daily | M | 92.25 | 65.75 | 29.50 | 14.33 | 4966.18 | 152.54 | 13.25 |
| | SD | 2.53 | 7.94 | 12.97 | 15.58 | | | |
| M.S. treatments F(df 4,17)[a] | | 133.23 | 390.98 | 173.53 | 91.18 | | | |
| | | 1.03 | 3.01 | 1.34 | .70 | | | |

[a] Error mean squares were derived from the original 2-factor analysis of variance. To determine the existence of significant differences among treatments and among days, the respective values were 129.87 and 32.56
[b] A mean difference greater than the critical difference was significant ($\alpha = .01$)

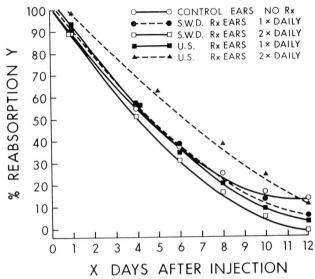

Figure 26–7. Comparison of different treatment groups. The plotted mean points are approximated with the best single smooth curves.

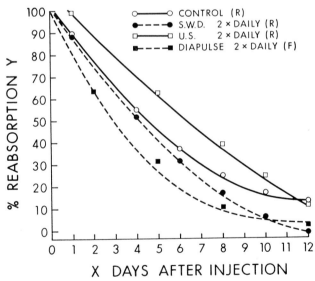

Figure 26–8. Comparison between treatment groups receiving a modality twice daily. The data from these groups was then compared with that from a study by J. Fenn. The plotted mean points are approximated with the best single smooth curve (R = Reid *et al.*) (F = Fenn).

take longer to be reabsorbed than the normal traumatic exudate. Perhaps the injected blood does not provide sufficient stimulation since tissue damage is at a minimum. However, the presence of superimposed tissue damage would have its own particular problems in terms of healing and if these facts are realized and accepted the conclusions drawn from this study may be viewed in the correct perspective and some useful information may be obtained. It may be that superimposed trauma could magnify the small statistical differences.

### Treatment by Ultrasound

The rate of reabsorption was increased in the group treated once per day at .8 watts/cm$^2$ for five minutes. In contrast, the group treated with the same intensity twice daily actually showed a slower rate of resolution, although at day twelve, it had reached the same point as the controls. This apparent reversal of results was due to burning of one of the rabbit's ears which greatly influenced the trend of the small group. The ear is thin and the cartilage interface probably presents a great deal of acoustic impedance and hence sheer waves which contribute greatly to heating. In retrospect, a dosage of 0.8 watts/cm$^2$ probably represents a relatively high dosage. In the rabbit's ear, it has been demonstrated that if the intensity is kept low, vasodilatation results whereas high dosages may cause spastic occlusion of the small vessels.[1,25] This may cause heat rise and hence burning.

If the curves are plotted using data only from the unburned animals there may be an increase in the rate of reabsorption of the treated group (U.S. twice daily) over the control group.

It has been clearly demonstrated that different dosages may have different effects on tissue healing, nerve conduction and cell permeability even within the short clinical range of 0.2–3 watts/cm$^2$.[10,17] The magnitude of intensity change needed for these different effects may in fact be as little as .5 watts/cm$^2$. There are other variables in using and evaluating ultrasound that must be considered. These include the nature of the tissue and its protein content, the blood supply to an area, the depth of penetration of the sound and the different effects of pulsed versus continuous therapy. These have been investigated to some degree but the clinical application of ultrasound and the prescription of dosage is still largely empirical, and is often based on supposition and trials with no controls.

To understand how ultrasound may aid in the resolution of hematomas, one must first be familiar with some aspects of wave motion.

Ultrasonic energy originating as mechanical vibration is transmitted through an elastic medium as a band of compression (acoustic pressure). Molecules of this medium are displaced and oscillate about their equilibrium points. The motion of the irradiated substance may be referred to as cyclic or acoustic motion. By virtue of the elastic properties of the medium, this molecular oscillation is transmitted from one layer to the next and the wave consequently progresses through the medium.

The forward motion of an oscillation produces compression whereas the reverse movement allows decompression. The forces involved in creating alternate density and rarefaction are not equal and the resultant imbalance is capable of moving particles of the radiated substance. This movement may be referred to as acoustic streaming and is a unidirectional motion of the particles which are free to move.[17,19,22] Acoustic or fluid streaming is directly proportional to the intensity of the ultrasound field and to the square of the frequency and inversely proportional to the coefficient of viscosity of the medium.

Heat is also produced along the radiation track as energy is transformed from one form to another. This is in proportion to the energy absorbed and the heat rise is dependent on the nature of the tissue, the presence of gas bubbles, colloids and the circulation. At inferfaces, where there is poor impedance matching, sheer waves play a part in producing heat.

Dyson and Pond[4] concluded that there were three principal mechanisms by which ultrasound could have an effect on tissue. These included thermal, cyclic and cycle averaging effects. The thermal effects arise as previously described. The cyclic effects are those tissue movements which are repeated at each wave cycle and the cycle averaging effects are those effects that do not average to zero over time, but actually accumulate.

It is tempting to attribute the therapeutic effects of ultrasound simply to thermal causes since metabolic activity and local blood flow usually increase in proportion to the rise in temperature. Lehmann *et al.*,[16] were able to demonstrate that the permeation of ions across membranes was increased during and after sonation beyond that which could be explained by heating effects alone. The increase in permeability was not increased to the same extent using controls whose tissue temperature was made to mimic the treated group. The acoustic streaming effect mentioned previously is probably one of the most significant features in reabsorption and is presently under investigation.[4,19,30] It may occur within, through and around cell membranes.

Observations with the aid of electron microscopy have revealed that fibroblasts may be stimulated to increase the synthesis of the molecular units of which collagen is composed. However, it is the polymerization of these units that is necessary to give mature collagen outside the fibroblast that may be inhibited throughout the period that ultrasound treatments are being given. This would have the effect of limiting fibrous adhesions, thus limiting the amount of scarring and allowing the elements of the hematoma to be completely reabsorbed.

Ultrasound has been shown to decrease the viscosity of colloidal substances, particularly hyaluronic acid.[5,11] *In vitro* conversion of a gel to a sol may take place with intensities of ultrasound as low as 0.4 watts/cm$^2$ in a period of two minutes at 800 k.c. frequency.[20]

The increased rate of resolution of subcutaneous hematomas with ultrasound treatment is probably due to an increase in circulation and permeability of the cellular elements. There is also a possibility of reduction of mature collagen synthesis and an influence on the viscosity of colloidal particles. These points are introduced as a suggested mechanism in the reduction of fibrous adhesions and residual scarring.[2,28]

---

### Possible Mechanisms of Increased Rate of Resolution due to Ultrasound

1. Vasodilatation and increased capillary exchange.
2. Oxidation and reduction processes increased.
3. Depolimerization of proteins.
4. Decreased viscosity of colloidal particles.
5. Agitation of cell content and mechanical strain on cell membranes.
6. Acoustic and fluid streaming of free particles.

---

### Treatment With High Frequency Apparatus

The curves showed a small increase in the rate of reabsorption in the group treated once daily with continuous short wave diathermy. This increased rate of resolution was magnified in the group treated with continuous shortwaves twice daily for twenty minutes. It should be noted that S.W.D. twice daily was the only series to demonstrate complete reabsorption in this study and this was statistically significant at the 95 percent level in the last time block, i.e. days nine to twelve.

Following each short wave diathermy treatment, the vessels of the ear were distended and the ear presented a flushed appearance for a varying period. Much of the reabsorption can probably be attributed to this increase in circulation. This is accompanied by increased metabolism of the area, decreased viscosity of the exudate, and a greater exchange of fluid at the capillary level. While this increase in circulation was desirable in a hematoma of the nature under investigation the danger of increased hemorrhage is apparent in the early stages of traumatic injury.

There are perhaps some effects that are directly related to the electromagnetic spectrum and not simply due to the heating of the tissue.[9,29] Recent experiments have shown an increase in blood flow and improved rate of healing which are not related to temperature rise in the tissues.[8,15] These nonthermal effects may be due to the group of kinins such as histamine, serotonin and related chemicals which have far reaching effects on blood flow and cellular metabolism. The blood level and tissue content of histamine is greatly increased after treatment with short-waves.[23,26,27]

Fenn's data showed pulsed shortwaves to be more effective than continuous S.W.D. in the early stages of treatment. A probable explanation is that much higher intensities of shortwaves may be administered without burning the tissues. Peak intensities of 1 kw may be administered with pulsed apparatus whereas the peak output of continuous shortwaves (560 watts) could not be approached.[3,21,24] The rest period in pulsed shortwaves prevents a build-up of heat. At maximum setting the pulse period is 65 microseconds with a 1600 microsecond rest period, i.e. a ratio of 25 : 1. Contrary to what has been reported, in the rabbit's ear there may be a drift of 0.5 to 5.0°C from the baseline even with the pulsed apparatus in a region of this nature.[6] The mode of action of pulsed versus continuous shortwave apparatus is still not clear but it is evident that they have different indications for use.

## References

1. Bauer, A.W.: *Brit. J. Phys. Med.* 17:97, 1954.
2. Conger, A.C.: *Genetics.* 33:607, 1968.
3. DeCamp, C.E.: *North American Veterinarian.* 23:785, 1942.
4. Dyson, M., and Pond, J.B.: *J. Chart. Soc. Phys.* 56:136, 1970.
5. Elpiner, I.E., and Bychov, S.M.: *Dokl. Akad. Nauk. SSSR.* 82:123, 1952.
6. Erdmann, W.J. II.: *Amer. J. Orthoped.* Aug. 1960.
7. Fenn, J.E.: *Canad. Med. Ass. J.* 100:251, 1969.
8. Fenn, J.E.: Personal Communication, June 1970, Dept. of Obstetrics and Gynecology, St. Michael's Hospital, Toronto.
9. Ginsberg, A.J.: Paper presented at N.Y. Acad. of Med. October 14–25, 1940.
10. Goldman, D.E., and Hueter, O.B.: *J. Acoust. Soc. Amer.* 28:35, 1956.
11. Griffin, J.E.: *J. Amer. Phys. Ther. Asso.* 46:18, 1966.
12. Hamdy, M.K., Konle, L.E., Rheins, M.S., and Deatherage, F.E.: *J. Anim. Sci.* 16:496, 1957.
13. Heath, J.L.: *J. Amer. Phys. Ther. Ass.* 47:9, 1967.
14. Joseph, J.: *The Medical Post.* Nov. 4: 33, 1969.

15. King, D.R., Hathaways, J.W., Reynolds, D.C.: *The Journal: District of Columbia Dental Society.* XLII: 1, 1968.
16. Lehmann: *Arch. Phys. Med.* 34:139, 1953.
17. Madsen, P.W., and Gersten, J.W.: *Arch. Phys. Med.* 42:645, 1961.
18. Moritz, A.R.: *The Pathology of Trauma.* Philadelphia, Lea Febiger, 1942.
19. Nyborg, W.L.: *Acoustic Streaming in Physical Acoustics.* (Ed. by W.P. Mason) New York, Academic Press, (1965).
20. Rauser, V.: *Arch. Phys. Ther. (Leipzig).* 10:469, 1958.
21. Reid, D.C.: Treatment by pulsating athermic shortwaves. Paper re-sented at the Annual Congress of the Canadian Physiotherapy Association. June 1970, Toronto, Ontario.
22. Selman, G.G., and Cource, S.J.: *Nature (London).* 172:503, 1953.
23. Shiffmann, M., and Safford, F. Jr.: *Physiother. Rev.* 23:6, 1943.
24. Silverman, D.R., and Pendleton, L.: *Arch. Phys. Med. Rehab.* 49: 439, 1968.
25. Stuhlfauth, K., Goelkel, A., and Mayer, L.: *Strahlentherapie.* 91, 629, 1963.
26. Valtonen, E.J.: *Amer. J. Phys. Med.* 47:4, 1968.
27. Valtonen, E.J.: *Amer. J. Phys. Med.* 47:2, 1968.
28. Wakim, K.G.: A Special Review. *Amer. J. Phys. Med.* 32:32, 1953.
29. Wildervanch, A., Wakim, K.G., Merrick, I.F., and Kruse, F.H.: *Arch. Phys. Med.* 40:45, 1945.
30. Wilson, W.L., Wiercinski, F.J., Nyborg, W.L., Schnitzler, R.M., and Siched, F.J.: *J. Acoust. Soc. Amer.* 40:1363, 1966.
31. Zulli, L.P.: *J. Amer. Podiat. Ass.* 58, No. 8, Aug. 1968.

# Chapter 27

# An Electromyographic Technique for Comparing the Relative Involvement of Skeletal Muscles During Exercise

G.B. Thompson

One fundamental limitation in the exercise specialist's ability to prescribe the most effective conditioning or rehabilitation exercise for a particular individual is his understanding of the exact muscular demands of each exercise. Researchers interested in conditioning and therapeutic exercises have found the myoelectric signal a useful diagnostic tool for determining phasic action, and for subjectively assessing the tension levels of participating muscles. It is now generally accepted that the electrical activity in human skeletal muscle bears a linear relation to the tension being exerted during an isometric contraction when experimental conditions are strictly standardized.[2,8,10,13] This relationship also applies to a muscle shortening at a constant velocity.[4,5]

Despite the obvious advantages in knowing the quantitative involvement of specific skeletal muscles in various exercises, most of the research has been confined to subjective assessment of action potentials. On the basis that the integrated myoelectric signal can be displayed as a deviation from the baseline proportional to the strength and duration of muscle contraction, a technique was developed in an attempt to permit a comparison of the quantitative involvement of a specific muscle for various exercises.

This paper describes the instrumentation and technique employed as well as some initial observations obtained when six

Note: The work was supported primarily by the Fitness and Amateur Sport Directorate of the Department of National Health and Welfare.

shoulder and arm muscles of forty normal male college subjects were compared for ten different variations of the shoulder flexion—elbow extension movement.

## Methods and Materials

Recognizing that the linear relationship between muscle tension and electrical activity are known to be individual and dependent upon the muscles studied, we decided to base any quantitative measure of the degree of involvement of a given muscle in a given exercise as a percentage of that muscle's "maximum" isometric contraction. Our approach is based on to work of Hill,[7] Bigland and Lippold[4] and Close, Nickel, and Todd,[5] which suggests that the myoelectric signal is proportional to the isometric tension of a muscle, and that in isotomic activity a linear relationship between muscle tension and electrical activity is possible only where there is constant velocity of muscle contraction.

The "pushup" exercise involving elbow extension and shoulder flexion was arbitrarily chosen for initial investigation. The triceps brachii, anterior deltoid, pectoralis major (clavicular and sternal portions), and the forearm extensor muscles were selected for monitoring.

Activity of the rectus abdominus was included in an attempt to assess the degree of trunk stabilization associated with each of the ten movements. Phasic activity for all six muscles was also recorded.

To obtain a myoelectric signal which represented the "maximum" force output of the muscle the cable-tension strength test techniques developed by Clarke and associates were used.[6] Maximum static contractions of shoulder flexion, elbow extension, and wrist dorsal flexion were obtained for this purpose (Fig. 27-1).

Each subject was asked to continue his effort for three seconds after an apparent maximum was reached. The integrated myoelectric signals from the six muscles were then obtained for each of the selected exercises. To minimize the influence of fatigue, the exercise order was selected at random for each subject.

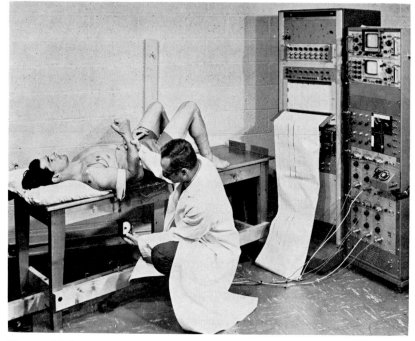

Figure 27–1. Measurement of "maximum contraction" of the shoulder flexors using the cable tension technique.

The following ten variations of the pushup exercise were performed by each of the forty subjects:

1. The "wall pushup" (subject stands with feet at arms length from wall, hands at shoulder height)
2. The "hip flex" pushup (subject pushes up to a kneeling position with hips flexed)
3. The "knee" pushup (a standard pushup performed with the knees flexed)
4. The "standard" pushup
5. The "wide" pushup (hands placed 10 inches wider than the normal position)
6. The "standard" pushup (hands placed 10 inches wider and ten inches forward from the normal position)
7. The "extended" pushup (hands placed 10 inches forward from the normal position)

8. The "bench" pushup (a standard pushup with subject's feet 18 inches above the floor)
9. The "circle" pushup
10. The "press up"

Because a linear relationship between muscle tension and electrical activity is possible only where there is constant velocity of muscles contraction, all movement during execution of these exercises was controlled by training the subject to move through the full range of movement of the exercise at a constant velocity (Fig. 27–2).

The portion of the record of a specific muscle's output during exercise which was selected for comparison with that during maximum output was that portion of the total signal representative of the largest amount of effort under conditions of constant velocity (Fig. 27–3).

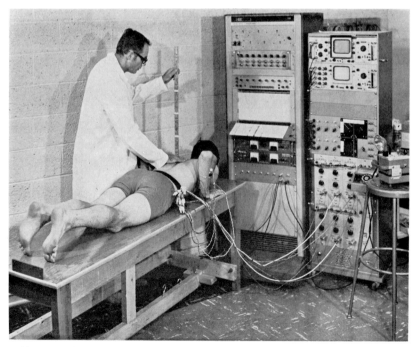

Figure 27–2. Training the subject for constant velocity movements.

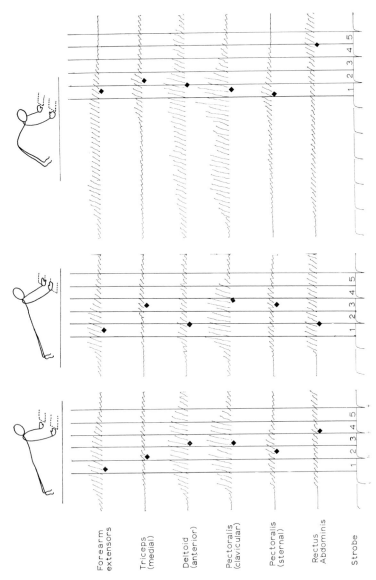

Figure 27–3. Integrated signals of three variations of the pushup exercise.

Instrumentation adapted at U.N.B. for both signal display and absolute mean level measurement was used.[15]

Myoelectric signal data was obtained by the use of a seven channel recording system including Bechman surface electrodes, TEKTRONIX 125 preamplifiers, buffer amplifiers, magnetic tape recorders (for signal storing) and a Hewlett Packard 7200 eight channel heat-writing recorder. Six channels recorded the myoelectric activity while the seventh was used to record the timing device and thereby link the arm position and angles of elbow and shoulder to the integrated signal during the exercise.

For measurement of the absolute mean level of the myoelectric signal a six-channel integrator system was used consisting of a low level full wave rectifier followed by an operational amplifier integrator. The period of integration, controlled by a multivibrator, was set to 0.1 seconds.

## Results

The mean "percentage-of-maximum" values of the six muscles for forty subjects obtained during the performance of ten variations of the pushup exercise is shown in Figure 27–4.

Statistical analysis employing the test show significant differences—in many cases to the .01 level—between mean levels of each muscle for the ten variations of the pushup exercise. No one variation required maximum demands for all muscles involved.

## Discussion

It would appear that under carefully controlled conditions the integrated myoelectric signal obtained from a muscle during the isotomic contraction of constant velocity can be given a quantitative value by being represented as a percentage of a determined "maximum" obtained by static contraction.

In this context, the quantitative involvement of a specific muscle can be determined and compared for various exercises as a means of objective selection of the most effective exercises for that muscle.

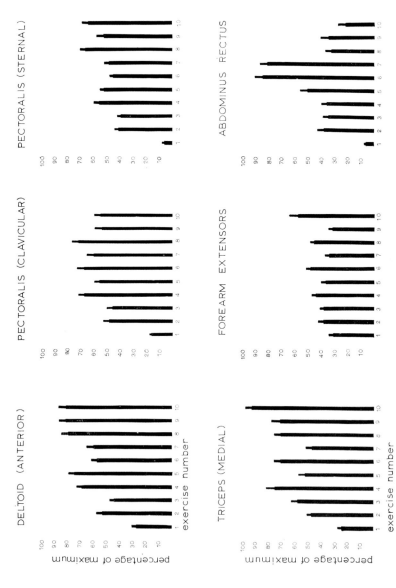

Figure 27–4. Mean "Percentage-of-Maximum" values for forty subjects for six muscles during ten variations of the pushup exercise.

# References

1. Basmajian, J.V.: *Muscles Alive—Their Functions Revealed by Electromyography.* Baltimore, Williams and Wilkins, 1967.
2. Bergstrom, R.M.: *Acta. Physiol. Scand.* 45:97, 1969.
3. Bierman, W., and Yamshon. L.J.: *Arch. Phys. Med.* 29:206, 1948.
4. Bigland, B., and Lippold, O.C.J.: *J Physiol.* 123:214, 1954.
5. Close, J.R., Nickel, E.D., and Todd, F.N.: *J Bone Joint Surg.* 42-A: 1207, 1960.
6. Clarke, H.H.: *A Manual of Cable-Tension Strength Tests.* Springfield, Springfield College, 1953.
7. Hill, A.V.: *Proc. Roy. Soc.* B:156, 1938.
8. Inmann, V.T., Ralston, H.J., *et al.: Electrocephalog. Clin. Neurophysiol.* 4:187, 1952.
9. Jonsson, B.: Electrode problems in electromyographic kinesiology, Paper delivered at 1st International Meeting of EMG Kinesiology, Montreal, August, 1968.
10. Jonsson, B., and Reichmann, S.: *Acta Morphologica, Neerlando—Scandinav.* 7:73, 1968.
11. Jonsson, B., Stein, B.: *Acta Morphologica, Neerlando—Scandinav.* 1965.
12. Liberson, W.T., Dondey, M., and Asa, M.: *Amer. J. Phys. Med.* 41:3, 1962.
13. Lippold, O.C.J.: *J. Physiol.* 117:492, 1952.
14. Pauly, J.E.: *Anat. Rec.* 155:223, 1966.
15. Scott, R.N. *et al.:* Myo-Electric control systems—Muscle function analysis, progress report No. 8. U.N.B. Bio-Engineering Institute Research Report 69.1, pp. 7–11, March, 1969.

Chapter 28

# Kinematics of the Standing Long Jump in Seven, Ten, Thirteen and Sixteen-Year-old Boys

BENOIT ROY

## Introduction

Many studies in the area of biomechanics have focused on locomotor skills, especially walking and running. The works of Eberhardt et al.,[5] Elftman,[9,10,11,12,13] Grieve et al.,[18] Murray et al.,[26] Ralston et al.[29] have been oriented toward the development of more functional prosthesis for handicapped people.

Other studies by kinesiologists like Clayton,[4] Eckert,[6,7] Ekern,[8] Felton,[15] Glassow et al.,[17] Halverson,[19] Hellenbrandt et al.,[22] Wilson[34] have dealt mainly with the analysis of basic skills like throwing, running and jumping. The object of these studies has focused on the evolution of these skills with age. Differences in terms of sex and levels of performance have also been considered.

Finally coaches and sports specialists like Fletcher et al.,[16] Hay,[20] Lascari,[24] Magel,[25] Payne et al.,[28] Karas et al.,[23] Hebbelinck et al.,[21] Wartenweiler et al.[33] have all contributed to bring a more scientific approach to sport skills.

Studies by Glassow et al.,[17] Halverson,[19] Roberts[30] tend to suggest that the kinematics of throwing, running, jumping and kicking are well established by six years of age.

According to Roberts, knee extension in the kicking skill of a 3½-year-old boy reaches an angular velocity of 1400 degrees/second, compared to 2000 degrees/second for an adult skilled

Note: This paper is part of a doctoral dissertation completed under the direction of Professor Elizabeth M. Roberts, Department of Physical Education, University of Wisconsin, Madison, U.S.A.

performer. Halverson,[19] Zimmerman[35] and Felton[15] report that good long jumpers reach greater joint angular velocities than poor performers. According to Wilson[34] knee extension during the flight phase of the standing long jump would tend to increase from four to twelve years of age. Other studies by Glassow *et al.*[17] and Eckert[6] have revealed that joint and segment angular measures tend to remain similar in boys six to twelve years of age. The present paper is part of a more complete investigation on the kinematics and kinetics of the standing long jump.[31] The present discussion will be limited to some kinematic factors of the jump.

## Methods and Procedures

Fifty male students, ages seven, ten, thirteen and sixteen were subjects for this investigation. All those who had not yet reached their next highest birthday were considered as eventual candidates for a given age group.

The middle 30 percent on the national norms of the standing long jump of the AAHPER[1] was used as a criterion of selection of the subjects in each age group. As the American norms do not include the seven-year-old category, the Canadian norms[3] were used to compute the equation of the regression line for this group. A correlation of .98 was found between the United States and Canadian norms at other age groups. The norms for the four groups were as follows: seven-year-old: 49 to 55 inches; ten-year-old: 58 to 64 inches; thirteen-year-old: 66 to 73 inches; sixteen-year-old: 81 to 89 inches.

Subjects were selected at random from the compiled listing of all those whose ages fell within the established categories of seven, ten, thirteen and sixteen. Those children whose average jump distance did not fall within the selected limits were excluded from the study.

Each group was finally made up as follows: seven and ten-year-old groups had fifteen subjects each; thirteen and sixteen-year-old groups had twenty subjects each. The following measures were taken as the subjects jumped from a force platform:*

* This platform was designed by Professor Ali H. Seireg from the Department of Mechanical Engineering of the University of Wisconsin, Madison.

the horizontal and vertical forces; the moment in a sagittal plane. A detailed description of this platform is given in Baz,[2] Patel[27] and Roy.[31]

At a second session, cinematographic records of the standing long jump were obtained from five subjects randomly selected from each group. Fig. 28–1 presents the testing situation. A 16

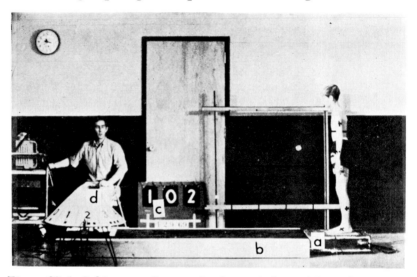

Figure 28–1. Subject standing on the force platform (a) until instructed to jump. Also identified are the landing platform (b), the subject's number board (c) and the electric clock (d).

mm camera was positioned laterally, forty to forty-five feet from the subject. The camera was set at sixty-four frames per second.

A model P-40 Recordak microfilm reader was used to enlarge (magnification 40) to the 16 mm film image so that the angular change could be measured at the metatarsophalangeal, ankle, knee, hip and shoulder joints. In principle, least-squares curve fitting, using Gauss elimination method was used to fit polynomials to the angular data points. Subsequently a fourth degree polynomial equation was generated. Thus the coefficients of the respective polynomial equations could be used to obtain velocity and acceleration measures at any point of the propulsive phase of the jump.†

† Special acknowledgment to Robert W. Schutz and Youngil Youm for their assistance in designing the computer program.

## Results and Discussion

Figures 28–2 to 28–6 present typical curves of angular velocity and acceleration for the different joints. Tables 28-I and 28-II present the means, standard deviations and coefficients of variation of the maximal angular velocity and acceleration values for all six articulations.

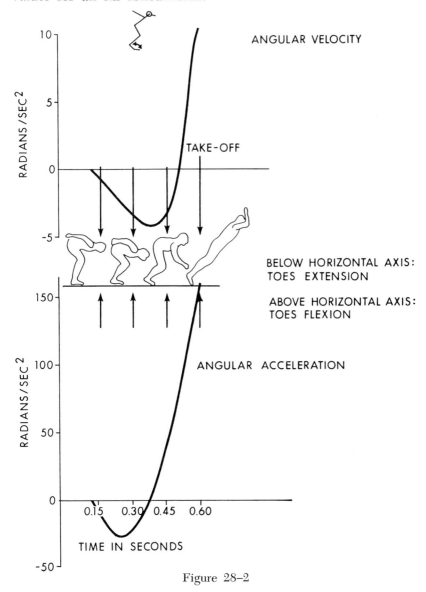

Figure 28–2

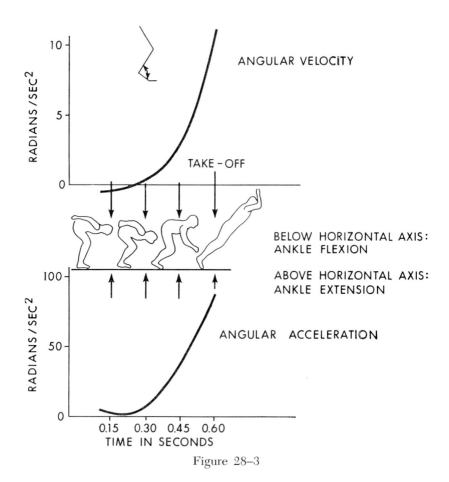

Figure 28–3

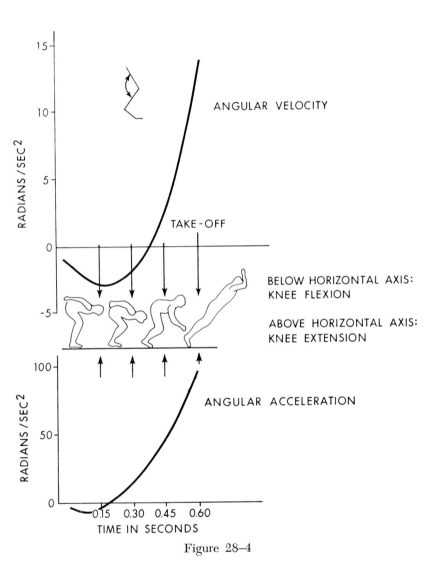

Figure 28–4

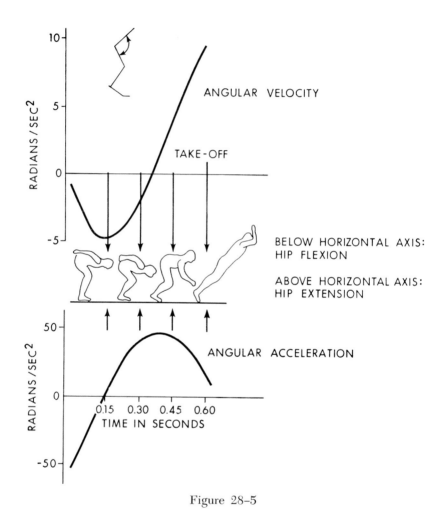

Figure 28–5

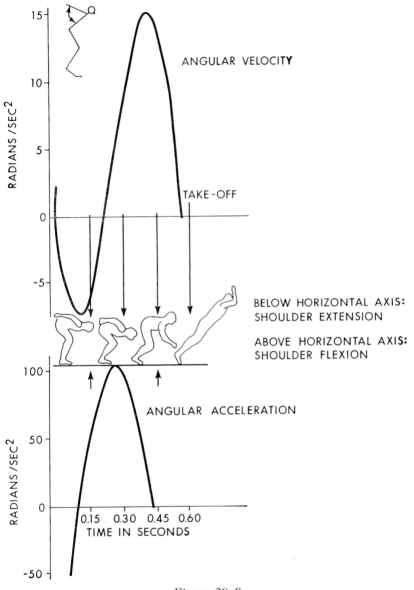

Figure 28–6

## TABLE 28-I
### MEANS AND STANDARD DEVIATIONS OF JOINTS' MAXIMAL ANGULAR VELOCITY (Radians/sec)

| Age | 7 (N = 5) | | | 10 (N = 5) | | | 13 (N = 5) | | | 16 (N = 5) | | |
|---|---|---|---|---|---|---|---|---|---|---|---|---|
| | M | σ | σ/M | M | σ | σ/M | M | σ | σ/M | M | σ | σ/M |
| Metatarsophalangeal | 8.6 | 2.7 | 31.3 | 7.1 | 1.3 | 18.3 | 10.6 | 3.7 | 34.9 | 8.8 | 1.6 | 18.1 |
| Ankle | 10.5 | 1.2 | 11.4 | 12.5 | 2.0 | 16.0 | 11.1 | 2.8 | 25.2 | 12.6 | 1.3 | 12.2 |
| Knee | 10.1 | 2.0 | 19.8 | 7.6 | 2.4 | 31.5 | 8.1 | 2.5 | 30.8 | 14.6 | 0.8 | 5.4 |
| Hip | 10.9 | 1.9 | 12.4 | 10.6 | 2.5 | 23.5 | 9.9 | 1.6 | 16.1 | 11.9 | 2.4 | 20.1 |
| Shoulder | 12.9 | 3.2 | 24.8 | 13.9 | 2.0 | 14.3 | 12.3 | 3.5 | 28.4 | 15.6 | 1.8 | 11.5 |

## TABLE 28-II
### MEANS AND STANDARD DEVIATIONS OF JOINTS' MAXIMAL ANGULAR ACCELERATION (Radians/sec²)

| Age | 7 (N = 5) | | | 10 (N = 5) | | | 13 (N = 5) | | | 16 (N = 5) | | |
|---|---|---|---|---|---|---|---|---|---|---|---|---|
| | M | σ | σ/M | M | σ | σ/M | M | σ | σ/M | M | σ | σ/M |
| Metatarso-phalangeal | 130.8 | 52.4 | 40.0 | 148.7 | 34.2 | 23.0 | 154.3 | 69.7 | 45.1 | 129.4 | 45.3 | 35.0 |
| Ankle | 71.7 | 28.3 | 39.4 | 108.8 | 23.6 | 21.6 | 92.2 | 37.5 | 40.6 | 98.4 | 18.3 | 18.5 |
| Knee | 65.0 | 22.6 | 34.7 | 48.6 | 14.2 | 29.2 | 45.8 | 16.5 | 36.0 | 123.6 | 13.9 | 11.2 |
| Hip | 50.6 | 4.5 | 8.8 | 60.6 | 14.7 | 24.2 | 49.6 | 12.3 | 24.7 | 56.7 | 20.5 | 36.1 |
| Shoulder | 80.8 | 20.9 | 25.8 | 98.9 | 22.7 | 22.9 | 85.5 | 26.3 | 30.7 | 95.4 | 17.8 | 18.6 |

TABLE 28-III

MEANS, STANDARD DEVIATIONS AND COEFFICIENTS OF VARIATION OF JOINT MAXIMAL VELOCITY

(Radians/sec)

Adapted from Eckert (22, 23)

| Age | 8 (N = 10) | | | 10 (N = 10) | | | 12 (N = 10) | | | Adult Males (N = 18) | | |
|---|---|---|---|---|---|---|---|---|---|---|---|---|
| | $M$ | $\sigma$ | $\sigma/M$ | $M$ | $\sigma$ | $\sigma/M$ | $M$ | $\sigma$ | $\sigma/M$ | $M$ | $\sigma$ | $\sigma/M$ |
| Hip | 11.0 | 2.9 | 26.3 | 13.0 | 3.0 | 23.0 | 14.0 | 2.8 | 20.0 | 13.5 | 2.5 | 18.5 |
| Knee | 10.1 | 4.3 | 42.5 | 10.2 | 2.0 | 19.6 | 12.0 | 3.9 | 32.5 | 13.9 | 2.6 | 18.7 |
| Ankle | 11.9 | 1.4 | 11.7 | 10.8 | 4.5 | 41.6 | 11.3 | 3.7 | 32.7 | 14.7 | 2.7 | 18.3 |

PRESENT STUDY

| Age | 7 (N = 5) | | | 10 (N = 5) | | | 13 (N = 5) | | | 16 (N = 5) | | |
|---|---|---|---|---|---|---|---|---|---|---|---|---|
| | $M$ | $\sigma$ | $\sigma/M$ | $M$ | $\sigma$ | $\sigma/M$ | $M$ | $\sigma$ | $\sigma/M$ | $M$ | $\sigma$ | $\sigma/M$ |
| Hip | 10.9 | 1.9 | 12.4 | 10.6 | 2.5 | 23.5 | 11.1 | 2.8 | 25.2 | 11.9 | 2.4 | 20.1 |
| Knee | 10.1 | 2.0 | 19.8 | 7.6 | 2.4 | 31.5 | 8.1 | 2.5 | 30.8 | 14.6 | 0.8 | 5.4 |
| Ankle | 10.5 | 1.2 | 11.4 | 12.5 | 2.0 | 16.0 | 9.9 | 1.6 | 16.1 | 12.6 | 1.3 | 12.2 |

A multivariate analysis of variance was used to determine if differences existed between the different groups in joint maximal angular velocity and acceleration. The sixteen-year-old group was the criterion to which the three younger groups were compared.

The statistical analysis revealed that only in knee extension did the sixteen-year-old group reach a higher velocity and acceleration than the other three groups. However only the ten and thirteen-year-old groups were significantly different from the sixteen-year-old group. Moreover, as shown in Tables 28-I and 28-II there was no systematic increase for any articulation from the seven through sixteen year old groups.

The results of this study confirm those of Eckert[6,7] as shown in Table 28-III. It is interesting to note that the maximal angular velocities for the adult subjects of Eckert's study are similar to the sixteen-year-old subjects of this study. On the other hand the maximal angular acceleration values, as shown in Table 28-IV are from three to seven times as large as those reported in this study. Eckert's technique of differentiation could be one of the reasons of the discrepancy between the two studies.

The results of this study confirm the work of Glasow *et al.*[17] who report that the kinematics of walking, running and jumping tend to remain constant between six to twelve years of age, especially in terms of joint angular velocities.

TABLE 28-IV

MEANS, STANDARD DEVIATIONS AND COEFFICIENTS OF VARIATION
OF JOINT MAXIMAL ANGULAR ACCELERATION
(Radians/sec²)

Adapted from Eckert (23)

| Age | 8 (N = 10) M | σ | σ/M | 10 (N = 10) M | σ | σ/M | 12 (N = 10) M | σ | σ/M |
|-----|------|------|------|------|------|------|------|------|------|
| Hip | 212.0 | 161.8 | 76.3 | 350.5 | 281.6 | 80.3 | 323.6 | 192.1 | 59.3 |
| Knee | 286.9 | 296.8 | 103.4 | 281.5 | 109.6 | 38.9 | 363.4 | 170.6 | 46.9 |
| Ankle | 251.2 | 110.1 | 43.8 | 311.7 | 192.2 | 61.6 | 432.8 | 300.0 | 69.3 |

PRESENT STUDY

| Age | 7 (N = 5) M | σ | σ/M | 10 (N = 5) M | σ | σ/M | 13 (N = 5) M | σ | σ/M |
|-----|------|------|------|------|------|------|------|------|------|
| Hip | 50.6 | 4.5 | 8.8 | 60.6 | 14.7 | 24.2 | 49.6 | 12.3 | 24.7 |
| Knee | 65.0 | 22.6 | 34.7 | 48.6 | 14.2 | 29.2 | 45.8 | 16.5 | 36.0 |
| Ankle | 71.7 | 28.3 | 39.4 | 108.8 | 23.6 | 21.6 | 92.2 | 37.5 | 40.6 |

There are no previous studies who have investigated the problem of occurrence in time of the maximal angular velocities and accelerations during the propulsive phase of the jump. As can be seen from Table 28-V, the differences between groups and individuals are small. Generally, knee maximal acceleration occurs .35 second prior to take-off and .10 prior to take-off for shoulder maximal acceleration. It is interesting to note that the maximal angular acceleration of the shoulder corresponds to the peak negative vertical deflection as recorded on the force platform. On the other hand the knee maximal angular accelera-

TABLE 28-V
TIME PRIOR TO TAKE-OFF THE JOINTS' MAXIMAL
VELOCITY AND ACCELERATION ARE REACHED*

| Subject Number | Shoulder | | Hip | | Knee | |
|---|---|---|---|---|---|---|
| | Vel. | Acc. | Vel. | Acc. | Vel. | Acc. |
| 072 | .292 | .496 | T.o | .116 | T.o | T.o |
| 073 | .090 | .300 | T.o | .150 | T.o | T.o |
| 076 | .219 | .394 | T.o | .131 | T.o | .073 |
| 078 | .120 | .300 | T.o | .240 | T.o | .210 |
| 079 | .150 | .330 | .015 | .240 | T.o | T.o |
| Mean | .174 | .364 | .003 | .175 | T.o | .056 |
| 101 | .189 | .335 | .043 | .219 | .073 | .248 |
| 103 | .175 | .350 | T.o | .204 | T.o | .146 |
| 104 | .248 | .452 | T.o | .219 | T.o | .102 |
| 105 | .146 | .292 | T.o | T.o | T.o | .058 |
| 106 | .146 | .321 | T.o | .175 | T.o | .116 |
| Mean | .180 | .350 | .008 | .163 | .014 | .134 |
| 132 | .175 | .379 | T.o | .146 | T.o | .146 |
| 133 | .165 | .375 | T.o | .175 | T.o | .150 |
| 134 | .160 | .335 | T.o | .180 | T.o | .160 |
| 135 | .165 | .345 | T.o | .195 | T.o | .135 |
| 136 | .116 | .321 | .029 | .204 | T.o | .146 |
| Mean | .156 | .350 | .005 | .180 | T.o | .147 |
| 162 | .160 | .365 | T.o | T.o | T.o | T.o |
| 163 | .160 | .335 | T.o | .248 | T.o | T.o |
| 165 | .160 | .365 | T.o | .277 | T.o | T.o |
| 166 | .175 | .379 | T.o | T.o | T.o | T.o |
| 168 | .146 | .350 | T.o | T.o | T.o | T.o |
| Mean | .160 | .358 | T.o | .105 | T.o | T.o |

* T.o = Maximal values reached at take-off
Metatarso-phalangeal and ankle joints' maximal values are reached at take-off
072–079 =   7-year-olds
101–106 = 10-year-olds
132–136 = 13-year-olds
162–166 = 16-year-olds

tion occurs at the maximal positive vertical deflection of the force curve.

The problems of the relative contribution of the upper extremities to the propulsive efficiency of the jump is treated more specifically in Roy.[32]

## Conclusions

The joint maximal angular velocities and accelerations tend to remain constant from seven through sixteen years of age in average performers in the standing long jump. The hypothesis that many of the basic skills have matured by six years of age seems to be verified as far as the jumping skill is concerned.

The time of occurrence of joint maximal velocity and acceleration seems also to exhibit a similar pattern among all subjects. The fact that not only the maximal values of velocity and acceleration are similar from one group to the next, but also their sequential occurrence in time, gives more weight to the hypothesis that most basic skills are mature before the beginning of schooling.

## References

1. American Association for Health, Physical Education and Recreation: *Youth Fitness Test Manual*. Washington, D.C., 1965.
2. Baz, A.S.: A Mathematical model for evaluation of supportive forces during human activities underwater. Unpublished master's thesis, Madison, University of Wisconsin, 1970.
3. Canadian Association of Health, Physical Education and Recreation: *Fitness Performance Test Manual for Girls and Boys Seven to Seventeen*. Ottawa, 1966.
4. Clayton, I.A.: A study of the evidence of the motor age based on technique of the standing broad jump. Unpublished master's thesis, Madison, University of Wisconsin, 1936.
5. Eberhart, H.D., Inman, V.T.: *Ann. N.Y. Acad Sci.* 51:1213, 1951.
6. Eckert, H.M.: Linear relationship of isometric strength to propulsive force, angular velocity and angular acceleration in the standing broad jump. Unpublished doctoral dissertation, Madison, University of Wisconsin, 1961.
7. Eckert, H.M.: *Res. Quart. AAHPER.* 39:937, 1968.
8. Ekern, S.R.: An analysis of selected measures of the overarm throwing patterns of elementary school boys and girls. Unpublished doctoral dissertation. Madison, University of Wisconsin, 1969.

9. Elftman, H.: *Amer. J. Physiol.* 125:359, 1939.
10. Elftman, H.: *Arbeitsphysiologie.* 10:477, 1939.
11. Elftman, H.: *Arbeitsphysiologie.* 10:485, 1939.
12. Elftman, H.: *Amer. J. Physiol.* 125:339, 1939.
13. Elftman, H. *Amer. J. Physiol.* 129:672, 1940.
14. Falize, J.L., Lucassen, J.P., Hunebelle, G.: *Kinanthropologie.* 1:25, 1969.
15. Felton, E.A.: A kinesiological comparison of good and poor jumpers in the standing broad jump. Unpublished master's thesis. Madison, University of Wisconsin, 1960.
16. Fletcher, J.G., Lewis, H.E., Wilkie, D.R.: *Ergonomics.* 3:30, 1960.
17. Glassow, R.B., Halverson, L.E., Rarick, G.L.: Improvement of motor development and physical fitness in elementary school children. Cooperation research project no. 696. Madison, University of Wisconsin, 1965.
18. Grieve, D.W., Gear, R.J.: *Ergonomics.* 5:379, 1966.
19. Halverson, L.E.: A comparison of performance of kindergarten children in the take-off phase of the standing broad jump. Unpublished doctoral dissertation, Madison, University of Wisconsin, 1958.
20. Hay, J.G.: An investigation of take-off impulses in two styles of high jumping. Unpublished doctoral dissertation, Iowa City, University of Iowa. 1967.
21. Hebbelinck, M., Borms, J., and Famaey, A.: *Kinanthropologie.* 1:311, 1969.
22. Hellenbrandt, F.A., Rarick, G.L., Glassow, R.B., and Carns, M.L.: *Amer. J. Phys. Med.* 40:14, 1961.
23. Karas, V., and Borms, J.: *Kinanthropologie.* 1:63, 1969.
24. Lascari, A.T.: The felge handstand—A comparative kinetic analysis of a gymnastic skill. Unpublished doctoral dissertation, Madison, University of Wisconsin, 1970.
25. Magel, J.R.: *Res. Quart. AAHPER.* 41:68, 1970.
26. Murray, M.P., Drought, A.B., Kory, R.C.: *J. Bone Joint Surg.* 46AI: 335, 1964.
27. Patel, D.V.: Supportive forces on the human body during underwater activities. Unpublished master's thesis. Madison, University of Wisconsin, 1969.
28. Payne, A.H., Slater, W.J., and Telford, T.: *Ergonomics.* 11:123, 1968.
29. Ralston, H.J., and Lukin, L.: *Ergonomics.* 12:39, 1969.
30. Roberts, E.M.: Mechanics: The role of physical activity in developing effective mechanics of movement. In: *The Encyclopedia of Sports Medicine,* L.A. Larson (Ed.). New York, MacMillan, 1971.
31. Roy, B.: Kinematics and kinetics of the standing long jump in seven, ten, thirteen and sixteen year old boys. Unpublished doctoral dissertation. Madison, University of Wisconsin, 1971.

32. Roy, B.: *Contribution relative du membre supérieur aux forces verticales et horizontales dans le saut en longueur, sans élan chez des garcons de 7, 10, 13 et 16 ans.* Kinanthropologie, in press.
33. Wartenweiler, J., Lehmann, G., and Wettstein, A.: *Kinanthropologie.* 1: 45, 1969.
34. Wilson, M.O.: Development of jumping skill in children. Unpublished doctoral dissertation, University of Iowa, 1945.
35. Zimmerman, H.: Characteristic likeness and differences between skilled and non-skilled performance in the standing broad jump. Unpublished doctoral dissertation, Madison, University of Wisconsin, 1951.

# Chapter 29

# Relationships Between Amplitude of Hip Movements and Jumping Performances

GINETTE HUNNEBELLE
JEAN PAUL MARÉCHAL
JULIEN FALIZE

Observations made by Laubach and McConville[17], Tyrance,[30] Broer and Galles,[1] Mathews et al.[20,21] and Falize[6,8] and Hunnebelle[12,13] leads us to conclude that articular flexibility is hereditary but that it is slightly influenced by individual morphology. Most of the authors agree that physical activity improves flexibility (s.22) or that it either increases or reduces it according to the type of training involved.[5,7,12,13,16,19]

We were unable to find studies aiming to establish the possible relationships between articular mobility of the hips and jumping performances.

A remarkable 8.90 meter broad jump achieved by Beamon at the last Olympic Games in Mexico leads us to believe that such relationships exist at least in champions. In this jump the hip movement consists of passing from a full extension at the take-off to an active flexion during flight and landing. The object of the present study is to bring out such relationships, if they exist, in a representative sample of sports adepts studying in physical education.

Since the hip and trunk movements are synergic we shall consider the articular flexibility of these two parts of the body. The technique used to measure flexibility will be that developed by Falize.[9] We shall measure the flexion and extension movements. We shall also add a third movement which we have called "flexion against resistance."

Since the regular broad jump requires a rather extensive

period of learning and advanced technique, the lack of style in our subjects was likely to complicate our studies. For this reason we also asked them to perform broad jumps and high jumps with both feet together, plus running forward high jumps. In this way the active hip and trunk flexion and extension movements would be easier to observe.

The articular flexibility and jumping performances are characterized and differentiated in male and female students. The statistical analysis of the results reveals the anticipated relationships.

## Material and Methods

*Subjects*

Thirty-eight male and twenty-eight female physical education students from the University of Liége were the subjects tested in this study. The age of the male students ranged from seventeen years and three months to twenty-five years and eight months, the mean age being twenty years and six months. The female subjects' age ranged from seventeen years and eleven months to twenty-four years and six months, the mean being twenty years and three months.

The subjects' standing height and weight were measured to the nearest mm and 50 gr respectively.

*Determination of the Articular Flexibility*

The techniques using linear measures or scores to estimate angular displacements were set aside, those of Cureton,[3,4] even adapted by Swalus,[29] those of Wells and Dillon,[31] and the "toe touch test," successful because of its easy and rapid application.[15,17,21]

Traditional goniometry,[14] currently used in kinesitherapy[2] gives rather inaccurate measures in view of the difficulty to locate the axis of the articular pivot and those of the mobilized body segments. Leighton's flexometer[18] eliminates the causes of errors but remains difficult to stabilize on certain body segments such as the hips and trunk.

We therefore used the photographic techniques developed by Falize.[9] Both positions of flexion and extension of the hips and trunk were retained as was also a third measure prompted by the movement of flexion. Each subject was photographed in the three positions. These are shown in Figure 29–1 (extension), Figure 29–2 (flexion) and Figure 29–3 (flexion against resistance). The direction of the body segments was drawn on each photograph as described by Falize.[9] We added a fifth direction on the flexion photographies: the tangent of the sacrum which we called "direction of the sacrum."

The following angles were measured to the nearest degree with a protractor:

—The angle formed by the direction of the upper middle dorsal region of the spinal column and by the direction of the middle lumbar region;

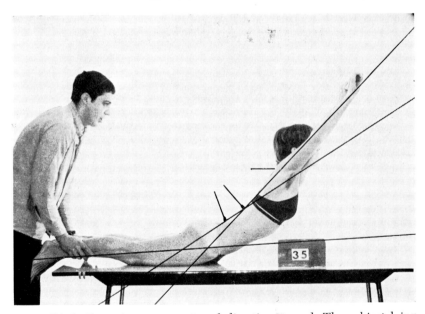

Figure 29–1. Extension movement and directions traced. The subject lying face downwards, arm extended along the axis of the body, holds an 80 cm ( ♂ ) or 60 cm ( ♀ ) stick in her hands. The cubital side of the hands remains in contact with two buffers fixed on the extremities of the stick which allows for proper arm spacing. The operator holds down the subject's legs against the table by pressing on her ankles. The subject makes a maximum trunk extension with her arms up. This position is held for one or two seconds, the time required to take the photography.

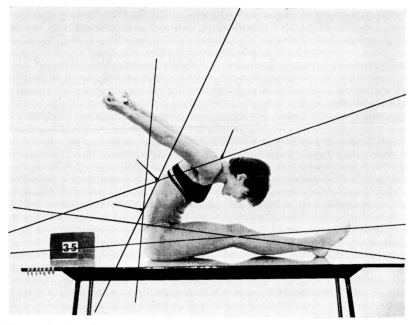

Figure 29–2. Flexion movement and directions traced. The subject is seated, legs extended along the table, arms extended over the head; she holds the stick as in the first position. She flexes her trunk on her legs, being careful to keep them extended as much as possible. The photography is taken at maximal flexion.

—The angle formed by the direction of the middle lumbar region of the column and by the direction of the thigh;
—The angle formed by the direction of the sacrum and by the direction of the thigh;
—When the subject's legs were not stretched all the way in exercises 2, we determined the contribution of the knee flexion in measuring the angle formed by the direction of the thighs and the direction of the legs. This value was subtracted from the hip flexion.

This method is reliable and repeatable (r = 0.960 with the test-retest technique); it is sufficiently accurate, the internal variance being smaller than the external variance.

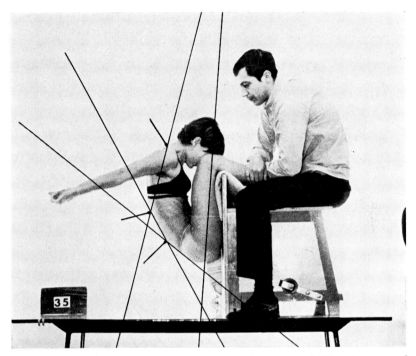

Figure 29–3. Flexion movement against resistance and direction traced. The subject is asked to make a trunk flexion on her legs against weight, without elongating her ischiatic muscles. The subject holds herself by her flexed knees to a vertical plane. The arm position is identical to that in the preceding position. From this position the subject makes a trunk flexion; the photography is taken at maximal flexion.

## Physical Tests

*Standing Broad Jump With Feet Held Together.* The length of the jump was the distance between the take-off line and the posterior part of the body nearest to that line after the jump. The best out of three performances was retained.

*Running Broad Jump.* The length of the jump was the distance separating the tip of the footprint left on the ground by the take-off foot and the nearest trace to it left by a part of the body after the jump. The best out of three attempts was retained.

*Running Forward High Jump With Joined Feet.* The transversal bar was raised 5 cm at a time and a maximum of three attempts were allowed. Any jump which was not absolutely made straight forward was discarded.

## Results and Discussion

### Characterization of the Samples

The mean values, the standard deviations and the coefficients of variation for both males and females are given in Table 29-I. The value of the variation coefficients shows that the variability of the characters is comparable for boys and girls. The extension movements were the most diversified; the trunk extension is particularly variable in the young girls. The other characters show a biological variability in the order of 10 percent, which is quite acceptable. The hip movements are less diversified than those of the trunk. The direction of the sacrum which is the most localized movement is also the least variable.

The elements of Table 29-II make it possible to compare the variables in both sexes: the mean difference, the ratio of the variances and the student "t" factor are calculated by applying the unpaired sample method.

Three ratios of variances are slightly above the significance threshold at the uncertainty level of 0.05. Therefore, trunk and hip extension movements and trunk amplitude movements must be compared with care because the samples cannot be considered as drawn from the same population.

Table 29-II clearly shows that only the trunk movements have comparable values between girls and boys. On the other hand, hip flexibility is greater in young girls, whereas height, weight and jumping performances are superior in young boys.

The results of flexibility in this study can be compared with those of Falize[9] and Swalus[28] obtained by Falize's method with physical education students (Table 29-III). However Swalus modified the extension exercise by making the weight agonist of the movement[28]; these results, which are not comparable to the others, are within parenthesis in Table 29-III. The mean values and their dispersion are comparable in the three studies except for the average hip flexion angulation which spreads from 86° (Falize) to 109.2° (Swalus), a spread of 25.2°.

TABLE 29-I

ESTIMATION OF THE MEAN, OF THE STANDARD DEVIATION AND OF THE COEFFICIENT OF VARIATION OF THE DIFFERENT VARIABLES STUDIED

| | | ♀ (n = 28) | | | ♂ (n = 38) | | |
|---|---|---|---|---|---|---|---|
| | | mean | stand deviation | coef var | mean | stand deviation | coef var |
| Trunk (In Degrees) | Flexion | 48.0 | 5.9 | 0.124 | 47.9 | 6.0 | 0.127 |
| | Extension | 21.3 | 13.2 | 0.623 | 17.2 | 8.6 | 0.498 |
| | Amplitude | 69.2 | 14.4 | 0.208 | 65.0 | 8.5 | 0.131 |
| Hips (In Degrees) | Flexion | 110.6 | 9.7 | 0.088 | 96.4 | 12.3 | 0.127 |
| | Extension | 35.8 | 10.9 | 0.305 | 23.4 | 7.3 | 0.313 |
| | Amplitude | 146.4 | 18.0 | 0.123 | 119.9 | 14.7 | 0.122 |
| | Direction of sacrum | 101.0 | 8.5 | 0.085 | 89.8 | 8.6 | 0.096 |
| Flexion Against Resistance (In Degrees) | Trunk flexion | 44.0 | 5.4 | 0.124 | 43.5 | 6.8 | 0.155 |
| | Hip flexion | 127.7 | 11.3 | 0.089 | 120.1 | 9.6 | 0.080 |
| | Direction of sacrum | 113.7 | 8.5 | 0.075 | 105.7 | 8.2 | 0.077 |
| Direct Measures | Height (cm) | 163.3 | 5.2 | 0.032 | 176.2 | 6.2 | 0.035 |
| | Weight (kg) | 55.9 | 5.7 | 0.102 | 72.0 | 6.5 | 0.091 |
| | Joined feet broad jump | 2.06 | 0.19 | 0.091 | 2.49 | 0.14 | 0.055 |
| Performances (In Meters) | Running broad jump | 3.85 | 0.39 | 0.101 | 5.03 | 0.47 | 0.093 |
| | Joined feet high jump | 0.82 | 0.08 | 0.101 | 1.00 | 0.09 | 0.093 |
| | Running forward high jump | 1.06 | 0.08 | 0.079 | 1.27 | 0.11 | 0.083 |

TABLE 29-II
MEAN DIFFERENCES ($\Delta\overline{m}$) BETWEEN THE VARIABLES STUDIED IN
THE FEMALES AND MALES; VARIANCE RATIOS (F) AND STUDENT
FACTORS

| | | | $\Delta\overline{m}$ | $t$ | $F$ |
|---|---|---|---|---|---|
| Trunk | Flexion | | +0,1 | 0,067 | 1,034 |
| | Extension | | +4,1 | *1,433* | *2,389* |
| | Amplitude | | +4,2 | *1,377* | *2,883* |
| Hips | Flexion | | +14,2 | *5,278* | 1,601 |
| | Extension | | +12,4 | *3,899* | *2,200* |
| | Amplitude | | +26,5 | *6,385* | 1,506 |
| | Direction of sacrum | | +11,2 | *5,258* | 1,015 |
| Flexion | Trunk flexion | | +0,5 | 0,100 | 1,541 |
| Against | Hip flexion | | +7,6 | *2,743* | 1,408 |
| Resistance | Direction of sacrum | | +8,0 | *3,846* | 1,086 |
| Direct | Height | | −12,9 | *9,214* | 1,438 |
| Measures | Weight | | −16,1 | *10,733* | 1,310 |
| Performances | Broad jump | joined feet | −0,43 | *10,750* | 1,867 |
| | | running | −1,18 | *11,238* | 1,426 |
| | High jump | joined feet | −0,18 | *9,000* | 1,246 |
| | | running | −0,21 | *10,500* | 1,600 |

$\Delta\,\overline{m}$ is obtained by subtracting the male values that is $\overline{m}\,♀ - \overline{m}\,♂$. Factor F is the ratio of the largest variance to the smallest variance (25). The ratio of the variances is significant (p 0.05) from 1.87 on, and the student t from 1.96 on(10). The significant values at this level of uncertainty are underlined.

Leighton[18] recommends that the flexometer be placed under the armpit to measure the trunk movement amplitude, and on the crista iliaca at the umbilicus level to measure that of the

TABLE 29-III
MEAN VALUES OF ARTICULAR FLEXIBILITY AND STANDARD
DEVIATIONS OBTAINED IN THREE COMPARABLE STUDIES
CONDUCTED WITH PHYSICAL EDUCATION STUDENTS

| | | | Our Study (n — 38) | Falize (n — 33) | Swalus (n — 209) |
|---|---|---|---|---|---|
| Trunk | Flexion | $\overline{m}$ | 47,9 | 49,0 | 44,0 |
| | | $\hat{s}$ | 6,0 | 5,67 | 5,6 |
| | Extension | $\overline{m}$ | 17,2 | 11,5 | (15,5) |
| | | $\hat{s}$ | 8,6 | 8,76 | 8,5 |
| | Amplitude | $\overline{m}$ | 65,0 | 62,0 | (60,0) |
| | | $\hat{s}$ | 8,5 | 9,45 | 9,8 |
| Hips | Flexion | $\overline{m}$ | 96,4 | 86,0 | 109,4 |
| | | $\hat{s}$ | 12,3 | 8,68 | 10,4 |
| | Extension | $\overline{m}$ | 23,4 | 30,5 | 45,6 |
| | | $\hat{s}$ | 7,3 | 7,28 | 10,1 |
| | | $\overline{m}$ | 119,9 | 117,0 | (154,5) |
| | | $\hat{s}$ | 14,7 | 13,6 | 15,0 |

The three authors are using Falize's method; however, Swalus modified the extenison exercise in making it a passive exercise; these results are within parentheses. Results are expressed in degrees.

hips. These landmarks correspond approximately to D2 and L2. They are slightly different from ours, but not enough to prevent any comparison, especially that of movement amplitudes.

Many authors have measured hip and trunk flexibility with this method; their results are shown in Table 29-IV. Although

TABLE 29-IV

HIP AND TRUNK MOVEMENT AMPLITUDE VALUES
AS DETERMINED BY DIFFERENT AUTHORS

| | Subjects | | | Movement Amplit | | |
|---|---|---|---|---|---|---|
| *Authors* | *Sex* | *N* | *Age (years, months)* | *Hips (°)* | *Trunk (°)* | *Observations on the Subjects* |
| Leighton (18) | ♂ | 56 | — | 109,4 | 63,0 | — |
| McCue (22) | ♀ | 130 | 19,06 | 140,49 | 106,35 | — |
| | ♂ | 35 | 20,00 | 106,14 | — | endomorphs |
| Tyrance (30) | ♂ | 35 | 20,00 | 113,20 | — | ectomorphs |
| | ♂ | 35 | 20,00 | 117,29 | — | mesomorphs |
| Laubach (17) | ♂ | 63 | 19,00 | 96,44 | 65,02 | — |
| Massey (19) | ♂ | 13 | 19,00 | 112,2 | — | — |
| | ♂ | 13 | 19,00 | 112,5 | — | weight training practice |

All used Leighton's flexometer. The values obtained by McCue cannot be compared to the others; the measures are taken by placing the flexometer at the tragus level.

the experimental conditions (fixed points, initial and final positions of movements) are slightly different from those used in our study, we end up with a trunk flexibility (65°) practically identical to that shown by Leighton (63°) and Laubach (65°). The hip flexibility of our physical education subjects is close to that attributed by Tyrance[30] to mesomorphs.

Table 29-V shows, as given by various authors, the jumping

TABLE 29-V

SOME BROAD JUMP MEAN VALUES TAKEN FROM THE LITERATURE

| | ♂ | | | ♀ | | |
|---|---|---|---|---|---|---|
| | *N* | *Running* | *Standing* | *N* | *Running* | *Standing* |
| Piéron (24) | 45 | — | 2,26 | — | — | — |
| Deproft cited by Ostyn (23) | 968 | — | 2,13 | — | — | — |
| Stakionene (26) | numerous | 4,31 | 2,26 | numerous | 3,34 | 1,78 |
| Vanderlinden (23) | 19 676 | 4,39 | — | — | — | — |
| Stemmler (27) | 2 505 | 4,59 | — | 1 619 | 3,60 | — |
| Hasegawa (11) | 1 368 | 4,42 | — | 1 000 | 3,13 | — |

All subjects are between eighteen and twenty-years-old; performances are expressed in meters.

performances of physical education students and of students not engaged in sports. The former have superior results.

### Relationships Between Different Variables

The correlations between the variables are presented in Tables 29-VI ( ♂ ) and 29-VII ( ♀ ). Trunk movements are intercorre-

TABLE 29-VI

PRESENTATION OF INTERCORRELATIONS

Male students (N = 38)

Legend:

Trunk — 1) flexion 2) extension 3) amplitude

Hips — 4) flexion 5) extension 6) amplitude 7) direction of sacrum

Flexibility against resistance — Direct measures — Performances

8) flexion trunk 9) flexion of hips 10) direction of sacrum 11) height 12) weight 13) standing broad jump 14) running broad jump 15) standing high jump 16) running high jump

The values are significant at the P<0.05 level

| | 1 | 2 | 3 | 4 | 5 | 6 | 7 | 8 | 9 | 10 | 11 | 12 | 13 | 14 | 15 | 16 |
|---|---|---|---|---|---|---|---|---|---|---|---|---|---|---|---|---|
| 1 | - | | | | | | | | | | | | | | | |
| 2 | -.3642 | - | | | | | | | | | | | | | | |
| 3 | .3439 | .7492 | - | | | | | | | | | | | | | |
| 4 | .0286 | .3860 | .4095 | - | | | | | | | | | | | | |
| 5 | .0235 | -.2109 | -.1959 | .0750 | - | | | | | | | | | | | |
| 6 | .0321 | .2219 | .2466 | .8478 | .5684 | - | | | | | | | | | | |
| 7 | .0074 | .0679 | .0738 | .7378 | -.0905 | .5694 | - | | | | | | | | | |
| 8 | .9413 | -.3808 | .2854 | .0215 | .0537 | .0473 | .0060 | - | | | | | | | | |
| 9 | -.0805 | .1862 | .1304 | .3907 | .2496 | .4420 | .3601 | .0862 | - | | | | | | | |
| 10 | .0031 | .2456 | .2499 | .3697 | .1114 | .3715 | .5156 | .1331 | .7930 | - | | | | | | |
| 11 | .0842 | .0695 | .1300 | .0845 | -.2400 | -.0428 | .2363 | .1121 | .0078 | .1581 | - | | | | | |
| 12 | .1604 | -.0993 | .0139 | .1338 | -.0920 | .1061 | .1978 | .1979 | -.1111 | -.0400 | .6359 | - | | | | |
| 13 | .3005 | .2173 | .4329 | .3819 | -.1298 | .2679 | .1715 | .3292 | .0179 | .1762 | .5916 | .5225 | - | | | |
| 14 | .1474 | -.0939 | .0100 | .0263 | .0459 | .0664 | .1378 | .2716 | .1296 | .2122 | .5092 | .5607 | .4355 | - | | |
| 15 | .2444 | .3384 | .5150 | .4293 | -.0814 | .3041 | .1426 | .2324 | .0520 | .1895 | .5750 | .3611 | .8022 | .3146 | - | |
| 16 | .1320 | .1786 | .2739 | .1777 | -.0960 | .1153 | .1044 | .1666 | -.0336 | .0809 | .5747 | .4284 | .6708 | .5944 | .6729 | - |

lated. The mobility of the trunk in extension seems to determine the amplitude of movement in the sagittal plane because the correlations among the corresponding movements are very high for both boys ($r = 0.749$) and girls ($r = 0.911$).

The amplitude of voluntary hip movements differs in the boys and girls as well by its angular value (Table 29-II) as by the relationships linking the different parts of the movement. In the male students movement amplitude depends mainly on their flexion ability ($r = 0.848$) while in the female students the degree of flexion as well as of extension are equally responsible ($r = 0.858$ and $0.890$ respectively) for the voluntary hip movement amplitude.

The fact that there are fewer high correlations in the exercise group called "flexibility against resistance" indicates that this test is a less exact measure of voluntary movement amplitude than the two preceeding ones. As a matter of fact it was not chosen to characterize it since it does not include a single measure of movement amplitude. The high correlation between hip

TABLE 29-VII

PRESENTATION OF THE INTERCORRELATIONS

Female students (N = 28)

| | | | | | Trunk | 1) flexion | Flexibility | 8) trunk flexion |
|---|---|---|---|---|---|---|---|---|
| | | | | | | 2) extension | against resistance | 9) hip flexion |
| | | | | | | 3) amplitude | | 10) direction of sacrum |
| 1 | | | | | Hips | 4) flexion | Direct measures | 11) height |
| 1 | - | 2 | | | | 5) extension | | 12) weight |
| | | | | | | 6) amplitude | Performances | 13) standing broad jump |
| 2 | -.0159 | - | 3 | | | 7) direction of | | 14) running broad jump |
| 3 | .3972 | .9112 | - | 4 | | sacrum | | 15) standing high jump |
| | | | | | | | | 16) running forward high jump |
| 4 | -.0453 | .2703 | .2294 | - | 5 |
| 5 | .4275 | .2601 | .4148 | .5299 | - | 6 | The significant values at a level of uncertainty of |
| 6 | .2342 | .3027 | .3743 | .8583 | .8899 | - | 7 | P <0.05 are underlined. |
| 7 | .2310 | .1765 | .2572 | .5888 | .6042 | .6821 | - | 8 |
| 8 | .8492 | -.1477 | .2141 | -.0531 | .3415 | .1780 | .2364 | - | 9 |
| 9 | -.1677 | .1985 | .1131 | .5783 | .1330 | .3915 | .3772 | .0205 | - | 10 |
| 10 | -.0353 | .1226 | .0980 | .4280 | .1843 | .3417 | .5743 | .1779 | .8313 | - | 11 |
| 11 | .1855 | .0165 | .0915 | -.0735 | -.1155 | -.1094 | .0351 | .0876 | .1344 | .0751 | - | 12 |
| 12 | .2242 | -.1854 | -.0778 | -.1905 | -.0872 | -.1552 | -.0306 | .0384 | -.5286 | -.5544 | .4739 | - | 13 |
| 13 | -.1394 | .2998 | .2178 | -.1017 | -.0585 | -.0901 | .1026 | -.1131 | .2282 | .2798 | .4207 | -.1530 | - | 14 |
| 14 | -.3216 | -.0374 | -.1668 | -.1052 | -.3614 | -.2752 | -.0551 | -.2061 | .4764 | .4125 | .1978 | -.3214 | .6647 | - | 15 |
| 15 | .0804 | .4338 | .4313 | -.0057 | .1193 | .0691 | .0038 | -.0183 | .0421 | .0339 | .2283 | -.1385 | .7179 | .4203 | - |
| 16 | -.3526 | .2906 | .1215 | .0277 | -.2457 | -.1337 | -.0343 | -.3386 | .2895 | .1385 | .0382 | -.3043 | .6158 | .6407 | .5440 |

flexion and sacrum direction (0.793 in ♂ and 0.831 in ♀ ) throws into relief the active role played by the pelvis in the accomplishment of this movement.

The high correlation value (0.941 in ♂ and 0.849 in ♀ ) between both trunk flexion movements (columns 1 and 8 of Tables 29-VI and 29-VII) is explained by the fact that these two motions, while being done in different positions, are quite similar. On the other hand the correlation is weaker between the two hip flexion movements. The correlation coefficient between both hip flexion movements (columns 4 and 9 of Tables 29-VI and 29-VII) is 0.391 in the boys' case and 0.578 in the girls' case. If we consider the sacrum direction in both positions (columns

7 and 10 of Tables 29-VI and 29-VII) we find a correlation of 0.516 in the boys and 0.574 in the girls. There is a big difference between these two movements: in one case the long ischiatic muscles are inhibitors and in the other case their action is eliminated.

As far as the performances are concerned, the results indicate that in general a good high jumper is equally a good broad jumper whether the jumps are running or standing jumps.

In the boys there is a correlation between the four jumps, height and weight. This could be attributed to the muscular development and the physical fitness of the subjects. But in the girls the only significant correlation lies between height and standing broad jump. This can be attributed to a lower degree of physical fitness in the female subjects, a fact corroborated by the negative correlation between weight and hip flexion against resistance $(r = -0.529)$, and to the sacrum direction $(r = -0.554)$ in this movement.

In the men we find significant correlations between voluntary movement amplitude and standing broad jump performances. In the latter, the speed gained from the run-up does not intervene as a favorable factor in their execution.

Trunk movement amplitude $(r = 0.433)$, flexion ability against resistance $(r = 0.329)$ and hip flexion $(r = 0.382)$ seem to have an influence in the standing broad jump. As for the joined feet high jump, it correlates with trunk extension $(r = 0.338)$, its movement amplitude $(r = 0.515)$, and with hip flexion $(r = 0.429)$. These trunk and hip movements depend on the very techniques of these jumps: active flexion and extension of the body.

These correlations cannot be found in the girls except for the influence of the extension $(r = 0.434)$ and of the trunk movement amplitude $(r = 0.431)$ on the standing high jump.

## Conclusions

Having observed jumping champions in action we are led to believe that there is a possible relationship between hip articular flexibility, and between synergy trunk flexibility and performances in jumps. We attempted to show this relationship in students engaged in sports.

Thirty-eight male and twenty-eight female physical education students performed running and standing high and broad jumps. The hip and trunk articular flexibility in the sagittal plane was determined by Falize's method.[7] Measures of flexion against resistance, height and weight were also obtained.

The analysis of the results shows that:

—Only standing jumps correlate with hip and trunk flexion and extension movements.

—The values of the coefficients are not sufficiently high to accurately predict whether a flexible subject will be a good jumper and vice versa.

—Highly significant correlations interrelating trunk movements on the one hand and hip movements on the other are an indication of the validity of the tests chosen.

—The test devised by Falize to estimate voluntary movement amplitude gives correlations of a higher degree of significance with jumping performances than do the measures of flexion against resistance.

—Hip voluntary movement amplitude is significantly superior in the female students. On the other hand at the trunk level it is quite similar in both groups.

—The results obtained are comparable to those of other studies which used the same techniques.

—The male students seem more fit than the female students if we consider the correlations between height, weight and jumping performances and flexibility tests.

Flexibility is certainly not the most important factor determining one's jumping skill. We are still believing that the relationship between jumping aptitude and hip voluntary movement amplitude must be more evident in champions and that a study conducted with champion jumpers would confirm this hypothesis. The results of this study lead us to think that it would be useful to consider this aspect in the preparation of jumpers.

318      *Training—Scientific Basis and Application*

## References

1. Broer, M.R., and Galles, N.R.G.: *Res. Quart.* 29:253, 1958.
2. Codreano, C., and Blanquier, B.: *J. Kinésith.* 124:7, 1964.
3. Cureton, T.K.: *Res. Quart.* 12:381, 1941.
4. Cureton, T.K.: *Physical Fitness of Champion Athletes.* Urbana, The University of Illinois Press, 1951.
5. Falize, J.: Recherche expérimentale sur l'amplitude des mouvements volontaires. Thèse de doctorat, Université de Liège, 1954, non publié.
6. Falize, J.: *L'Homme Sain.*
7. Falize, J.: *Rev. Educ. Phys.*
8. Falize, J.: *Wychowanie Fizyczne i Sport.* 3:567–572, 1959.
9. Falize, J.: *I.N.E.P.S. Bruxelles,* 1959.
10. Fisher, R.A., and Yates, F.: *Statistical tables for biological agricultural and medical research.* London, Oliver and Boyd, 1963.
11. Hasegawa, J.: Physical fitness statues of Japonese youth through sport test. *Proceedings of International Congress of Sport Sciences,* K. Kato, Tokyo 1966, 326.
12. Hunebelle, G.: Détermination et analyse des courbures antérieures de la colonne vertébrale. Thèse de doctorat, Université de Liège, 1967–68, non publié.
13. Hunebelle, G.: Essai d'établissement des bases scientifiques d'un cours de gymnastique de redressement vertébral. *Communication au 2me Congrès Européen de médecine sportive,* Bucarest 30 sept. –3 oct. 1969, RApport des Communications, sous presse.
14. Hunebelle, C.: *American Academy of Orthopedic Surgeons,* 1965.
15. Kraus, H.K., and Hirschlaod, R.P.: *Res. Quart.* 25:178, 1954.
16. Kusinitz, Y., and Keeney, C.E.: *Res. Quart.* 29:294, 1958.
17. Laubach, L.L., and McConville, C.E.: *Res. Quart.* 37:241, 1966.
18. Leighton, J.R.: *Res. Quart.* 13:205, 1942.
19. Massey, B.H., and Chaudet, N.L.: *Res. Quart.* 27:41, 1956.
20. Mathews, D.K., Shaw, V., and Woods, J.B.: *Res. Quart.* 30:297–302, 1959.
21. Mathews, D.K., Shaw, V., and Bohnen, M.: *Res. Quart.* 28:352, 1957.
22. McCue, B.F.: *Res. Quart.* 24:316, 1953.
23. Ostyn, M., Simons, J., Vanderlinden, B.: Variabilité des valeurs somatiques et fonctionnelles chez les jeunes d'âge scolaire. Atti VI Congresso della societa latine di medicina della sport, Minerva Medica Tirino, p. 268–274.
24. Piéron, M.: Evaluation de la valeur physique individuelle par la mesure de l'énergie utilisée dans les épreuves athlétiques. Thèse de doctorat, Université de Liège, 1969, non publié.
25. Schwartz, D.: *Flammarion,* Paris 1963
26. Stakionene, V.: Izmenenie fizitcheskoi-pedgovlennosti outchachtchikh-

sia pod vozdeistviem razlitchnykh faktorov. XI Meznarodni kongres o tel esne zdatnosti mladeze, Praha 1967, p. 93.
27. Stemmler, R.: *Wiss. Z. DHFK.* 4:47, 1962.
28. Swalus, P.: *Hermès, Rev. Inst. Educ. Phys. Louvain.* 2:15, 1967
29. Swalus, P., and George, F.: *Hermès, Rev. Inst. Educ. Phys. Louvain.* 3:13, 1968
30. Tyrance, H.J.: *Res. Quart.* 29:349, 1958.
31. Wells, K.F., and Dillon, E.K.: *Res. Quart.* 23:115, 1952.
32. Willgoose, C.E.: *Evaluation in Health Education and Physical Education.* New York, McGraw-Hill, 1961.

# Chapter 30

# The Effects of Isometric, Isotonic, and Speed Conditioning Programs on Speed of Movement, Reaction Time, and Strength of College Men

Stephen Mendryk

The interest in and subsequent investigation of the relationship between the static strength of a particular group of muscles and the speed with which these muscles could move a limb is a direct result of a critical appraisal of the role of static strength in general motor ability, motor performance and physical fitness tests.

A review of studies on the relationship between static strength and speed of limb movement indicates that substantial amounts of relationship are infrequent, and unimportant for predictive purposes. The majority of investigators,[1,2,3,4,5,6,7,8] have found nonsignificant relationships between strength and speed of limb movement. Contradictory findings have been reported by Clarke,[3] Clarke and Glines,[9] Kerr,[10] Nelson and Fahrney,[11] and Macintosh.[12] Generally the correlations have been significant but low, ranging from —.50 to .36. Fahrney and Nelson, however, report high positive correlations of .74 to .79 between strength and speed of an elbow flexion movement.

The most recent trend in experimentation on the static strength-speed of limb movement relationship has been the study of the effects of an increase in static strength on the speed of limb movement by means of strength training programs. Endres,[13] Smith,[14] Whitley and Smith,[15] and Clarke and Henry[16] all reported that significant limb strength increases were associated with significant gains in speed of limb movements.

However, Pierson and Rasch,[17] Kerr,[10] and Macintosh[12] found that significant increases in limb strength were not accompanied by concomitant increases in speed of limb movement.

## Purpose

The purpose of this study was to examine:

1. The interrelationship between changes, if any, in hip flexion strength, hip flexion strength/mass ratios, speed of hip flexion movement, and the reaction time of the preferred leg.

2. The effects of the three training methods on hip flexion strength, speed of hip flexion movement, and the reaction time of the preferred leg.

## Methods and Procedures

Seventy-four volunteer subjects from the men's physical education service program at the University of Alberta were tested for effective leg mass, leg reaction time, maximum static strength of hip flexion, and speed of hip flexion movement. The subjects were assigned at random to four groups. One group of nineteen subjects served as a treated control group. The treatment was administered three times a week, and consisted of an exposure to a "pseudo ultra-violet lamp" for a period of one minute. The control group did not engage in any physical activity during the experimental period. A second group of nineteen subjects engaged in an isotonic exercise program designed to strengthen the muscles that flex the hip as they are used in the actual speed test movement. Each subject in the isotonic group moved a weight with a hip flexion movement through an arc of 70° a minimum of five and a maximum of eight times per bout of exercise. When a subject was able to complete eight repetitions with a given weight, the weight was increased until five repetitions was again maximal. A third group of eighteen subjects participated in an isometric exercise program designed to strengthen the hip flexors throughout the total range of leg movement in the speed of movment test. Five maximal isometric contractions at positions approximating 0, 17,

34, 51 and 70 degrees with a thirty second rest between each contraction constituted one exercise bout for this group. A fourth group of eighteen subjects practiced maximal speed of leg movement in order to improve neuromotor skill in the movement. Each exercise bout consisted of five speed movement trials with a thirty second rest period between trials. The subjects of the control and experimental groups received treatment and exercise respectively, three times per week for a period of six weeks. Seventy-four subjects were retested for leg mass, leg reaction time, maximum static strength of hip flexion, and speed of hip flexion movement at the end of the six week experimental period.

### Measurement of Leg Mass

The effective leg mass was measured with the subject in a prone back-lying position on a testing table. The leg of each subject was placed so that the midline of the lateral malleolus rested on the midpoint of a scale platform. The scale platform was attached to a Toledo Scale Model No. 15594 that was suspended from the ceiling. The average of two leg mass readings was used as the leg mass measurement. The two leg mass readings were taken immediately after the first test of maximum static hip flexion strength. The scale was checked for accuracy of measurement prior to each testing period. A reliability coefficient computed for the two postexperimental leg mass measurements of the first thirty subjects to be retested was .97.

### Measurement of Hip Flexion Strength

A cable tensiometer (Model T 601001 —C8— 18) was used to measure the static strength of hip flexion according to a procedure developed by Clarke.[18] One week prior to actual initial testing, all subjects were given the opportunity of becoming familiar with the testing procedure and with exerting a maximal hip flexion force on the apparatus. In the actual test, two maximal strength trials were given to each subject, and the highest raw score reading was converted to pounds by means of a conversion table. The tensiometer was checked for accuracy after each testing period on a six hundred pound capacity chatillon dynamometer scale. A reliability coefficient computed for the two postexperimental scores of the first thirty subjects retested in this study was .86.

### Measurement of Reaction and Movement Times

The subject stood erect, grasping a two inch steel bar which could be adjusted horizontally and vertically so that the arms of the subject were outstretched and nearly completely extended at shoulder height. The use of the bar standardized the testing position for each subject and enabled the subjects to maintain balance while completing a straight-legged hip flexion movement with the preferred leg through and beyond the target cord. The apparatus and testing procedure were described in a previous paper.[19] The split–half method of computing reliability coefficients was used for reaction and movement time. They are .88 and .92 respectively.

### Changes in Reaction Time Relationships with Changes in Speed of Movement

Correlations between percentage and absolute changes in reaction time and percentage and absolute changes in speed of movement for both the total sample and for the four subgroups are presented in Table 30-I. Four of these correlations were significant, two at the .05 level and two at the .01 level.

The correlation for the total sample between percentage changes in reaction time and percentage changes in speed of movement was —.305; when corrected, this correlation was —.355. This correlation was significant at the .01 level. The only subgroup to show a significant relationship with these variables was the control group. The correlation between percentage changes in reaction time and percentage changes in speed of movement for this group was —.490; when corrected for attenuation, the correlation reached —.539. This correlation was significant at the .05 level.

TABLE 30-I

PRODUCT-MOMENT CORRELATIONS BETWEEN PERCENTAGE AND ABSOLUTE CHANGES IN STRENGTH, STRENGTH/MASS, REACTION TIME AND PERCENTAGE AND ABSOLUTE CHANGES IN SPEED OF MOVEMENT

| Variables Correlated | Total Sample | | Control Group | | Speed of Movement Group | | Isometric Group | | Isotonic Group | |
|---|---|---|---|---|---|---|---|---|---|---|
| | Raw | Corrected | Raw | Corrected | Raw | Corrected | Raw | Corrected | Raw | Corrected |
| Percentage Change in Strength with Percentage Changes in Speed of Movement | .059 | .063 | −.316 | −.338 | .251 | .269 | .018 | .019 | −.061 | −.065 |
| Percentage Changes in Strength/Mass with Percentage Changes in Speed of Movement | .084 | .090 | −.148 | −.159 | .032 | .034 | .312 | .334 | −.147 | −.157 |
| Percentage Changes in Reaction Time with Percentage Changes in Speed of Movement | −.305** | −.335** | −.490* | −.539* | −.195 | −.214 | −.304 | −.374 | −.167 | −.184 |
| Absolute Changes in Strength with Absolute Changes in Speed of Movement | .104 | .111 | −.238 | −.255 | .190 | .203 | .112 | .120 | .007 | .082 |
| Absolute Changes in Strength/Mass with Absolute Changes in Speed of Movement | .138 | .148 | −.091 | −.097 | −.063 | −.067 | .447 | .497* | −.032 | −.034 |
| Absolute Changes in Reaction Time with Absolute Changes in Speed of Movement | −.332** | −.365** | −.471* | −.518* | −.248 | −.273 | −.382 | −.420 | −.179 | −.197 |
| Degrees of Freedom | 72 | | 17 | | 16 | | 16 | | 17 | |
| Correlation Required for Significance | | | | | | | | | | |
| at .05 | .229 | | .456 | | .468 | | .468 | | .456 | |
| at .01 | .302 | | .575 | | .590 | | .590 | | .575 | |

* Significant at the .05 level
** Significant at the .01 level

For the total sample, a correlation of —.332, significant at the .01 level, was obtained between absolute changes in reaction time and absolute changes in speed of movement; when corrected for attenuation, the correlation was —.365. For the subgroups, only the control group showed a significant relationship between these variables at the .05 level. This correlation was —.471; when corrected for atteunuation, it became —.518.

## Changes in Strength and Strength/Mass Relationships with Changes in Speed of Hip Flexion Movement

The correlations between percentage and absolute changes in strength and percentage and absolute changes in speed of movement and between percentage and absolute changes in strength/mass and percentage and absolute changes in speed of movement for the total sample and for the four subgroups are presented in Table 30-I. With one exception, the correlations between these variables for the total sample and for the subgroups were found to be nonsignificant. The exception was a corrected correlation of .479, significant at the .05 level, between absolute changes in strength/mass with absolute changes in speed of movement for the Isometric Group.

## The Effects of the Three Experimental Conditions on Strength, Strength/Mass, Reaction Time and Speed of Movement

*Movement*

An examination of the preexperiment strength, strength/mass reaction time, and speed of movement means of the four randomly assigned subgroups used in this experiment revealed preexperiment mean differences between groups for these variables . Therefore, the postexperiment subgroup means in strength, strength/mass, reaction time, and speed of movement were evaluated for significant differences by means of an analysis of covariance. This statistical technique made allowances for differences of the preexperiment subgroup means in determining whether or not there were significant differences between the postexperiment subgroup means. The postexperiment means for the four subgroups were adjusted for differences in preexperiment means, and the differences between adjusted postexperiment means were tested for significance by the Newman—Keuls Test.[20] A one-way Analysis of Covariance, designed by Stephen Hunka, and on file at the Division of Educational Research Services of the University of Alberta under Program AC-1000 (August, 1965) was used to perform the analysis of covariance involving one preexperiment and one postexperiment mean for each of the four subgroups for each of the following variables: strength, strength/mass, reaction time, and speed of movement time.

The .05 level was established as the criterion for significance of the $F$ ratios obtained by the covariance analyses. With G-1, or three degrees, of freedom for the numerator, and N-G-I, or sixty-nine, degrees of freedom for the denominator and $F$ ratio of 3.98 is required for significance at the .01 level.

### The Effects of the Three Experimental Programs on Strength

The analysis of covariance $F$ ratio derived for significant differences in post experiment strength means, adjusted for differences in preexperiment strength means was 19.31. This $F$ ratio was significant beyond the .05 level. Therefore, postexperiment strength means for each of the four subgroups were adjusted for differences in preexperiment means by the procedure presented in McNemar.[21] The results of the tests of significance between adjusted postexperiment strength means, using the Newman—Keuls method, appear in Table 30-II. Only the Isometric and Isotonic groups exhibited significant gains in hip flexion strength after the six-week training program.

### Effects of the Three Experimental Programs on Reaction Time and Speed of Movement

The analysis of covariance $F$ ratios for adjusted postexperiment reaction and movement time means were .91 and .96

TABLE 30-II
NEWMAN-KEULS TEST ON ORDERED MEANS OF ADJUSTED
POSTEXPERIMENT STRENGTH

| Treatments in Order | Control | Speed | Isometric | Isotonic |
|---|---|---|---|---|
| Means | 182.23 | 185.02 | 207.11 | 214.96 |
| Control | | 2.79 | 24.88* | 32.73* |
| Speed | | | 22.09* | 29.94* |
| Isometric | | | | 7.85 |
| Isotonic | | | | |

* Difference significant when greater than Truncated Range r for that order

| | | | |
|---|---|---|---|
| Truncated Range r | 2 | 3 | 4 |
| 9.05 (r,69) | 2.82 | 3.39 | 3.72 |
| $9.05\ (r,69)\sqrt{\dfrac{MS\ error}{n}}$ | 10.57 | 12.71 | 13.95 |

respectively. These *F* ratios were not significant at the .05 level. Thus, it was assumed that there were no significant differences in either the postexperiment reaction or movement time means.

## Discussion

In this study, significant correlations were not obtained between changes in strength and in strength/mass and changes in speed of hip flexion movement, either for the total sample or for three of the four subgroups. The absence of a relationship held true for percentage changes as well as when changes were presented as absolute values. A correlation of .479 between absolute changes in strength/mass and absolute changes in speed of movement exhibited by the Isometric Group was significant at the .05 level only after correction for attenuation. Clarke and Henry[16] obtained a correlation of .405, significant at the .05 level, between changes in strength and changes in speed of movement for the total sample in their study. Macintosh[12] reported that the Isotonic Exercise Group in his study demonstrated significant relationships between percentage changes in strength and strength/mass and percentage changes in speed of forearm flexion. These relationships were respectively, −.414 and −.412 significant at the .05 level. Smith[14] reported significant mean increases in pretensioned arm speed accompanying significant increases in mean arm strength. Nelson and Fahrney[11] reported high positive correlations of .74 to .79 between strength and speed of an elbow flexion movement. On the other hand, studies conducted by Rasch and Pierson[17] and Kerr[10] revealed no significant mean increases in speed of movement occurring concomitantly with significant increases of mean strength.

The computed correlations for the total sample for the three of the four subgroups between changes in strength or in strength/mass, and changes in speed of hip flexion movement were nonsignificant at the .05 level. The absence of a relationship indicated a high degree of specificity in the relationship between increases in static hip flexion strength and the speed of hip flexion movement.

The results of the correlational and covariance analyses indicated that significant increases in hip flexion strength are not accompanied by corresponding significant increases in speed of hip flexion movement. Practice of maximal speed of hip flexion movement by the speed of movement subgroup in this study did not result in a significant increase in speed of hip flexion. The nature of the speed training program in this study might have been the limiting factor in attaining significant gains in speed of hip flexion movement.

## References

1. Rasch, P.J.: *Res. Quart.* 25:328–332, 1954.
2. Henry, F.M., and Whitley, J.D.: *Res. Quart.* 31:24–33, 1960.
3. Clarke, D.H.: *Res. Quart.* 31:570–574, 1960.
4. Smith, L.E.: *Res. Quart.* 32:208–220, 1961.
5. Henry, F.M.: *Res. Quart.* 31:440–447, 1960.
6. Henry, F.M., Lotter, W.S., and Smith, L.E.: *Res. Quart.* 33:70–84, 1962.
7. Whitley, J.D., and Smith, L.E.: *Res. Quart.* 34:379–395, 1963.
8. Smith, L.E., and Whitley, J.D.: *Res. Quart.* 34:489–496, 1963.
9. Clarke, H.H., and Glines, D.: *Res. Quart.* 33:194–201, 1962.
10. Kerr, B.A.: *Res. Quart.* 37:55–60, 1966.
11. Nelson, R.C., and Fahrney, R.A.: *Res. Quart.* 36:455–463, 1965.
12. Macintosh, D.: *Res. Quart.* 39:138–148, 1966.
13. Endres, J.P.: "The effect of weight training exercise upon the speed

of muscular movement." Microcard Master's Thesis, Madison, University of Wisconsin, 1953.

14. Smith, L.E.: *Res. Quart.* 35:554–561, 1964.
15. Whitley, J.D., and Smith, L.E.: *Res. Quart.* 37:132–142, 1966.
16. Clarke, D.H., and Henry, F.M.: *Res. Quart.* 32:315–325, 1961.
17. Pierson, William R., and Rasch, Philip J.: *Percept Motor Skills.* 14: 144, 1962.
18. Clarke, H.H.: *Cable-Tension Strength Tests.* Springfield, Mass., Murphy, 1953.
19. Mendryk, Stephen: The relationship of leg strength and strength/mass ratio to speed of a hip flexion movement of the preferred leg. Unpublished paper presented at the Research Section of C.A.H.P.E.R. convention at Montreal, Quebec, June, 1967.
20. Winer, B.J.: *Statistical Principles in Experimental Design.* New York, McGraw-Hill, 1962.
21. McNemar, Quinn: *Psychological Statistic.* New York, Wiley, 1962.

# D. STATISTICS AND COMPUTERIZATION

# Chapter 31

# Statistical Analyses of Hockey

R.T. Hermiston

Coaches often infer that learning occurs when practice sessions improve the performance of a particular skill. Presumably the coach excludes the improvement in performance attributed to physical condition, muscular strength, alteration in motivations toward the sport, etc . . . Likewise, the coach should consider the decrements in performance caused by fatigue.

Scientific analyses of human performance must make a distinction between learning and performance. Positive learning implies an improvement whereas performance is simply a score at a particular time. In order to improve sports skills coaching, the direction and emphasis of research must be based on a variety of performance measurements. No single measure is capable of assessing all aspects of any particular performance. Armchair quarterbacks are aware of the statistical analysis of a game which shows one team winning on the statistics board yet their opponents winning on the scoreboard. In particular, you might reflect on the 1969 NHL playoff series between Boston and Montreal. Boston won the games statistically but Montreal put the puck in the net more often and were declared the Stanley Cup Champions.

Ideal measuring systems have four characteristics[1]:

1. The sensitivity of the input-output relationship and the balance between the two components of this relationship is important. Consider the goal production of a hockey player; in order to understand the meaning of this goal production, one must understand the meaning or quality of the input. Who is he facing? The St. Louis Blues in their own league were the

best but against the original teams in the NHL they were unable to score as many goals.

2. Measuring systems must be appropriate for the type of task which is being measured. Tasks can be divided into three categories:

a. Discrete tasks—the task has a definite beginning and end, such as a face-off;

b. Serial tasks—the task has a beginning and an end identified by a series of events following one another in rapid succession, such as dumping the puck into an opponent's end and then regaining possession in the opponent's end;

c. Continuous tasks—the task is presented as a moving object and continuous information is constantly being presented to the subject. He must make corrections to keep the system in a balanced state. An example is the offensive shots taken at a goaltender.

Any measuring system should allow meaningful comparisons within these three categories.

3. Measuring systems must be sensitive to the accuracy of the responses made by the subjects. If one considers offensive shots and does not look at the shots off the net and the blocked shots, the measuring system omits the accuracy of the players.

4. The final characteristic must take into account the length of time taken to perform the skill in relation to the accuracy with which the skill is performed. For example, all defensemen can shoot a moving puck at the net—but can they do it fast enough to avoid the charging defender?

### Methods and Materials

Keeping these four characteristics in mind, several statistical records were kept on hockey teams during the 1969–70 hockey season. Many different statistics were attempted. They varied from total number of passes to total number of minutes a team had possession of the puck. Needless to say, the end-result of the initial trial and error period did not lend itself to statistical analysis. Based upon the 1969–70 season, the following set of statistics emerged:

*Offensive shots*—shots off the net, blocked by the defense, on the net, and goals.

*Icing the puck*—when the team is full and also short-handed.

*Dumping the puck*—dumping the puck into the offensive corner, from outside the blue line and recording whether or not it is retained by the offensive team.

*Long shots*—shots from outside the blue line and their retentions.

*Goals against*—while teams are equal, short-handed, or in power-play condition.

*Goals for*—under the same conditions.

*Face-offs*—offensive, neutral and defensive.

*Face-offs*—puck direction.

*Face-offs*—puck receiver.

*Face-offs*—puck retention.

In addition, this year the crew is attempting to add an analysis of violation of tactical pattern, and puck turn-overs (similar to the basketball turnover criterion).

One of the main reasons that these statistics were selected is based on interindividual consistency. The correlation between observers was greater than 0.90 for all statistics except the face-off winners (0.72). None of the paired "t" tests was significant. However, the addition of the puck receiver and puck retention statistics has moved this descrete task into the continuous task group and still has not violated the model of performance measurement.

## Offensive Shots

The offensive arena area is divided into sixteen squares. This technique was used to make puck location more accurate. The codes for the shots are shots off the net represented by the player's sweater number; shots blocked, represented by the sweater number underlined; shots on the net, shown with a double underline; and goals with the sweater number circled. The + sign beside a number means that the shot was taken when the offensive team had a man advantage. These data are being fed into computer programs to compute detailed percentages of total shots, percentage of shots from the sixteen offensive segments and player evaluations per period and per game. The running total is also kept for each team throughout the period.

## Icings, Dump-ins, Long Shots, Players on the Ice for Goals

One statistician handles the detailed analysis of icings, dump-ins, long shots and players on the ice when goals are scored. Running totals are also kept for each team along with the running totals for face-offs.

## Face-offs

Another statistician handles the detailed face-off analysis phase. The face-off sheet diagrams the puck direction from the face-off position to both the receiver and the next player, who retains the puck if the receiver passes immediately. These data are also fed into the computer for analysis and probable play patterns after the face-off. Between periods, this statistician transfers the basic data on all the individual face-off shots to a sheet showing face-off wins and losses.

Between periods, the statistical crew sum the running totals for entry on the summary sheets for the coach. These data as well as the tactical errors and the offensive shots are given to the coach within five minutes of the end of the period. Between periods, all data are added to the cumulative game sheets. As a result, a fourteen-page xeroxed report is handed to the coach thirty-five minutes after the game. The original sheets are taken back to the computer facility for trend analyses computations. Accumulated records are printed for the coach each week. These records are for all opponents as well as for each opponent over the six games.

## Results and Discussion

In order to present the statistical results for the team totals in all categories, seven games have been used, and both the means and standard deviations shown:

### Offensive Shots

Total 55±11 Off Net 12±3 Blocked 15±5 On Net 26±7
Goals 2±1

### Dump-Ins

Dumps 21±7        Retentions 9±4        Face-offs 1±0.8

### Icings

Teams equal 4±2                         Short handed 7±4

### Long Shots

Shots 6±4                               Retentions 1±0.8

### Face-Offs

Total 73±15       Offensive       43±4       Neutral 30±7
Defensive

Individual player statistics for counseling sessions and player improvement, although calculated, cannot be presented at this time because of agreement with the team used in the project.

## Reference

1. Fitts, P.M., and Posner, M.I.: *Human Performance.* Belmont, California, Brooks/Cole, 1967.

# Chapter 32

# Application of a Computer Retrieval System for Exercise Physiology

R.R. WALLINGFORD

The spiralling of knowledge has left the modern faculty member deluged with an ever-increasing amount of literature. He has difficulty keeping current in his specialty, let alone his whole field of instruction. This, coupled with the multiplicity of demands made on a faculty member poses a serious threat to the effectiveness of the instructional situation. Synthesizing the voluminous research into a body of knowledge relevant to the needs of the students presents an ever increasing problem. If one accepts a prediction that "The new scientific knowledge of the next fifteen years is likely to be equal in volume to all the knowledge which has so far been acquired in the whole history of mankind"[3] and one appreciates the growing educational pressure for greater individualization of instruction, it would appear crucial that some concerted efforts be made to systematize the available knowledge into a functioning instructional situation with some consideration for individual differences.

One possible solution, considering the fantastic sorting ability of the electronic computer, could be in harnessing the computer to assist the instructor in selecting the appropriate instructional information for students. Harnack,[2] in Buffalo, has attempted just this by directing the computerization of a pool of knowledge in such a way as to make possible the withdrawal of specific instructional information at a level commensurate with the individual interests and backgrounds of the students.

The culmination of amassing a weath of instructional knowl-

edge and coding it to specific teaching objectives became known as a computer based resource unit.
Development of a computer based resource unit entails the following steps:
1. Collecting summary statements of major facts, concepts or findings from recent research.

370. BECAUSE OF THE VASODILATORY EFFECT OF ALCOHOL ON PERIPHERAL BLOOD VESSELS BODY HEAT IS LOST MORE QUICKLY AFTER THE CONSUMPTION OF ALCOHOL.

371. THERE IS NO NUTRITIONAL JUSTIFICATION FOR TRAINING TABLES. B RICCI, PHYSIOLOGICAL BASIS OF HUMAN PERFORMANCE, (PHILADELPHIA. LEA AND FEBIGER, 1967), P. 220.

373. SOME STUDIES AFTER GRUELLING EXERCISE HAVE SHOWN THE PH LEVEL OF THE BODY TO GO BELOW 7.00. B. RICCI, PHYSIOLOGICAL BASIS OF HUMAN PERFORMANCE (PHILADELPHIA. LEA AND FEBIGER, 1967), P. 221.

374. THE FEEDING OF ALKALIES TO INCREASE THE BUFFERING ACTION OF THE BLOOD IS STILL A DEBATABLE POINT. B. RICCI, PHYSIOLOGICAL BASIS OF HUMAN PERFORMANCE (PHILADELPHIA. LEA AND FEBIGER, 1967), P. 222.

375. AMPHETAMINE (BENZEDRINE) HAS NOT BEEN PROVEN TO ASSIST ATHLETIC PERFORMANCE. B. RICCI, PHYSIOLOGICAL BASIS OF HUMAN PERFORMANCE, (PHILADELPHIA. LEA AND FEBIGER, 1967), P. 222

376. GELATIN IS OF NO ERGOGENIC BENEFIT TO ATHLETES. B. RICCI, PHYSIOLOGICAL BASIS OF HUMAN PERFORMANCE, (PHILADELPHIA. LEA AND FEBIGER, 1967) P. 224.

377. IN THE ACCUMULATIVE SENSE OXYGEN CANNOT BE STORED IN THE BODY.

378. OXYGEN AS AN ERGOGENIC AID IS EFFECTIVE IF ADMINISTERED DURING AN ACTUAL PHYSICAL EVENT.

379. ATHLETIC PERFORMANCE BY THE FEMALE APPEARS TO HELP PARTURITION BY CUTTING DOWN ON THE TIME OF LABOR AS WELL AS DIMINISHING THE NUMBER OF CESAREAN SECTIONS IN THE ATHLETE MOTHER.

380. AN ATHLETE BEFORE COMPETITION MAY SUFFER PAIN AND DISCOMFORT ON PASSING URINE, THESE SYMPTOMS ARE A NATURAL PART OF A HEIGHTENED AUTONOMIC ACTIVITY ASSOCIATED WITH THE FIGHT AND FLIGHT REACTION. J. G. P. WILLIAMS, MEDICAL ASPECTS OF SPORT AND PHYSICAL FITNESS, (OXFORD, PERGAMON PRESS, 1965), P. 93.

Figure 32–1. Content.

2. Gathering of reference materials of instruction in the form of tables, charts, diagrams, illustrations, graphs, models and films.

118.    GRAPHS OF MAXIMAL OXYGEN UPTAKE OF NOMADIC LAPPS
        COMPARED WITH OFFICE WORKERS. M. KARVONEN AND A.
        BARRY, PHYSICAL ACTIVITY AND THE HEART,
        (SPRINGFIELD, ILL. C. C. THOMAS, 1967) P. 13.

119.    ILLUSTRATION OF AEROBIC CAPACITY OF NORWEIGIANS, AGED
        20-30 YEARS AND AGED 50-60 YEARS. M. KARVONEN
        AND A. BARRY, PHYSICAL ACTIVITY AND THE HEART,
        (SPRINGFIELD, ILL. C. C. THOMAS, 1967) P. 14-15.

121.    DIAGRAM ILLUSTRATING EFFECT OF SHORT TERM TRAINING UPON
        THE SIZE OF THE HEART OF YOUNG MEN, HEART VOLUME
        IN RELATION TO MAXIMAL OXYGEN UPTAKE. M. KARVONEN
        AND A. BARRY, PHYSICAL ACTIVITY AND THE HEART,
        (SPRINGFIELD, ILL. C. C. THOMAS, 1967) P. 16.

123.    DIFFERENT SLOPES OF LINEAR RELATIONSHIP BETWEEN HEART
        RATE AND WORK LOAD AT LOW AND HIGH METABOLIC
        LEVELS. M. KARVONEN AND A. BARRY, PHYSICAL
        ACTIVITY AND THE HEART, (SPRINGFIELD, ILL. C. C.
        THOMAS, 1967) P. 27.

124.    TABLE OF NORMAL DISTRIBUTION OF CARDIAC OUTPUT. M.
        KARVONEN AND A. BARRY, PHYSICAL ACTIVITY AND THE
        HEART, (SPRINGFIELD, ILL. 1967) P. 70.

125.    SCHEMATIC DIAGRAM OF THE ULTRAFLOW FREQUENCY
        BALLISTOCARDIOGRAM AND ITS METHOD OF OPERATION. M.
        KARVONEN AND A. BARRY, PHYSICAL ACTIVITY AND THE
        HEART, (SPRINGFIELD, ILL. C. C. THOMAS, 1967) P. 85.

126.    A COMPARISON OF BALLISTOCARDIOGRAMS OF THREE DISTANCE
        RUNNERS WITH THOSE OF THREE ABNORMAL BALLISTOGRAMS
        FROM MEN IN THEIR SIXTIES. M. KARVONEN AND A. BARRY
        PHYSICAL ACTIVITY AND THE HEART, (SPRINGFIELD,
        ILL. C. C. THOMAS, 1967) P. 86.

127.    BALLISTOGRAM CHANGES DURING A SIX-MONTH TRAINING
        PERIOD. M. KARVONEN AND A. BARRY, PHYSICAL ACTIVITY
        AND THE HEART, (SPRINGFIELD, ILL. C. C. THOMAS,
        1967), P. 288.

Figure 32–2. Reference materials.

## 3. Listing several classroom demonstrations or laboratory experiments as possible instructional activities.

64. MEASURE ANY CHANGES IN HEART RATE BEFORE AND AFTER SMOKING A CIGARETTE.

65. MEASURE THE STRENGTH DECREMENT THAT TAKES PLACE AFTER A WORK BOUT. (STRENGTH, - WORK BOUT, - STRENGTH DECREMENT).

66. MEASURE P W O 170 ON THE MONARCH CICYCLE ERGOMETER AND TELEMETER ELECTROCARDIOGRAMS. RECTAL TEMPERATURE, BLOOD PRESSURE, AND RESPIRATION RATE CAN BE MEASURED DURING RECOVERY ON THE PHYSIOGRAPH.

67. TAKE PULSE IN STANDING POSITION, SITTING POSITION AND PRONE POSITION, HAVE SUBJECTS, ONE FIT AND ONE UNFIT, RUN UP AND DOWN STADIUM STEPS TWICE, RETAKE PULSE IN ABOVE MENTIONED POSITIONS.

68. STUDY THE EFFECTS OF BREATHING AIR, OXYGEN AND CARBON DIOXIDE, WHILE WORKING ON THE BICYCLE ERGOMETER. USE THE DOUBLE BLIND FOR THIS EXPERIMENT.

69. MEASURE THE EFFECTS OF WARM TEMPERATURES, HOT ROOM AND WEARING RUBBER SWEAT SUITS, ON BODY TEMPERATURES.

70. MEASURE THE EFFECTS ON SNORKEL BREATHING OF ALTERING THE POSITION OF THE SCUBA BREATHING COMPONENTS IN THE DEPTH OF THE WATER.

71. SIMILATE HIGH ALTITUDES BY USING LOW OXYGEN MIXTURES AND PERFORM EXERCISE WHILE BREATHING THESE MIXTURES.

72. EVALUATE COMMON SPORT ACTIVITY ENERGY COST BY USING TELEMETERED HEART RATE, DOUGLAS BAG COLLECTION OF EXPIRED GASES, OR POST BREATH-HOLDING MEASUREMENTS.

73. COMPARE THE HEART RATES OF THE SAME INDIVIDUAL WORKING IN A HOT HUMID ENVIRONMENT AND DOING THE SAME WORK IN A RELATIVELY COOL ENVIRONMENT IF POSSIBLE ALSO HAVE INDIVIDUAL PERFORM IN A COLD ENVIRONMENT SO HE IS SHIVERING AS WELL, NOTE ANY CHANGES IN HEART· RATE.

74. STUDY THE EFFECTS OF HYPERVENTILATION AND OXYGEN INHALATION UPON THE BREATH HOLDING TIME AND ON RECOVERY TIME.

Figure 32–3. Instructional laboratory activities.

4. Developing teaching objectives as goals to which the above information is coded.

85. ANALYZE THE CONTRIBUTIONS MADE BY EXERCISING IN PRESERVING THE BODY FROM PREMATURE AGEING.

86. MAKE STUDENTS FAMILIAR WITH THE CONVENTIONS OF EXPRESSING DATA IN SYMBOLIC FORM IN RESPIRATORY PHYSIOLOGY.

87. CONVEY KNOWLEDGE OF CRITERIA FOR THE EVALUATION OF TRAINING PROGRAMS.

88. DEVELOP SKILL IN THE ABILITY OF PREDICTING PERFORMANCES FROM CERTAIN PHYSIOLOGICAL TESTS.

89. SKILL IN EVALUATING THE ACCURACY OF PUBLISHED ARTICLES IN PHYSIOLOGY OF EXERCISE.

90. COMPARE AND CONTRAST THE DIRECT AND INDIRECT METHODS OF CALORIMETRY.

91. ANALYZE THE RELATIONSHIP OF GREATEST FORCE TO JOINT ANGLE FOR ELBOW FLEXION AND EXTENSION.

92. ANALYZE THE FACTORS WHICH MAY LEAD TO OR MAGNIFY ATHLETIC INJURIES.

93. ANALYZE FACTORS WHICH HAVE A CRITICAL BEARING ON MAXIMAL PERFORMANCE EFFICIENCY IN ATHLETICS.

94. IDENTIFY THE PHASES OF RESPIRATION.

95. COMPARE THE MALE AND FEMALE ADAPTATION TO ATHLETIC TRAINING.

96. ANALYZE THE CLIMATIC EFFECTS ON EXERCISE.

97. ANALYZE THE FACTORS WHICH DECREASE THE CAPACITY FOR HIGH ATHLETIC ACHIEVEMENT WITH AGEING.

98. EVALUATE THE USE OF ERGOGENIC AIDS IN SPORT.

99. ANALYZE THE RELATIONSHIP BETWEEN EXERCISE AND WEIGHT CONTROL.

Figure 32–4. Teaching objectives.

5. Amassing evaluative questions for the objectives so as to provide the instructor and students with some guidance as to what is expected to be achieved by a given objective.

86. DISCUSS THE EFFECTS OF HEAT ON THE CIRCULATORY SYSTEM.

87. DESCRIBE THE ADVANTAGE OF STORING GLYCOGEN IN THE MUSCLES.

88. DIFFERENTIATE BETWEEN ISOTONIC AND ISOMETRIC CONTRACTIONS.

89. DISCUSS ADVANTAGES AND DISADVANTAGES OF SURPLUS BODY FAT IN SPORTS.

90. DISCUSS THE POSSIBLE INFLUENCE OF THE ADRENAL CORTEX ON THE TRAINING INTENSITY OF AN INDIVIDUAL.

91. DESCRIBE HOW CLIMATE MAY EFFECT HEART RATE.

92. DISCUSS FACTORS WHICH CONTRIBUTE TO A SUSTAINED HIGH HEART RATE AFTER EXERCISE.

93. DISCUSS ADVANTAGES OF TAPERING OFF GRADUALLY (WARMING DOWN) AFTER SEVERE EXERCISE.

94. DISCUSS LIMITATIONS OF THE BICYCLE ERGOMETER AS A MEANS OF ASSESSING THE MAXIMUM OXYGEN UPTAKE.

95. SET UP A TRAINING PROGRAM FOR RUNNERS THAT WOULD INCORPORATE THE PRINCIPLES OF GRADUAL ADAPTATION.

96. DISCUSS THE SIGNIFICANCE OF THE INTERMITTENT CONTRACTIONS OF THE DIAPHRAGM MUSCLE IN BREATHING.

97. DISCUSS THE CONCEPT OF HOMEOSTASIS.

98. DESCRIBE THE PHENOMENA OF EXTENSIBILITY IN MUSCLE.

99. DISCUSS THE FACTORS WHICH INFLUENCE THE SHAPE OF BONE TISSUE DURING GROWTH.

100. DISCUSS HOW THE RESISTANCE TO THE FLOW OF BLOOD CHANGES IN THE DIFFERENT PARTS OF THE CIRCULATORY SYSTEM.

Figure 32–5. Evaluative questions.

## 6. Coding material to the teaching objectives.

OBJECTIVE NO. 85 ---
   ANALYZE THE CONTRIBUTIONS MADE BY EXERCISING IN
   PRESERVING THE BODY FROM PREMATURE AGEING.

   CONTENT OUTLINE

      EMOTIONAL REACTIONS CAN CAUSE VERY GREAT CHANGES IN THE
         BLOOD PRESSURE.

      ONE FUNDAMENTAL TRUTH ABOUT TRAINING IS THAT IT IS A
         CONTINUOUS PROCESS - IT IS FOOD AND DRINK TO
         PHYSICAL FITNESS AND WITHOUT IT FITNESS DIES.

      THE HEART OF A SUBJECT WITH AN ABNORMALLY HIGH BLOOD
         PRESSURE MUST WORK MUCH HARDER THAN THAT OF THE
         NORMAL SUBJECT.  THE RESTING HEART RATE IS HIGHER
         WHILE DIGESTIVE PROCESSES ARE IN PROGRESS THAN IN
         THE POST ABSORPTIVE STATE.

      EMOTIONAL STRESS BRINGS ABOUT A CARDIOVASCULAR RESPONSE
         THAT IS QUITE SIMILAR TO THE RESPONSE TO EXERCISE.

      SOMETHING ASSOCIATED WITH WEIGHT LIFTING PROGRAMS AND
         RUNNING SEEM TO CONTRIBUTE TO A MORE YOUTHFUL
         TYPE OF HORMONE SECRETION. F. E. ABBO, AGEING
         EXERCISE AND ENDOCRINES, (JOURNAL OF SPORTS
         MEDICINE, VOL. 6, NO. 1, MAR. 1966), P. 62.

      GYMNASTICS PRACTICED HABITUALLY SEEMS TO HAVE A
         FAVORABLE EFFECT ON RETARDATION OF AGEING AS
         MEASURED BY RATIOS OF COMPONENTS EXCRETED IN THE
         URINE.  EFFECTS OF HABITUAL PRACTICE OF
         GYMNASTICS IN MIDDLE AND OLD AGE. (JOURNAL OF
         SPORTS MEDICINE AND PHYSICAL FITNESS, VOL. 6, NO.
         1, MAR. 1966), P. 69.

      WELL SPACED PERIODS OF REGULAR LIGHT EXERCISE ARE OF
         BENEFIT TO THE INDIVIDUAL BY INCREASING THE
         NONSPECIFIC RESISTANCE TO SUCH UNFAVORABLE
         STRESSES AS OVERHEATING, COOLING, HYPOXIA,
         IRRADIATION, AND INFECTION.  L. MOREHOUSE AND A.
         MILLER, PHYSIOLOGY OF EXERCISE, (ST. LOUIS. C.V.
         MOSBY COMPANY, 1967), P. 283.

Figure 32–6. Example of content coded to an objective.

OBJECTIVE NO. 99 ---
    TO ANALYZE THE CLIMATIC EFFECTS ON EXERCISE.

  CONTENT OUTLINE

    EXERCISE HEART RATE IS INCREASED IN TEMPERATURES
        ABOVE 30 DEGREES CENTIGRADE, THE EFFECT IS
        SLIGHT AT 33 DEGREES CENTIGRADE, BUT CONSIDERABLE
        AT 37 DEGREES CENTIGRADE.  RESEARCH UNIT REPORT
        5 M 1967, UNIVERSITY OF ALBERTA, EDMONTON.

    CLOTHING IMPEDES EVAPORATION BY CREATING POCKETS OF
        STILL AIR WITH A HIGH VAPOR PRESSURE, AND BY
        VIRTUE OF THE VAPOR IMPERMEABILITY OF THE
        MATERIAL.

  REFERENCE MATERIALS

    DIAGRAM ILLUSTRATING THE EFFECT ON HEART RATE OF
        SUBJECTS EXPOSED TO EXERCISE AS WELL AS TO HEAT.
        E. JOKL, HEART AND SPORT, (SPRINGFIELD, ILL. C.
        C. THOMAS, 1964), P. 53.

    HUNTINGTON'S CLASSIFICATION OF CLIMATE ACCORDING TO
        ITS EFFECT ON THE ENERGY AND EFFICIENCY OF
        HUMAN BEINGS IN THE PRESENT PHASE OF CIVILIZATION.
        E. JOKL, PHYSIOLOGY OF EXERCISE. (SPRINGFIELD,
        ILL. C. C. THOMAS, 1964), P. 26.

  ACTIVITIES

    DEMONSTRATE THE EFFECTS OF HEAT AND COLD UPON EXERCISE
        HEART RATE ON THE BICYCLE ERGOMETER BY
        SUBJECTING THE PERFORMER TO HEAT BY INFRA RED AND
        COLD BY A LARGE FAN

    COMPARE SURFACE BODY TEMPERATURES IN THE RESTING AND
        ACTIVE STATE USING COPPER-CONSTANTAN
        THERMOCOUPLES APPLIED WITH TAPE TO THE SKIN

  EVALUATIVE DEVICES

    DISCUSS THE EFFECTS OF HEAT ON THE CIRCULATORY SYSTEM.

Figure 32–7. Example of content, reference material, activities, and evaluative questions coded to an objective.


The computer based resource unit is thus a reservoir of instructional support, providing for teachers assistance in the instructional process. It is not a substitute for instructional effort but rather a means of assistance which can multiply by unusual magnitude the ability of the instructor to devise appropriate means for directing the learning process of individuals and groups.[1]

The computer-based resource unit can be used to assist the

instructor in preparing the lecture and directing the learning process of the individual or group or it may be used by the student as an independent study guide. A particular feature of this system is that it makes allowances for individual differences in students. This is accomplished by having students check the appropriate areas on the Student Variable Sheet and then listing the teaching objectives for which they desire information. In this way an individual print-out for each student

UNIVERSITY_____STUDENT NAME_____

INFORMATION ON THIS SHEET WILL BE USED TO OBTAIN A "TAILOR

MADE" PRINT-OUT OF OBJECTIVES FROM THE MASTER LIST.  THE

INFORMATION RETRIEVED WILL BE SELECTED FOR EACH STUDENT

ACCORDING TO THE BELOW DESIGNATED AREAS.

INSTRUCTIONAL ACTIVITY                    ATHLETIC ENVIRONMENT

01   PROBLEM SOLVING              22   WATER SPORTS
02   STUDENT PRESENTATION         23   WINTER SPORTS
03   STUDENT LED DISCUSSION       24   SUMMER SPORTS
04   ACTUAL EXPERIMENT
05   INDEPENDENT STUDY            ATHLETIC CHARACTERISTIC

STUDENT PREPARATION AREA(S)            25   STRENGTH
                                       26   ENDURANCE
06   SOCIAL SCIENCES              27   SKILL
07   LANGUAGE ARTS
08   PHYSICAL EDUCATION           ATHLETIC INVOLVEMENT
09   MATHEMATICS
10   BIOLOGICAL SCIENCE           28   COACHING
11   PHYSICAL SCIENCE             29   PARTICIPATION
12   ELEMENTARY EDUCATION         30   ADMINISTRATION

SPECIALIZED PROFESSIONAL INTEREST     SEX

13   THE ATYPICAL CHILD           31   MALE
14   PRE-SCHOOL CHILD             32   FEMALE.
15   PRIMARY CHILD
16   INTERMEDIATE AGE CHILD
17   PRE-ADOLESCENT CHILD
18   ADOLESCENT
19   ADULT

ATHLETIC INTEREST

20   TEAM SPORT
21   INDIVIDUAL SPORT

                    OBJECTIVES SELECTED ___ ___ ___ ___

Figure 32–8. Student variable sheet.

can be procured which is tailor-made to the student's background and interests. For example, a student who has a background in biochemistry would retrieve physiology of exercise information for any given teaching objective with more emphasis on the biochemical aspects than would someone not indicating this background.

Since information for a computer-based resource unit is first stored on cards and then transferred onto magnetic tapes, old information can be purged and new information included by adding or deleting cards rather than redoing the whole unit. The updating process is being constantly improved. These refinements have expedited the updating process immensely.

One immediately expects that a system such as the aforementioned would entail costs which would be rather prohibitive. On the contrary, this system is set up as a nonprofit system and all the person wishing to capitalize on it must do is pay the administrative costs of processing plus computer time. The information returned which is selectively retrieved can be produced for less than the cost of the same amount of printed material in the usual textbook. The computer cost amounts to about two cents per sheet of print-out provided there is a sufficiently large request.

One of the major limitations of this system is in the lack of adequate materials which have been compiled. As this is a nonprofit venture the collector is only given mention as a contributor to the unit and hopefully gets his return in the satisfaction of making a contribution to his students and colleagues.

Anyone wishing to compile his own resource unit in another area, or wishing to make use of the current information which is available in physiology of exercise, or wishing to assist with the pending revision of the current unit in physiology of exercise may contact the writer for further information. The Center for Curriculum Planning, Faculty of Educational Studies, State University of New York at Buffalo has the master tapes and provide services as requested at the present time. It is hoped that duplicate tapes can be made so that information can be supplied directly from Laurentian University in the future.

# References

1. Fall, Charles R.: *Individualizing University Instruction*. Buffalo, Inter-University Project One, State University of New York at Buffalo, n.d.
2. Harnack, Robert S.: *The Use of Electric Computers to Improve Individualization of Instructor Through Unit Teaching*. Buffalo, New York, State University of New York at Buffalo and Research Foundation of the State of New York, Cooperative Research Project No. D-112, 1965.
3. Urquhart, D.J.: *Times Literary Supplement*. 519, May 7, 1970.

# Chapter 33

# Closing Remarks

CLAUDE BOUCHARD

In Canada we are presently experiencing an important development in the sector of sports for mass participation and sports for the elite. Many motivation elements contribute in fact to this rapid evolution. Among these we can note the fact that Canada will be in 1976 the theatre for the great Olympic Games.

The Canadian Association of Sport Sciences is not and does not want to stay away from these important stages. By its annual assizes and more specifically this year by a symposium on "training," our Association continues to manifest itself in this sector.

We have centered our efforts on *training: its scientific basis and its applications.*

## A Model

Training can represent various things. But in our context training represents first of all a group of practices and directives that athletes will follow to eventually realize sport feats. In this sense training must conform itself to the exactingness of every specific performance. But sports performances are numerous and very diversified. There is not only one single performance but there are effectively as many sports performances as sports activities.

It is possible to extract general factors on which all performances rely. And it is here that is found the key to a system. On what exactly do these sports performances rely? On what are they based? What makes an athlete capable of high performances?

To answer this question we must turn towards research. And, this question cannot be answered properly without a convenient system that will allow us to integrate the elements of the answer. Consequently we are proposing a *model for the identification of the determinants of a sport performance.* With it, it seems possible to approach more efficiently the problems of training.

---

S  P  O  R  T      P  E  R  F  O  R  M  A  N  C  E


P      =      H  ,  D  ,  C  ,

---

Our theoretical model is made up of the following cells. (Fig. 33–1). The sport performance (P) is determined by the contribution of three sets:

H = the invariable determinants of performance.
D = the variable determinants of performance.
C = the determinants of organization and controls in view of a performance.

What exactly is H in this system? In the following illustration (Fig. 33–2) we can identify the factors of H. If H represents the invariable determinants of performance,

Hm = the hereditory factors related to the morphological structures of the physical value.

THE INVARIABLE DETERMINANTS

H = Hm, Ho, Hp, Hps, ...,

Ho = the hereditory factors related to the organic structures of the physical value.
Hp = The hereditory factors related to the perceptual
structures of the physical value.
Hps = the hereditory factors related to the psychological
characteristics of personality.

What are, on the other hand, the variable determinants of a
sport performance (Fig. 33–3)? If D = the variable determi-

THE VARIABLE DETERMINANTS

D = Et, Is, Dpg, Dps, Pps, Vs, Fc, R, ...,

nants of a performance, the determinants that are influenced by training,

Et = technical efficiency in the activity concerned.
Is = strategic intelligence in the activity concerned.
Dpg = the general physical condition of the athlete.
Dps = the specific physical preparation of the athlete for the activity concerned.
Pps = the psychological preparation of the athlete for his performance.
Vs = the social milieu of the athlete and its influences on his training and performance.
Fc = complementary factors acting directly on the performance, such as atmospheric conditions, warm-up, equipment condition, etc.
R = the influences of relaxation techniques, of recreation, of leisures on the preparation of the athlete.

Finally, how could we define factor C (Fig. 33–4)? If C = the determinants of organization and controls of training in view of a performance, we could say that:

Cr = critical decisions which direct the champion preparation.

DETERMINANTS   OF   ORGANIZATION

AND   CONTROLS

C = Cr , Ce , Emg , Edg , Eds , Ss , . . . ,

Ce = training notebook of the trainee.

Emg = preventive or corrective general medical examination.

Edg = evaluation of the variable general determinants.

Eds = evaluation of the variable specific determinants.

Ss = the role of every sport science specialists in the preparation of the champion.

## A Summary

With this system in mind, it is now possible to summarize what we have done during this symposium. Through about fifteen presentations we were able to partly stake out three objectives.

Firstly we drew general summaries concerning either the physiological characteristics of highly trained athletes or psychological facts concerning these same athletes.

Secondly, we obtained interesting conclusions from researches, in progress or completed, on very precise aspects of one or another of the determinants of a sport performance. As in all scientific society, we made important investments.

Lastly, many new work hypotheses were formulated. The questions raised by those scientists who presented papers ask for future projects that we must realize in order that the science of training can progress normally.

We can note however that the studies presented converge mainly toward the variable determinants of a performance (D). Effectively, the majority of the researches presented at this symposium dealt with the physical and psychological aspects of the factors influenced by training. This is somewhat normal and shows that studies are strongly progressing in some sectors, but it also shows that there is place for greater activity in the direction of the other sport performance determinants.

# Index

## A

Acidosis, 18, 60, 66, 67, 68
Adipocytes, 22, 35, 63
Adipose cell, 22, 23
Adipose depot, 22
Adipose tissue, 22, 23, 24, 25, 32, 34, 35
Aerobic, 70, 72, 107, 108, 113
Age, 10, 46, 52, 116, 139, 168, 181
Aggressive behavior, 222, 228, 233, 234
Altitude, 15, 16
Amplitude, 305
Anabolic steroids, 175
Anaerobic, 70, 72
Angina, 39, 48, 54
Angina pectoris, 39, 48, 54
Arrhythmias, 40
Arteriovenous difference (avD), 8, 9, 10, 131
Attitudes, 198, 225, 242, 258, 259

## B

Behavior patterns, 198
B-receptor, 12
Bicarbonate, 60
Bilirubin, 117
Blood flow, 131, 136
Blood volume, 136

## C

Capillarization, 123, 124
Carbohydrate, 23
Cardiac output, 8, 13, 17, 87, 89, 131, 132, 134, 136
Cardio respiratory fitness, 97, 100, 101, 133, 141, 144, 146, 149, 152
Cardiovascular disease, 5–20
Catecholamines, 166, 171
Cells, 24–31, 60
Cell proliferation, 35
Cholesterol, 40, 46, 47, 181, 184
Circulation, 70, 83

Coding, 344
Computer analysis, 41
Computer receival equipment, 338
Coronary heart disease, 124
Coronary insufficiency, 11
Cutaneous vaso constriction, 131
Culture, 222

## D

Danabol, 175, 176, 177, 178
Diastolic pressure, 13, 117
Discrimination, 197, 198, 200, 201, 202, 205, 206
DLCO, 139, 140, 142
DNA, 24, 25, 32, 34, 35
Dp/dt, 12
Dyspnea, 62

## E

ECG, 14, 39, 47
Edema, 270
Ejection fraction, 10
Electrocardiography, 39, 40, 41, 42, 43, 44, 50, 52, 53, 54, 55, 56, 97
Electromyography, 14, 282
Enddiastolic volume, 11
Endsystolic volume, 11
Epicardial fat, 11
Epididymal fat pads, 21, 23, 24, 28, 30, 32, 34
Epinephrine, 171

## F

Fat, 22, 24, 35
Fat cell, 22, 34
Fat metabolism, 22
Fat tissue, 32
Flexibility, 107, 305, 316
Free fatty acids, 21, 22, 24, 25, 28, 33, 34, 36
FFA mobilization, 23, 33, 34

**G**

Glucose, 22
Growth, 22

**H**

Heart rate, 6, 7, 8, 9, 50, 52, 53, 70, 77, 82, 89, 100, 110, 118, 139, 140, 151, 154, 163, 170, 210
Heart volume, 5, 6, 10, 14, 17
Heart weight, 10, 11
Hematocrit, 111, 117
Hematoma, 267, 269, 273
Hemoglobin, 15, 11, 117
Hemorrhage, 267
High frequency apparatus, 267, 279
Hyperhaptoglobinemia, 184
Hyperplasia, 22
Hypertension, 48, 55
Hypertrophy, 10, 14, 22, 35, 46, 136
Hyperventilation, 43, 60, 82, 160, 164
Hypoxia, 16, 17, 18, 60

**I**

Immunoglobin, 184
Infarct, 55
Interval training, 149, 160
Ischemia, 35, 42, 50, 53, 55, 56
Isometrics, 320
Isotonics, 320

**K**

Kinematics, 290, 300

**L**

Lactate, 42, 50, 60
Lactic acid, 42, 50, 60
Leisure participation, 213, 214
Lipid, 22, 23, 33, 36, 64
Lipidectomy, 23, 24, 28, 30, 32, 33
Lipolysis, 33–35

**M**

Maximal angular velocity, 302
Maximal oxygen uptake, 5, 6, 7, 8, 13, 15, 16, 65, 71, 72, 74, 77, 79, 82, 87, 98, 100, 132, 170
Maximum heart rate, 6, 8, 13
Maximum stroke volume, 13
Mechanical efficiency, 133

Mental health, 213, 214, 220
Minute ventilation, 92
Movement time, 320
Myocardial fiber capillary ratio, 123, 124, 127, 129, 130
Myocardial ischaemia, 40

**N**

Need achievement, 207, 209
Norepinephrine, 171

**O**

Ordinal position, 235
Oxygen consumption, 44, 77, 163
Oxygen debt, 74
Oxygen deficit, 71
Oxygen pulse, 151
Oxygen transport capacity, 10, 17
Oxygen uptake, 44, 46, 50, 70, 76, 107, 119, 133, 151, 168

**P**

Personality, 193, 235
Personality factor test, 106, 109
pH, 62, 63, 68
Physical training, 10
Potassium, 42
Prejudice, 197, 198, 205
Proliferation, 35
Propranolol, 12
Psychology, 159, 190, 193, 236, 237
Psycho-neurotic systems, 220
Pulmonary artery, 13, 14, 16, 17
Pulmonary circulation, 9
Pulmonary diffusion capacity, 139, 141
Pulmonary function, 139
Pulmonary hypertension, 16
Pulmonary vasoconstriction, 17, 18
Pulmonary veins, 5
Pyridine, 176

**R**

Race, 198, 201, 203, 205, 242
Reaction time, 106, 320
Regeneration, 21, 22, 23, 25, 28, 30, 32, 34
Respiration, 83
Respiratory quotient, 63, 110
Right bundle branch block, 14

**S**

Sex, 181, 235
SGOT, 176, 177, 178
Siblings, 236, 237, 239, 240
Socio-economic status, 226
S-T segment, 42
Speed, 320
Statistical analysis, 333
Strength, 320, 327, 328
Stroke volume, 8, 9, 10, 17, 89
Superior athlete, 189, 190, 193
Sympathetic activation, 14
Sympathetic nervous system, 34, 166, 167
Sympathetic stimulation, 12, 13
Systolic pressure, 9, 117

**T**

Temperature, 70
Test anxiety, 207
Tomography, 5
Training, 5, 8, 10, 21, 23, 24, 28, 32, 34, 35, 36, 50, 53, 97, 100, 101, 103, 108, 110, 115, 124, 136, 139, 142, 154, 166, 170, 180, 194, 200, 349

Training model, 349–353
Trauma, 267, 276

**U**

Ultra sound, 267
Urine, 166, 169, 170, 171, 173

**V**

Vagotonia, 14
Values, 225
Vanilmandelic acid, 166, 167, 169, 171, 172, 173
Vascular resistance, 14
Vaso-dilatation, 276
Ventilation, 62, 64, 65, 77, 110, 163, 164, 168, 170
Vital capacity, 46
VMA, 166, 167, 169, 171, 172, 173

**W**

Warm-up, 70, 71, 72, 74, 163, 164
Wenchenbach phenomena, 14
White fat, 22